SHAPING
Your Baby's
FOUNDATION

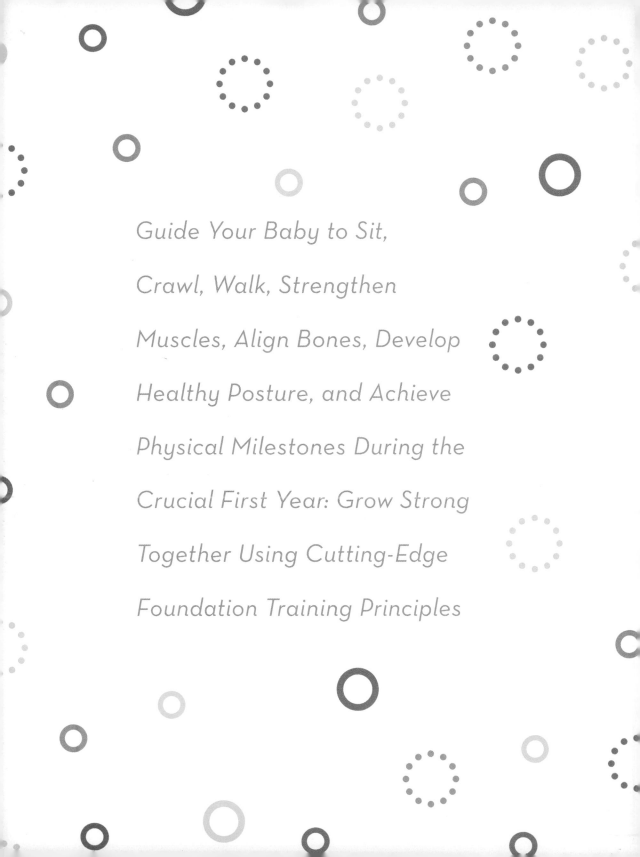

Guide Your Baby to Sit,

Crawl, Walk, Strengthen

Muscles, Align Bones, Develop

Healthy Posture, and Achieve

Physical Milestones During the

Crucial First Year: Grow Strong

Together Using Cutting-Edge

Foundation Training Principles

SHAPING
Your Baby's
FOUNDATION

JEN GOODMAN, PT, MSPT
WITH HY BENDER

HARPER WAVE

An Imprint of HarperCollinsPublishers

SHAPING YOUR BABY'S FOUNDATION. Copyright © 2021 by Jeanene S. Goodman. All rights reserved. Printed in Canada. No part of this book may be used or reproduced in any manner whatsoever without written permission except in the case of brief quotations embodied in critical articles and reviews. For information, address HarperCollins Publishers, 195 Broadway, New York, NY 10007.

HarperCollins books may be purchased for educational, business, or sales promotional use. For information, please email the Special Markets Department at SPsales@harpercollins.com.

FIRST EDITION

Designed by Elina Cohen

Library of Congress Cataloging-in-Publication Data has been applied for.

ISBN 978-0-06-267121-9

21 22 23 24 25   LSC   10 9 8 7 6 5 4 3 2 1

JEN GOODMAN

To all the unique characters who have helped shape my own foundation—my parents, Sandy and Jess; the brothers I was lucky to grow up motivated and challenged by; various special branches of my giant family tree; my love and life partner, Eric, and our delightful daughter, Sunora—you all mean the world to me.

To all the special teachers, doctors, and therapists with whom I've had the honor of learning or working; and, to all the kiddos whose care I've been involved in—it's been a joy and privilege. Thank you all for enriching my life, inspiring my career, and being part of what led to this book.

To all the wonderful Docs out there caring for kids and guiding their families—thank you for considering this resource and sharing these important aspects of growth and health.

And, last but certainly not least, to all the little ones and caretakers out there whom we hope this book reaches and helps. The collective team behind this book wishes you well!

HY BENDER

This book is dedicated to you, our reader, and the endless love you have for your baby. Please know these pages were created with love, and with the hope that they help your baby grow strong, agile, fit, and joyous.

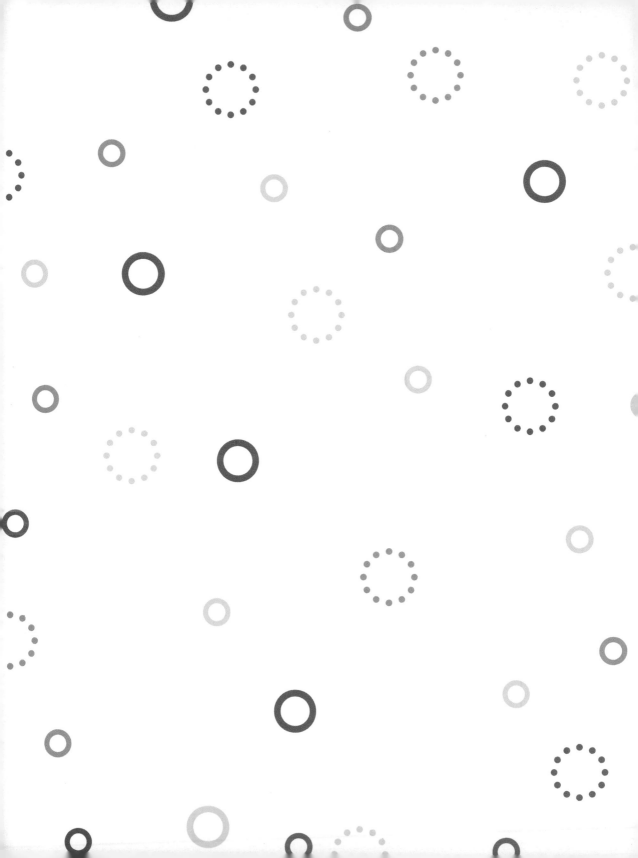

Preventive pediatrics recognizes the importance of both genetics and the environment of the patient. The interaction between these two factors has been likened to a dance that sets the stage for how a child will blossom into adulthood, and what is a dance if it doesn't include movement? Movement is crucial for healthy childhood development, from the earliest intrauterine calisthenics performed by the baby to the critical kinesthetic milestones that occur after birth in the first year of life. Unfortunately, our fast-paced culture tends to underestimate these delicate milestones, as more babies are sequestered in their first year of life into car seats, strollers, or carriers. Babies need to be allowed to go through the milestones of rolling, crawling, sitting, and standing with a watchful eye for support and stability.

In our increasingly sedentary society, most people recognize how important movement is for our older children, but fewer appreciate just how important it is in the earliest stages of life. The first year of life is an especially critical time of neural development, and proper movement stimulates both neural pathways and cognitive function. Supporting a baby in achieving kinesthetic milestones is an increasingly important need, an essential investment in your baby's future well-being, and a priceless opportunity to join your little one in their earliest "dance" of life.

IRIS CASTANEDA-VAN WYK, MD, FAAP
*Member of the Section on Integrative Medicine,
American Academy of Pediatrics*

Contents

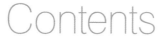

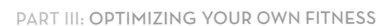

PART III: OPTIMIZING YOUR OWN FITNESS

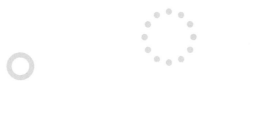

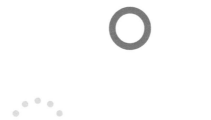

Foreword

As a new parent or caregiver, there is so much to learn about how to care for your little one. How do you trim or file their nails and clean their ears? How do you give them a bath? What is the best way to nourish them? How should you hold them when nursing or bottle-feeding them? There is so much to think about that we often overlook some of the most basic parts of a baby's life: how they're positioned when in your arms, lying down, or sitting up in a car seat, and how their muscles are strengthened to reach all their expected physical milestones. Babies do not come hardwired for perfect movement, nor do they come with a manual, and one could spend a lot of time wondering about whether a new baby's postures, reflexes, and movements are normal.

As parents, we are fortunate to have the possibility of making profound effects on our child's development. This is perhaps most true during a baby's first year.

That's in part because the connections between your baby's brain and the rest of their body aren't fully formed at birth. These connections grow with your help. Baby's world outside the womb is expansive and full of new sensations; and it is up to us to effectively help them explore their potential for movement.

There is a lot going on when a baby performs basic movements such as lifting the head (which is a major challenge for newborns). The brain must connect to thirty-one pairs of spinal nerves to do that! These nerves play a critical part in your baby's physical movement, as well as their sensations and things like heart rate, respiratory rate, digestion, and various other aspects of underlying health. Depending on the action the baby is working to achieve, some of the nerves will be firing more actively for movement while others will be working to keep various segments of the body still. Every attempt at movement is teaching these nerves, the muscles, and your baby's brain. And every position of the body can either allow smooth conductive flow of information through the nerves or it can compress them and potentially complicate movement, or worse.

During the first year of life, a critical area of the baby's body to take note of is the posterior chain—that is, the muscles along the backside of the whole body, from head to feet, which includes the muscles of the neck, back, bottom, and legs. The posterior chain is the primary focus of the process I created called Foundation Training, which has been used by people of various ages all around the world, from full-time moms to the elite of Special Forces, to Olympic athletes, to NASA scientists, to folks with spinal, hip, and other injuries— obviously all with different body shapes, sizes, and movements—to help treat and prevent injuries by reeducating and reprogramming the body with strong and healthy movement patterns.

It's fascinating how this area of the body truly seems to wake up and begin to strengthen when baby emerges from the womb and experiments with movements that work these important muscles against the new-to-them force of gravity.

When it comes to babies, the posterior chain is challenged by activities such as tummy time, which is the best way to get it firing. Tummy time puts babies on their stomachs in a position that encourages them to lift their heads while also providing them with a firm surface to push into as they learn to control their movements. This gradually builds strength and endurance in the muscles of a baby's whole body, from their head and neck downward, as they learn to come up higher and higher and eventually push back to all fours and other more vertical positions. Caregivers would do well to consider that tummy time not only helps develop a baby's movement, but also their sensory skills, as it gives them another view and position from which to experience and engage with their environment. For your baby, the whole world is new, and full of so many lights, sounds, smells, and textures to touch. Be mindful of how you help babies to fully experience their environments (in the home, out of the home) through their senses. Practice type, position, quality, and quantity all count here. Frequent bits of focus on movement, coupled with steady focus on quality support being provided in every position, and attention to the shape and angle (concave versus flat versus incline versus decline) of the surface your baby is on, all come together to build necessary muscles to contribute to healthy spinal curves and limb alignment as well as symmetrical head shape (flat spots in the skull are a warning sign!).

When your baby's body is in motion, it's experiencing a series of changes in position (as well as some muscle recruitment for the sake of stabilization) at the head, neck, shoulders, elbows, wrists, hands, chest, abdomen, back, hips, knees, ankles, and feet. Coordinating these movements between the brain, spine, nerves, and body as a whole is no small thing. We hope to impress upon you just how big a deal this actually is, how much is actually going on in your child's brain and body. Learning and refining skills takes months (and continues for a lifetime) as the baby builds endurance, strength, control, and coordination, all while other learning and growth is simultaneously and perpetually occurring within this multidimensional little creature.

Over time patterns of movement for your baby get established. This occurs regardless of whether you take an active role in guiding your child's movement. Any particular pattern can benefit or subtly injure your baby's body. Movement patterns that take the body out of balanced alignment of their joints can eventually lead to serious pain, which is why you need to take an active role in shaping your baby's movements and posture. In adults, and even in teenagers and young children, untreated negative patterns can persist, almost as if growing with the body, and predispose it to injuries. The vast majority of my adult patients came to me suffering from repetitive pattern-based injuries. My patients, much like me, were not taught good movement and posture habits, which led to flaws forming in their physical foundation; and those flaws gradually grew over years or decades, until they caused pain severe enough to make many of these patients consider dangerous medications or high-risk surgery before they discovered the alternative solutions to create lasting changes to the root of their issues provided by Foundation Training.

Too many people think of physical problems (like back pain, neck pain, hip pain, TMJ issues, tension headaches, sciatica, carpal tunnel syndrome) as unavoidable, and just a price we pay for getting older; but they're mistaken. This is why a baseline of healthy movement habits is so necessary—and it is important to initiate this developing from the very start. If you regularly perform the activities in this book with your baby, and you conscientiously make small adjustments, as necessary, to optimize their position in space, wherever they are throughout the day, over time your baby is likely to develop a healthy spinal curve, great alignment, and powerful coordination between their muscle groups as they learn how to move. And this is likely to be beneficial for them not only during their first year, toddlerhood, and childhood, but throughout their life.

My wife, Jen, has spent more than a decade helping babies and children achieve optimal movement, through physical therapy, and this book is full of essential information she has found parents need. Within the course of her career and patient care, she was asked (by more than one of the local pediatricians who repeatedly referred their patients to her for physical therapy) for a resource they could point new parents to so they could help their kids on the path to growing well, physically, before they developed any need for "rehabilitation." Not knowing of one, she was inspired to help where she felt she could.

Jen has simplified and hidden the serious work to be done with your baby within playful activities that are likely to be fun for both you and your little one, keeping your kiddo engaged and challenged, while at the same time bolstering their development. These activities are laid out through hundreds of carefully selected photos that show you what to do and what responses to look for from your baby, along with concise descriptions that highlight any key information in each photo. They're your outline to build upon and make playtime uniquely stimulating and fun for your unique child.

Focusing on your baby's fitness doesn't mean neglecting your own. Be aware of your own body as you're doing what you're doing, and be kind to it. The things you do for your baby daily—kneeling, bending, reaching, lifting, holding, feeding, burping, changing diapers, giving baths—can take a lot out of you. Your movements have the potential power to either build you up or break you down. That's why this book ends with a chapter describing over a dozen Foundation Training exercises and poses for you as well. The chapter covers the importance of decompression breathing, how to strengthen your own posterior chain, and more. These additions can help us to stay strong, reflexive, coordinated, and overall better prepared for the ever-present physical demands of life, which now include the safety, care, and education of a tiny, dependent human. And they can be especially helpful in the postpartum physical journey as a mom's center of gravity is shifting (along with her organs) as it heals and reconfigures.

I appreciate this book from more than a professional perspective. I lived it, because I (clumsily) helped Jen apply its principles and activities with our daughter, Sunny (who, as I write this, is three years old, has remarkable movement and reflexes, and is already such a bright, thoughtful, chatty young girl). This allowed me to see firsthand the enormous benefits of guiding a baby's movements and overall development from her very first day earthside.

I hope that you end up living this book, too, and that it helps you create a solid foundation of healthy movement for your baby from which they can grow strong, coordinated, and joyously prepared for the physical demands of toddlerhood and beyond.

—Dr. Eric Goodman, founder of Foundation Training

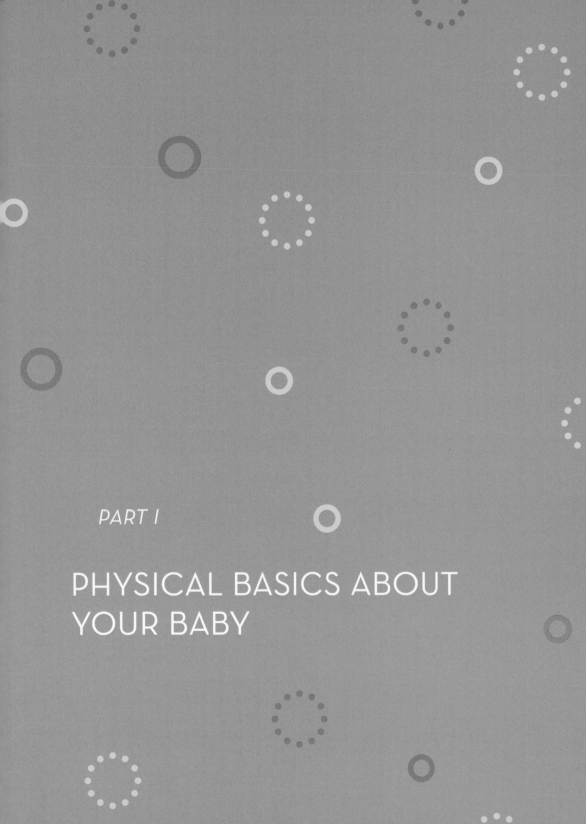

PART I

PHYSICAL BASICS ABOUT YOUR BABY

Introduction

Your baby's first year will start mostly horizontal and end mostly vertical.

In between will be endless wondrous challenges as your baby works to develop the strength, coordination, and skills to lie faceup, lie facedown, reach, roll, sit, crawl, kneel, stand, cruise the furniture, and eventually walk.

Along the way, as they are experiencing and exploring the world through all their senses, babies will pick up many abilities that are intimately tied into the development of their movement skills, such as visually tracking things with their eyes, turning their heads in response to sounds, bringing their hands together in the midline of their bodies, purposeful grasping and releasing, and so much more. The different exposures and learning opportunities babies have will help them to steadily engage and interact more physically as they grow in their understanding of the world, their place in it, and how to negotiate moving their bodies within it.

The first year is a vibrant period of growth. Your baby will, barring any limiting health conditions, develop a remarkable neural network conveying messages between body parts and the brain; a well-shaped spinal curve with smoothly communicating nerves; beautifully aligned bones that create a powerful structure for their body; and strong muscles with functional symmetry that allow them to confidently physically interact within the world. These developments over the first twelve months will establish the early foundation of the body's physical structure.

And there are numerous ways things can go wrong along the way.

A newborn's body is 100 percent dependent on you. It has soft spots in its skull, and has yet to develop any muscular strength. Once outside the womb, the baby has to struggle against gravity, and they lack sufficient strength to hold up their head with any sort of endurance (it might only be for *one* second at first). This is all normal, but it's important to understand that the bones of a baby's body can actually shift out of alignment under the force of gravity and at the mercy of whatever surface the baby is atop. If your baby is sleeping in a less-than-ideal position, sitting crooked in a car seat or swing, being held in an awkward position, or suffers an abrupt jolt or twist, irritation to the nerves and muscles can result. The effects can be short-lived or persist in your baby's body, leading to actual imbalances in alignment, asymmetry of skull shape and/or facial features, issues or delays with developing motor skills, or perhaps even a predisposition for early breakdown of healthy structures.

Modern conveniences you may depend on with the best intentions for hands-free parenting—such as the car seat, the bouncer, the carrier, and the swing—can create physical stresses that nature never anticipated. Such devices can cause your baby's body to slump, twist, roll, and basically scrunch into compromised positions that do not encourage good posture, allowing gravity to drag your little one's body parts into misalignment.

If you've ever tried to soothe a baby who's fussy for no apparent reason, you know how upsetting this can be for everyone involved. If you eliminate all the baseline potential causes (e.g., hungry/thirsty, tired, teething, dirty diaper, hot/cold, sensory system overloaded by too much stimulus like noise or bright lights, or simply needing affection) and baby is still fussy, then there's a fair chance the problem is something structurally off base—say, a pinched nerve or a tight muscle. One small kink in the spine can result in significant discomfort. What's worse, though, is the reality that if such a problem isn't properly addressed, it can lead to imbalances, delays, or potentially even injuries that occur as early as childhood.

Your baby will undergo physical challenges over the first year that lead to profound changes in the developing curvature of their spine and alignment of their body's structure. Your ability to guide them physically, in their positioning and movements, both at rest and as you introduce incremental, stage-appropriate challenges, will help determine how stable and efficient (biomechanically speaking) a mover your child becomes.

We all know adults who complain of stiffness and pain in the lower back or neck, tenderness in the joints, nerve-related issues, and sore muscles. It cannot be ruled out that any of these ailments could be related to a lack of structural integrity in the body or faulty movement mechanics stemming from missed opportunities during their first twelve months.

As any engineer will tell you, when a heavy load—such as a baby's body weight pulled by the compressing force of gravity—is added to a weakened or misaligned structure, that structure can give way.

So between the damage caused by modern conveniences and caretakers being inadequately prepared to guide their infant through the physical challenges of the first year of life, many babies' bodies aren't growing as well as they could be. This doesn't have to be. There are things you can do to help facilitate healthy movement as a child grows.

As a physical therapist dedicated to pediatrics, I've observed and worked with countless patients from as young as one week old up to teenage years; and, I also had the experience of working with adults of all ages while in my student years. The simple yet insanely dynamic reality that little bodies grow into the big bodies that adults move around in fascinates me. Healthy movement is not a guarantee and so much can shift and change through a lifetime as the body changes, grows, and moves. My husband's work, Foundation Training, has been dedicated to the other end of the spectrum. Through exercise, he helps adults experiencing pain and dysfunction. As he teaches someone how to muscularly shift their way to new strengths and postures, he is also helping them to rewrite their movement patterns in their brain, to change their habits. Coming from the pediatric side of the spectrum, professionally, I can't help but wonder, at what stage did these folks' dysfunctional movement habits really, *truly*, begin? I feel it is often much sooner than most folks might consider: during formative stages. Then, with years of less-than-ideal body usage, people wind up breaking down their body and end up in pain. I've seen this in preteens with severe back pain, whose parents could recall their baby showing some sort of funky movement pattern, like habitual tiptoe walking, for example. Young kids breaking down should not be the norm, but sadly it is more common than you might think, so this needs to be considered. Looking at it simply, a baby is at the very baseline of this spectrum, from zero to adulthood. The starting baseline sets the stage for the structural foundation that everything else builds upon. As the baby grows and weight gets added onto their structure, muscles strengthen and the body begins to move in new ways. And the body is steadily adapting, in some way or other, depending on how it is moving and positioning. This is going to continue happening through life, and attention to creating a functionally strong baseline is crucial.

When I was still a student therapist I had a deeply formative experience during my final clinical internship in a setting that specializes in helping children with special needs. In addition to traditional therapies, which are typically thirty to sixty minutes, one or two times weekly, this center offers "intensive" therapy sessions for those whose systems need a different approach. Typical intensive sessions are three weeks long and they consist of five therapy days a week, during which the child is seen for three to four hours a day. I was blown away to see the results of this approach. In my mind it was akin to training intensely for a sport, practicing with dedication to form, and seeing gains come from those efforts. I saw remarkable resilience and the power of the brain and body to create change with hard work. I saw big efforts and big results. And I came away from the experience inspired with pure joy, knowing that just about *any and every body can improve its quality of movement and structural alignment with the right focused guidance, challenges, and practice time.* I left inspired to help kids because they have their whole lifetime of moving ahead of them. In my mind it was this simple: move well, grow well—and be healthier for it.

When I passed my board exams and got my PT license, I sought mentors with long careers of experience effectively helping kids, and I took jobs that allowed me to work as part of comprehensive rehabilitation teams beside occupational, behavioral, and speech therapists. I communicated directly with pediatricians and other specialists, like orthopedists, neurologists, and orthotists, about the care of our mutual patients. I worked with children of all ages and abilities and found, over and over, that regardless how minor or major a child's structural imbalances or limitations, guided movements can truly make a profound difference in how movement skills are learned. Furthermore, the sooner (read: younger) an imbalance is identified and addressed, the easier it is to intervene and make lasting changes to movement habits.

This is what led me to working solely in early intervention, which is specifically with ages birth to three, typically in the home, and sometimes in their daycare. The experiences this brought me reinforced that, by far, the best practice is creating daily guided movement exposures for little ones that help strengthen their bodies in ways that prevent misalignments from ever happening in the first place. Also, physical guidance toward the right muscle usage can actually promote achieving the expected motor milestones babies should be hitting and building upon in their first year.

I feel compelled to share that in my years of clinical practice, something I encountered that I found upsetting was how frequently parents reported noticing an imbalance during their child's first few months or years and either never considered doing something about it or were told "they'll outgrow it." Some of these kids were only five, seven, nine years of age at the time they were being referred, coming in for evaluation with issues like slipped vertebrae in their spine, chronic neck, back, and other specific joint pain (knees, ankles) from repeated muscle use with poor alignment. This was painful for everyone involved; and, it was heartbreaking for me as I wondered (1) how the warning signs could seemingly be overlooked so frequently and (2) why no one was being taught how to help their young ones to exercise their muscles from the start.

I also feel compelled to share that I've encountered many parents who unknowingly assumed postural imbalances, like a head tilting to one side, to be part of "nature's plan," or a "quirk" of their baby's individuality. It is out of genuine concern that I bring to light the reality that most folks are completely naive to the fact that such a tilt could actually be causing changes to their child's head shape or the pressure in their sinuses and on their brain. Also, beyond knowing they are supposed to do tummy time, most don't actually know how to best go about it, nor do they give much thought to focusing on their baby's alignment. Baby exercises and their postural health are simply not common conversation or thought. There is no shame or judgment, just a call to awareness, because most people have not gone into advanced study of anatomy, development, or health.

I mean no judgment or shame on anyone when I share that there have been numerous well-meaning parents who have brought their injured, delayed, and/or pain-afflicted little ones to be evaluated and proceeded to share comments that hinted to muscle imbalances or other physical issues. Comments such as:

"My sweet baby shows so much personality, whenever her dad holds her she shyly leans her head to the left."

"My little one HATED tummy time, so we never did too much of that."

"My baby loved to roll, but only to the right."

"My amazing baby crawls super fast and uses just one hand and one side of their butt."

"I just knew she would be a lefty, I could tell by eleven months!"

"My child was so ready he entirely skipped crawling and went straight to walking."

I found it sad to encounter this gap in knowledge and understanding so often; and, it inspired a desire to help bridge the gap. There are many simple practices that parents and caretakers can weave seamlessly into their days to help babies thrive physically. They would benefit from understanding the path ahead for the little body when it comes to their movement. Learning some key details about how babies move will help parents and caregivers to notice shifts away from what is normal and ideal and then take action to improve their child's experience.

For example, when a baby consistently favors one side over the other while in a "container" like a car seat, crib, or baby carrier, that device could be forcing their little body into positions that are somehow skewed, encouraging them to look and move asymmetrically. This could end up compromising their joint alignment, muscle length, or, worse, potentially compressing and damaging delicate underlying structures. Favoring one side over the other could also be the result of the crib simply being positioned in the room in a way that encourages the baby to look in one particular direction, for instance, toward the doorway once they begin to recognize this is where caregivers enter the room. Either situation has simple solutions if caregivers are privvy to what is going on. If they are not, negative consequences can result over time.

Habitually holding an asymmetric alignment or showing discrepancies of movement from one side of the neck to the other is almost always a clear sign of muscular imbalances (called torticollis), and this can lead to changes in a baby's head shape (called plagiocephaly) like flat spots and asymmetrical facial features.

It's also problematic if a baby is moving with faulty patterns, using more or fewer limbs than is usual at a certain age—for example, if at ten months she's still sitting with both hands planted on the ground to avoid falling over, or if she's crawling without using both arms and both legs equivalently and it looks more like a scoot than a hands-and-knees crawl.

Paying attention to your baby's posture is good, but you're not expected to know how to assess it. Sometimes things aren't always how they appear, so recognizing when something appears off-kilter and checking in with your kiddo's pediatrician is important.

For example, it's entirely possible that a child experiencing stomach discomfort will present with head tilting that appears to be true torticollis when the reality is the child is physically leaning away from the source of discomfort, as if to take pressure off their stomach.

It is also possible that head tilting can be the result of baby shifting to accommodate for issues with their vision.

These sorts of things can be assessed further with the help of a pediatric physical therapist. This is shared to highlight the importance of open dialogue with your child's pediatrician as early as possible so they can properly refer you for further testing. When it comes to asymmetric posturing, regardless of the cause, it can result in further damage and delays in movement skill acquisition. Determining the underlying cause(s) will help direct any necessary treatment interventions.

If a baby skips a key developmental stage, whether due to muscular weakness or simple lack of exposure, it robs the baby of the opportunity for muscle strengthening, endurance building, increased movement control, and patterning practice that they'd normally gain by time spent within that stage. For instance, babies who skip crawling are rushing less prepared into more advanced movements such as walking, and they're also missing out on weight-bearing practice through their arms and hands. This creates a risk for muscle weakness, instability, faulty movement patterns, and misalignments of the limbs and spine.

We don't believe this lack of parental and caregiver understanding is for lack of caring. We assume that most all parents deeply love their children, want only the best for them, and fight hard to shield them from the dangers that they're aware of. The problem is most folks haven't been taught that a blanket trust in "nature," genetics, or instinct is an inadequate substitute for an informed parental focus on movement.

The truth is, the first year of your baby's physical development is too crucial to leave to chance. It's not enough to simply hope nothing goes wrong; or that if something does, it'll be obvious enough for you to recognize it, or for your child's pediatrician to correctly identify and effectively treat it the second it begins. Furthermore, as a word of caution, if there is the need for a pediatric physical therapist, depending on where you live and what kind of access to health care you have, finding one can sometimes be difficult. Not every physical therapist specializes in the same area, and if your typical patient is someone coming for treatment of low back pain or a hip or knee replacement, for example, a six-month-old with a developmental delay is a completely different ball game. This is all the more reason to empower yourself to assist your child as they grow. Abate the need for intervention as best you can by giving this your attention as your child develops (and not just during their first year).

Instead, *what is required is a parental approach that's proactive, in which you steadily keep a mindful practice of assisting your child into healthy alignment in whatever position they are in and you guide them to perform movements geared to their current stage of development.* It's as simple as exercise hidden in play. If your baby is having fun, they aren't going to think twice about how challenging it might be. *Parents and caregivers can make strategic tweaks to any environment their child is in to establish a purposeful play session.* Doing so will help strengthen your baby's muscles, improve their skeletal structure, enhance their range of motion, and help prepare them to achieve the expected motor skills that their pediatrician will be looking for during their visits. It will also stack the odds in favor of your baby enjoying optimal posture with functionally healthy alignment.

On top of these perks, it may encourage you to know that research studies over the years have actually shown that there is a positive correlation between physical activity and both cognitive and language development! *Simply put—helping your baby's muscles also helps their brain!*

Of course, a baby doesn't come equipped with a manual explaining how to raise a tiny body. In fact, there's a surprising lack of mainstream information for parents on how to guide a little one's physical development.

The content of this book is based on years of studies of anatomy, physiology, human movement, and all aspects of physical rehabilitation during my formal education, clinical affiliations (aka internships), and years of continuing education related both to pediatric and adult PT practice, including certification courses in infant massage instruction, Pilates, and Foundation Training; and of course all the observations and experiences I've had working with patients and their families.

This book is also the indirect result of a pediatrician asking me to create a resource for parents. This particular doctor, who had been sending me his patients for physical therapy care for years, humbly shared that pediatricians simply do not have the time or expertise to teach parents all the ins and outs of movement when they often have less than thirty minutes to assess every system of the body. He kindly referred to pediatric physical therapists as "movement experts" when it comes to assessing and treating children's physical development. That request was like a call to action for me. I started to really think about the things I found myself repeatedly sharing with parents, what details about a baby's development could be helpful for parents to know as they guide them toward acquiring motor skills and overall healthy structural development.

From further communication with other local pediatricians and patients' parents, a few of whom were specialist doctors and medical practitioners in different fields, I heard more than once the complaint about a lack of resources on the subject. And this was upsetting to me because this stuff really isn't complicated, but if you've never studied it, how are you to know? It's not exactly common knowledge; therein lies the problem. And it's a problem most folks don't realize even exists.

So this book is a call to awareness as much as it's a call to action. It will give you a toolset to utilize, a framework to follow and build from to make your baby's play sessions appropriately challenging. This allows you to focus more of your energy on keeping things FUN as you're engaging-motivating-stimulating-supporting-challenging and bonding with your unique child.

This book will help you guide your baby through their first twelve months. It will teach you how to optimally position your baby, how to use your hands to support and strengthen their muscles, and how to create play sessions that spur your kiddo's skill development. Our intention with the multitude of images is that their descriptions will not only provide guidance but also offer explanations for some of what you may already see your child displaying during their efforts.

As you endeavor forward, we encourage you to keep in mind that a child's development consists of so much more than just movement. Each child is on their own timeline and trajectory based on their unique makeup—genetics, nutrition, energy, and body structure—and, of course, what they are exposed to for practice experience. Some will hit milestones sooner than others. We encourage a mind-set of lovingly and positively meeting babies where they are, and playfully hiding the "work" for the muscles in the play and tasks of the day.

These pages are also enriched by what my husband, Eric, and I have been learning every day in the process of raising our own daughter (whose presence was a joyful surprise in the midst of this book project). I wholeheartedly consider her my muse. She has literally been living this book from her very start. Observing her growth, development, and responses to this level of attentiveness has been fascinating. She joins four other adorable babies as the models in this book.

By setting up gentle physical challenges for your baby at their own pace and in the safety of your home, you'll help them learn and hone numerous movement skills, such as optimal ways to sit, stand, crawl, walk, and how to strongly shift from one position to another. You'll also be priming your child to eventually meet real-world physical challenges—such as being shuffled around in a car seat, held in a less-than-ideal position by a well-meaning relative, confined for a bumpy ride in a stroller, or walking over uneven surfaces like mulch in a park.

Movement develops progressively, always building on the strengths gained and skills learned in previous stages. With the help of this book, I hope you feel empowered to confidently guide your baby to meet the challenges at every stage during the critical first year. Your dedication to this aspect of development is a labor of love that will help them create a solid foundation upon which to continue to build as they grow.

How This Book Is Organized

This book is organized into three parts that provide you with important information about your baby's anatomy and movement development, show you how to guide their physical skill progression through the first year using strategic play-based activities, and help you to boost your own strength and spinal health in the process by incorporating Foundation Training.

Part I: Physical Basics About Your Baby: This part introduces the WHY behind this book. Here you will find fundamental info about your baby's physical structure, including what it was like for them positionally in the womb and how their experience changes with the introduction of gravity. You'll find information about some of the reflexes a baby exhibits in their first year, as well as a general outline of the physical skills you should see them develop. You'll learn how those movements relate to developing the natural curves of their spine.

This section introduces important things to keep in mind to help you supportively guide your baby and minimize risks (you may not have considered) as you introduce movement.

Part II: Guiding Your Baby from Horizontal to Vertical: Armed with an understanding of important fundamentals from Part I, this section provides activities to, essentially, build your baby up. Where Part I answered WHY, Part II is your HOW.

In these pages you'll find guidance for how to most safely hold and position your new baby on flat surfaces and in devices like carriers, car seats, high chairs and other kinds of seats, and standers. The activities provided here include hundreds of full-color photos, accompanied by descriptions that highlight key details, making it easier for you to understand where to place your hands and focus your energy.

Each activity should be introduced in its presented order and progressed at your baby's individual pace, as sequential activities will rely upon the strength and skills your baby will gain from repeated practice of earlier activities. If you're jumping in with an older baby, no worries; most activities identify the age at which your baby is likely to be ready to tackle them, expressed as a range of months (many of which, you will notice, overlap). Simply start where you feel confident, based on their current age and skill set, your child can comfortably begin. If they are able to participate as described, build from there. If the activity is too difficult or they become upset with each attempt, consider spending time there and supporting your baby as necessary to help them find success, strength, and independence with the physical skill before progressing onward. Work backward in the preceding activities to help your child build strength in areas they might have previously missed.

As you go, you're encouraged to observe your baby's reactions, do your best to tap into their experience, meet them where they are, and guide them with positivity and support.

Part III: Optimizing Your Own Fitness: This part changes the focus from your baby's body to your own; and it will help in your rise to the physical demands of parenthood. We carefully selected several Foundation Training (FT) exercises to prime your muscles for everything from holding and carrying a baby whose weight is steadily increasing (and often wiggling), to changing diapers at all hours (read:

when you're completely spent and the last thing on your mind is your posture), to all the shifting up and down from the floor as you engage your child. These exercises are your preventive medicine against the very real threat of exhaustion and caring for your baby pulling your posture into poor positions that predispose you to pain. Taking these strategies into your day can strengthen your muscles, change how you move, improve your posture, energy, and overall health—all of which can absolutely help you thrive as a parent and caretaker.

And since this journey should be fun, we've included a chapter to end the book called "Growing Stronger Together" that shows parents doing FT alongside their little ones—wearing them, tending to them, and moving and grooving with them. Hopefully you skip ahead to view some of this adorableness before you dive into the activities. Consider this a little creative inspiration as you gear up to get started.

At the back of this book you'll find a supplemental summary of other fine motor and sensory skills that should also be developing in the first year. This is included because of how interrelated these areas are to the development of gross motor skills. Created with the help of pediatric occupational therapists, this is helpful information for optimizing your kiddo's development.

Last you'll find a glossary with definitions of many of the terms used in this book. If you come across a word or phrase that is unclear within the context of the section you're reading, please check here. Terms are listed in alphabetical order.

Baby Fundamentals

Before you begin the activities in Part II, and *ideally* before your baby even arrives, you would do well to know some important and formative things about your little one's body. This chapter covers a variety of topics, including the challenges and benefits of gravity, the importance of neutral alignment, how your baby learns through movement, and what physical developments to expect during the first year. Being knowledgeable about your baby's anatomy, physical abilities, and needs will help you make informed choices while you're guiding this important aspect of their development.

Weightless in the Womb: Gravity and Unfurling

While in the womb, your baby's body is essentially floating, surrounded by amniotic fluid that keeps it safely cushioned.

As the baby grows larger and the womb space grows smaller, their body is curled up, resembling the letter C. This is called *physiologic flexion* and is characterized by the head and limbs being flexed

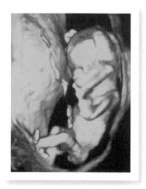

20 weeks. The midpoint of pregnancy and perfectly showing physiologic flexion

and tucked in toward their body's center. Because the womb has increasingly limited space for the baby during the third trimester, their body assumes an even more compact position (which isn't necessarily symmetrical) within this space. This all changes dramatically after birth.

It should be noted that the birthing process can be considered physically traumatic for the baby (and for a mom, too, which is part of why we've included Part III of this book). For baby to be vaginally birthed, they must negotiate their body through the pelvis and the birth canal, squeezed by muscles and contorted by forces. Unfortunately, sometimes injuries can happen during the process. The bones of the skull naturally shift, which assists the baby in squeezing their way through, but sometimes a shoulder or arm, for example, won't move through as seamlessly. Sadly, babies can experience an array of different injuries, including fractured bones. Some might experience microscopic muscle tears or damage to their nerves—which could go undetected for several days, weeks, or even months until discrepancies in posture or movement are more visibly noticeable. This is all the more reason to focus on healthy practices that call the muscles to rise to action and support overall physical development. *Teaching and guiding the muscles from the start can minimize the necessity for future therapeutic intervention, whether there are traumatic birth injuries or not. If there are known injuries, licensed medical professionals can help guide necessary adaptations for positioning, holding, and other activities.*

The greatest force your newborn grapples with is gravity.

As adults we seldom think about gravity, because our bodies have adapted to it.

Gravity doesn't play a major role in the womb, either, as the amniotic fluid makes your baby buoyant and their experience is relatively weightless as they move around (though not exactly "weightless" from the perspective of the pregnant mama carrying them). They will eventually take up more space and push into their mother's body more, which gives their body some sense of pressure.

When your baby is born, though, their body has an instant

confrontation with gravity that is abrupt and dramatic. Your infant is suddenly slammed with their body's full weight. This new responsibility, having to work so hard just to lift their head, is also a blessing.

That's because *one of your baby's first acts on earth is to resist the force of gravity; and this instinctual response is what activates your little one's muscles to begin to unfurl and elongate* from their in-utero flexed and bound-up positions. Your baby isn't *weak*, in a weak versus strong sense, so much as they just haven't encountered gravity *yet*—they don't know how to actively engage their muscles *yet*. This is why we are using hands-on techniques to guide them through the developmental process and really want to help ensure they are finding strong alignment in each new position they encounter. Babies gain strength from top to bottom (head to feet) as they begin to lift their heads. At the same time, they are also developing strength from their core outward toward their limbs, their arms and hands, legs and feet. More on this to come.

As babies' muscles lengthen, with each move they pull on the bones to which they're attached. This generates force, leading to the muscles becoming stronger and more coordinated over time with practice. This begins to create a more mature postbirth alignment of the bones, as babies gradually pull out of their physiologically flexed predispositions through their repeated muscle usage.

Attention to the spine's alignment and (current absence of) curves is of significant importance because of just how formative this is. *Every attempt at movement, every position baby is in, can impact their structure.*

Spinal Curves and Neutral Alignment

As babies continue to unfurl over time, opportunity to practice movement in various positions will provide what their muscles need to stretch, elongate, and engage, which allows their body to posture differently as they grow and gain strength. Bones will move as a result of the forces generated by the contraction of the muscles attached to them. As this happens throughout the body, strength is developed and leads to stability development and structural shifts. We feel it's important to highlight the significance of this occurring along the backside of the body, referred to as its *posterior chain*, because it plays a key role in helping determine how the dozens of bones in your little one's spine will align (and much more).

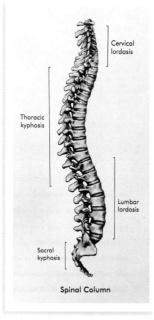

Cervical lordosis

Thoracic kyphosis

Lumbar lordosis

Sacral kyphosis

Spinal Column

The early action of the muscles of the posterior chain literally pulls the body out of physiologic flexion. This is fundamental in terms of setting the stage for the spine's curvature.

It should develop such that the neck (cervical spine) is predominantly in a lordosis, the upper back (thoracic spine) is in a kyphosis, and low back (lumbar spine) is in a lordosis with the sacrum in a kyphosis. Here is a profile of an adult spine showing these curves, to help you get a sense for what these words mean. A baby's spine has yet to develop this alignment. These curves do not fully mature for years, essentially not until growth stops; *but* they can be impacted for better or worse, throughout life. The first year is setting important groundwork for this curve. *You must question what happens to the body structure, the spine, the nerves, if an imbalance occurs early in life, before the body is vertical against gravity. If there's some sort of kink in the spine that doesn't get remedied, as the body grows and more weight and force are applied to those faulty zones, what happens to the spine's curve?* Shifts in its alignment can affect nerves, sensation, and movement.

Healthy spinal curvature is something we should all want because it helps create a body structure that has ample *space* for nerves, blood, and lymph vessels to function without impedance. This is important for systemic health of the whole body, as a baseline for physical skills, and to help ensure that movement skills express the same from one side of the body to the other. These illustrations show you the complexities of how these structures weave throughout the skeletal structure.

A FEW WORDS OF CAUTION REGARDING COMMON "CONTAINERS" YOU MAY CONSIDER PURCHASING . . .

. . . such as cribs, swings, wraps, carriers, slings, and seats. If you should come across products that offer a cozy feel "like in the womb," be judicious.

You want to be cognizant about what babies are lying upon and how their bodies react to each surface. It isn't helpful for their spines to round and their limbs to remain flexed as they were in-utero. What's more desirable are firm, flat surfaces that encourage your baby to unfurl and experiment with movement.

This provides the opportunity to resist gravity as they push into the surface below them and feel the pressure generated by each move. At rest, a flat surface means there are no slopes or bumps that could potentially contort a segment of the baby's body. Beware of thick blankets and excessive cushions that allow the body to sink into the surface. It's better for the body's weight to be supported on flat surfaces that disperse relatively uniform pressure across the portions of the body upon it. Basically, while the body of the little one is unstable, the surfaces they rest and "play" upon should be extra stable.

While it is not completely visualized here, these vessels run on top of, around, and through muscles. Some pass directly to the brain, some directly to the heart, and others to the body's various organs. *This is the same in a baby's body; and attention to this space is important from the very start of life. While the mature curvatures of the spine won't be fully set for several years, as a baby begins moving their body's segments against the force of gravity, the formation of these curves is being initiated.*

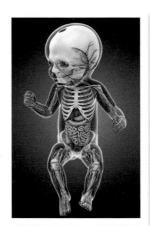

The first experiences of lifting the head are essentially like a baby's posterior chain waking up, igniting. This initiates the cervical "lordosis" between the base of the skull and the top of the shoulders, which is a concave curve that is more or less like a backward C shape.

As the baby comes up higher from the surface, pushing their arms into the floor with their upper back rounding up away from the floor initiates their thoracic "kyphosis," a convex curve in the upper to midback.

In months to come baby will press up higher from the surface with their low back extending on their pelvis and the muscles at the front of their hips stretching farther out of physiologic flexion, resulting in the pelvis resting lower to the ground and giving shape to the lumbar lordosis and the sacral kyphosis as they gain the ability to pull their legs underneath their body in an all-fours position. And all this is further defined as they learn to come up on two limbs versus four.

Your ability to name these curves is not what is important here (hence the very cursory explanation, which may already feel like information overload—bear with us and don't attach to names!), so much as recognizing that *it's crucial to keep a watchful eye on the positions your child is in both at rest and when moving.* The development of these curves can be impacted at any age or stage by habitually resting in or moving from a poor alignment (i.e., in the car seat, swing, stroller, or sling), or by using muscles on one side of the body more than the other. Also keep in mind that these curves continue to develop and can be impacted by our posture as we age, not just during this formative early stage. *For children to begin to achieve a baseline of nicely functioning spinal curves by the time they're upright and walking, it's important to pay attention to what they are doing throughout the first year as their bodies establish their relationships with gravity and begin to support themselves.*

And this is all critical because the spine plays such key roles as supporting the upper body's weight; providing the structure needed for movement and flexibility; and protecting the spinal cord, which coordinates signals between the body and the brain.

Furthermore, how the spine sits also dictates how the head is held, and therefore how the eyes are aligned within the head as the child visually takes in the world. Without getting in depth to ponder the potential long-term complications that could ensue, a word of caution about this: we have six small muscles around each eye that help direct the visual path. Perpetually tilting the head means that these muscles are functioning asymmetrically and altering the visual-perceptual input the brain receives. Posture, ergonomics, muscle use—it's important to pay attention, this is all intimately intertwined in the developmental processes.

If muscle usage is perpetually off-kilter, the bones of the body's limbs or spine can become misaligned and the spine can end up curving in ways that lead to pain and further physical compromise, such as compression of vital nerves, blood, and lymphatic vessels, or can even lead to changes in head shape and facial features. The unfortunate reality is that any of these issues can contribute to physical delays or imbalances in a baby's movement skill acquisition.

Now please take a moment to consider a baby's skull's "soft spots." These delicate zones are actually open areas of connective tissue between the bones and they exist until the bones grow together and become solid at their "suture" lines (the place where the two bony plates meet). In that last anatomy image of the baby, you have a view of one of the six soft spots with which a baby is typically born. Soft spots allow the bones to shift and the shape of the head to accommodate the tight spaces as the baby passes through the birth mother's pelvis and birth canal during delivery. Their solidification begins early in the first year and typically completes by the later part of a child's first year; however, this can also occur sooner or later, and into the second year.

This is important because this means that your baby's skull shape can change until this occurs—and "perfect" head shape is not a guarantee.

Activity of the muscles pulling on the neck and skull, as well as pressure experienced directly through the head while lying down, can make visible impacts on skull shape. This means that if your baby spends too much time lying on their back, instead of experiencing a variety of positions, there is a chance they could have a flat spot along the back of their head (or any other portion of their skull depending on where their weight is held). This is a condition called plagiocephaly and it tends to go hand in hand with another condition called torticollis (which is an imbalance in the length of the muscles in the neck). Both issues can lead to other developmental delays.

To help promote healthy neck alignment and symmetrical head shape and facial features, the muscles need experience working at different angles, pulling on the neck and skull in different ways, and the weight of the head needs to be dispersed through various portions of the skull throughout the day. *And this is for far more than cosmetic appearance. Changes in skull shape can impact the pressure within the skull and upon the brain, the effects of which might never be felt or could be dramatic, depending on what portions of the brain are under pressure. There's no knowing exactly how this could impact cognitive capabilities, let alone physical.* This is one of the biggest reasons why it is so important to know how to position your child and how to both support and challenge them within each position. You are both protecting them against gravity and preparing their muscles to do this on their own.

Without getting into detail about how to treat problems that could arise (because that would be unique to each individual case), we want to make clear that *asymmetries can be treated, improved upon, and some can even resolve completely.* Assessment is a time-sensitive issue (because sutures become solid by the later part of the baby's first year of life AND there are conditions where this can happen sooner) that should be discussed as early as possible with a child's pediatrician for efficient cross-referrals (which hopefully include a physical therapy evaluation to ensure mobility in the neck and that movement skills are not limited).

This might all seem overwhelming or scary, and leave you wondering: What's a parent to do?

To avoid such concerns, the ideal goal is for all caretakers to keep a watchful eye on the positions your child takes throughout the day, both at rest and in active, awake times. Understand that their spinal curves can be affected at any age by habitually resting in a poor alignment, or using muscles on one side of the body more than the other. The most common visual telltale signs of this occurring are asymmetries, such as a baby tilting their head and looking one particular direction more than others; developing a bald spot, flattened portion of their skull, and/or facial asymmetries with eyes, ears, cheeks, or corners of the mouth; favoring one side over the other with head turning and/or rolling skills; difficulty propping up on both arms while on the belly; differences in reaching or grasping skills and hand strength; and this is all before baby is coming upright from the floor and meant to be developing more advanced movement skills. Early detection and intervention of such issues will help put a halt to delays in movement skill development.

All that said, it's also important to note that there are times when an asymmetry doesn't necessarily represent a structural problem. For example, a baby in a crib might prefer looking toward one particular side because of the way the crib is positioned in the room, or because the little one is aware of and most interested in the door where Mom and Dad enter. Another example is a baby only rolling over one side. This may simply be because they are motivated to turn their head and neck to that particular side because there is an interesting item of furniture catching their eye in that direction. If their upper spine rotates, their lower spine will follow; but, if there is nothing of interest in the other direction to get them to first turn their head and neck, the rest of the spine is going to be a lot less likely to rotate that direction for baby to effectively initiate a rollover. Those two examples are scenarios easily corrected by simple changes in the child's environment and attention to ensure that they have variety to their visual and positional perspectives. If left unresolved, however, a case like this could absolutely lead to developing structural asymmetries because of habitual posturing and imbalanced muscle usage. If you find yourself concerned, don't hesitate to consult with your pediatrician, chiropractor, and/or pediatric physical or occupational therapist. Trust your eyes, gut, intuition, and that another set of eyes assessing your child can potentially direct you to helpful practices specific to your child's needs.

Because not all practitioners have the same backgrounds and toolsets with which they approach patients, open dialogue is encouraged with your pediatrician and all those participating in your child's care. If interventions are encouraged, be sure every caretaker, babysitter, family member, and/or daycare teacher is on board with a unified approach to help create new habits and lasting changes.

The goal for each baby, with longevity of healthy movement in mind, is to meet gravity, unfurl while being gently physically challenged and dutifully supported, and develop a healthy spinal alignment with healthfully moving, stable spinal curves, and unimpeded nerve conduction, blood flow, lymphatic circulation, and digestion/elimination. All these aspects of physical health coming together, including the ability to breathe well, promote movement being its most optimal, which increases the likelihood of expected movement milestones being reached with strength and stability. You help your baby achieve these goals by presenting loving challenges throughout the day, in the form of positioning and play. We encourage steady monitoring and helping to alleviate discrepancies before they lead to bigger issues.

Over time, baby should develop a fairly neutral alignment of their body, both at rest and hopefully throughout movement as well. When the bones in the spine and the joints are lined up well, in their most congruent positions with the least amount of force and no twisting, bending, or compressing, this allows for important aspects of conduction, circulation, digestion occurring in the body's various systems. This helps to keep things moving and functioning well.

To visualize neutral alignment, imagine standing with tall, strong posture:

- Head and neck are lined up with the torso's midline.
- Chin points to the center of the chest.
- Ears are level with each other and stacked over the tops of the shoulders with even space between them when comparing sides.
- Shoulders are in a straight line across the body, forming a T with the neck, and aligned (in a top-to-bottom sense) directly above the hips.
- Hips are level and stacked over the knees.
- Knees are level and stacked over the ankles.
- Feet are flat on the ground, with toes pointing relatively straight ahead, and weight evenly dispersed among the heel, the ball of the big toe, and the pinky toe.

This is a general description for a more mature body, and while it is the goal to achieve as close to this as possible when a baby is positioned on their back or belly, their body simply is not ready to do so yet. The activities to come will guide you to align your child optimally for each task to facilitate strength building and establish control that will take their body toward more neutral alignment as their resting habit.

It's easily overlooked but so important to note—the posture a baby's body rests in will speak to the alignment of their bony structures—this helps caregivers to see how their young body is handling all the forces upon it. Baby's body steadily receives varying degrees of input from all the forces and sensations they experience, whether awake or asleep, in your arms, or on some other surface. Gravity is always present and every position counts as baby tests out using their muscles, shifting and repositioning in a game of active learning. As they go, movements will naturally take their body out of neutral; and, part of the challenge of the first year is handling that with balance and an increasingly more stable body.

In pages ahead, you'll learn the path of development, which body segments are called to rise when and how. You'll learn how to best support and guide your baby to optimal alignment during floor time, while in your arms, while in containers, and while moving. In general, activities are arranged in an order that helps the baby toward gaining postural strength, stability, and mobility together as they unfurl, grow, and begin moving.

Another important note: *Skipping fundamental segments of strength building can lead to weaknesses or lagging strands of movement throughout the body. Poorly aligned posture left uncorrected is essentially being reinforced with any additional "strengths" then lined up to be built upon a less stable foundation.* Not the start you want for your baby, who has their lifetime ahead. Make it as physically sound as possible. These are important considerations and your baby's body segments won't all strengthen and stabilize at the same pace. This is covered in more detail next.

Directions of Development

When your baby is performing less-than-smooth motions that appear uncoordinated and random, that's typically not actually wasted movement. Your baby is trying out the different parts of their body, and in the process developing greater muscle strength, endurance, control, and coordination.

This doesn't occur in all areas of the body at the same pace. It proceeds in a top-down manner referred to as "cephalocaudal," which is Latin for "head to tail." Your baby will first work on the muscles attached to the head, neck, and upper spine as they work to lift their head. The actions and efforts of their body to press up farther from the surface will then work the muscles farther down their body. The upper trunk, the lower trunk, the hips, and so on, segment by body segment, all the way to the feet.

At the same time, your baby's body works hard to develop control of the areas near their midline before then proceeding outward to the limbs. For example, the upper body develops control from the head and neck to the shoulders, to upper arms to forearms to wrists, and finally to the tiny muscles of the hands. Similarly, the lower body develops from the abdomen, pelvis and hips, to the buttocks and down the leg, to the feet. This helps to first stabilize the core and larger joints, while leaving precise control of smaller appendages (wrists and hands, ankles and feet) farther from the body's core until later development.

During the first several weeks, your baby's muscles are so uniformly weak that they require your full support everywhere, especially at the head and neck. Over time, being aware of how their body is developing and challenged in each position can help you decide where and when to allocate support, and how to best position your baby to maximize their experiences.

For more on why your baby's seemingly haphazard movements are actually highly beneficial, please read on.

Learning Through Senses and Movement

An alert, awake baby is seldom still. Their senses are waking up, day by day, moment by moment, experience by experience. The input that the baby's senses register within their brain cause responses and reactions; and, new patterns or "neural pathways" of information are formed for future use in executing movement. The senses of sight, hearing, touch (temperature, pressure, tickle, itch, pain), taste, and smell are waking up and *baby is learning so much, daily, through the process of processing all this new information.* Information comes in—via the senses, the nerves, and signals travel through the spinal cord to the brain—and the brain responds by sending signals back with orders for how to physically respond. In the beginning these happenings are anything but organized or controlled. The brain is continuously forming pathways and connections, developing not only movement patterns for muscles, but also increasing body and spatial awareness that will later contribute to more refined movement skills, balance, and eye-hand coordination.

Especially during the first few months, just the experience of having a body that's constantly pushing against gravity, and limbs that can move outside the constraints of a womb, is an exciting adventure. Depending on how your baby is positioned—on their belly, their side, their back, or positioned somehow in your arms—they can use any combination of muscles to move. Some segments of the body will move together until other areas are sufficiently strengthened and movement then becomes more controlled and separated.

You're encouraged to develop a keen eye to observe the details of your baby's body postures and motions. Consider details like: When their head lifts, how is it positioned during that motion? Is it rotated to one side? Is it tilting? And if so, to which side? Can they lift their head and turn their neck both to their left and right sides pretty equivalently in measures of both how much movement as well as quality of movement? Can both arms move through the same arcs of motion while on their back, sides, belly? Are both fists loosening and opening? Are both legs bending and straightening, kicking, and pushing? Can they turn their head and roll to their left side the same as they can to their right? Every body is different and exposure and practice experiences will provide strength-building opportunities for your baby.

As basic as it sounds, don't forget to consider that movement requires energy. It's crucial to pay attention to the amount and quality of sleep a baby gets, and to their feeding, nutrition, digestion, and elimination. Sleep is a vital ingredient in the recipe for baby's happy and healthy growth. Each time babies sleep, it's like a small reset for them; their brains get to reboot with all they have experienced and learned, and they're basically storing notes to apply to future movements. In our own day-to-day experience, we saw the best carryover of skills from one play session to the next when our daughter was well rested and happily fed. It all boiled down to how fresh and alert she was at any given play session. If she was tired, we consistently saw less control, less endurance. Along the same lines, if her tummy was full or hungry, gassy or constipated, then willingness to move or put pressure through her stomach decreased.

Babies will naturally experience different windows of energy during the day, and there will be optimal times when they are receptive and excited to move. When they are awake, alert, and energetic, they will be better able to "work" (read: *play*). It's one of the challenges of the caregiver to recognize these windows and creatively capture the daily potential.

These "windows" of energy are NOT when a baby has a full tummy or a messy diaper. The wrong position and pressure on the tummy right after eating is a recipe for losing the contents of the stomach before it even has a chance to move along in the digestive tract (said differently: spitting up, reflux). *Aim to wait at least forty-five minutes after eating before putting the baby horizontal, and especially atop their tummy.* This can mean being held upright in your arms, sitting in a bouncer seat, or even using a positioning wedge so they are lying at an incline versus flat. As for soiled diapers—some babies are more sensitive than others about this. Cleanliness and germs aside, just ask yourself how comfortable you would be moving about with a wet, messy, bulky diaper squishing about under you. *You may want to consider allowing your baby to experience some diaper-free movement time so there are no restrictions* (a tight diaper at the front of the hips may be a reason some babies self-limit their movements).

DON'T FORGET TO CONSIDER THE QUALITY OF BABY'S "FUEL"

From breast milk to formula to purees to solid foods and supplements . . . what is providing the energy for baby's growth and movements? A few words that you may want to consider from a nutritionist whose work focuses on maternal and baby health:

"Nutrition plays a critical role in early development starting from the time before a baby's entry into this world. Without proper nutrient, antioxidant, omega, fatty acid, and amino acid levels, development suffers. Nutrition in pregnancy and the first year of life is incredibly impactful on the outcome of a baby's health for years to come. So many systems are initially supported in these early months; for example, gut bacteria are inoculating for the first time into the colon wall, and the brain, nervous system, and neurochemistry building blocks are all laid out. This all directly relates to the baby's energy, strength, growth, and therefore physical skill development."

—Dani Rhoades, NC, cofounder of Happy Healthy Littles

Movement can be an emotional matter at times for new little systems trying to figure it all out. Try to stay tapped in to your baby's wavelength, so to speak. Watch their nonverbal reactions and facial expressions, listen to their sounds, their grunts, their breathing. If the baby is resistant or upset, pause and see if you can guide the situation to make it calm and enjoyable for baby so that it registers in their mind as a positive experience. If you can't, don't force it as that could create a negative association, activity resistance, and upset the baby with future attempts of the same movements. There is some level of psychology to this and, though it's not the direct subject matter of this book, I bring it up because truly observing and listening in this way has proven so vital a piece to connecting with and guiding each unique child.

Watch for sensory overload. If there is some sort of sensory stimulus that is overwhelming for your baby, like too loud of a room (a dog barking, a loud relative, competing noises of the television and someone on a phone call, a siren), it can make it hard for the baby to focus on whatever task is at hand and it can create an upsetting or overwhelming experience for them. Attention to volume is important; watch how your baby responds. If the baby is melting down, we encourage you to reroute to another task without skipping a beat. Stay positive, calm, comforting, and engaging, rather than waste time pushing for completion of the task and potentially upsetting the baby further. Reapproach again later, and make an effort to attempt your positions and activities more than just once or twice in a day.

Along similar lines, be mindful of your own facial expression, tone of voice, and chosen words as you engage your baby. They may not understand every word you say, but they can often read and mirror facial expressions and emotions, and respond to changes in tone. Do your best to tune in to your baby's willingness to engage and participate.

We encourage you to look at the whole of the day as full of various opportunities to rotate through each of the positions the baby should be in, including spending time in different devices or "containers" like bouncer seats and carriers. You can make the analogy to this being like a little rotisserie. Keep turning baby so they experience the heat to cook thoroughly. In this case, the "heat" is the challenging work the baby's muscles experience in each position. It's a crude analogy, but one that seems to make sense to most folks. A little time spent in each position, all the way around (belly, to side, to back, to other side, and also upright), helps the baby's muscles learn to engage with stability regardless of where their body is in space. Too much of just one position can lead to imbalances and delays.

When a baby is energetic, you might consider beginning their awake sessions first with a calm, enjoyable activity as a warm-up before going for the activities that are more challenging for them. You may find that this can help prepare them to meet the challenges of a position versus being potentially overwhelmed or upset (which can happen if they are tired, hungry, fatigued). Basically, it's a balancing act of finding available windows of energy and rotating through a few different positions during those windows. During one wakeful window, for example, you may start out on their back (since they woke up there), then switch to sitting upright in a bouncer, then return to the floor for tummy time.

You may find it helpful to aim to pair baby's activities with your own tasks throughout the day. For example, as you're folding laundry or loading a dishwasher, doing so in a solidly decompressed Foundation Training hinge or a strong kneeling position is a way you can layer in extra boosts for yourself throughout the day. And it's a great time for baby to be working too—flat on their back or propped in side-lying atop the floor or some other flat surface, safely exploring their own subtle movements. Diaper changes present another opportune time to engage your body mindfully. Since you'll be doing them often, why not do them in a way that is beneficial to you? Doing these in a hip hinge offers you a few solid moments to use a strong position versus a weak one that could lead to pain. Once the diaper is changed and you're cleaning things up, while the baby is waiting, they can benefit from a few minutes atop their tummy in a safe, flat spot like the floor or your bed. Perhaps while you do a few of your own morning exercises to start your day feeling good, baby is upright in their bouncer seat, exploring a rattle with their hands.

The realities of life, jobs, and schedules don't always make it easy, but—as much as possible—when it comes to how you switch up the rotation between positions and challenges, try to go with the flow of the day and let baby's energy lead the way. This might look like creating a loose written schedule or checklist of the positions you want the baby to experience throughout the day. And consider taking notes for how many seconds they did x-y-z. This can be a thrilling way to keep accountability and note the little progressions. Sharing a list like this with all baby's caregivers can be extremely helpful too.

As a baby's movements bud and grow, it's important to be realistic with your expectations. Skill development takes time. For example, don't expect the baby to be able to keep their head up for long at first. This skill may start out as just a few seconds here and there; and, over time, you should see dramatic gains in their abilities as their endurance grows. In the first three months alone, the baby begins to control lifting their head and turning it, visually tracking with their eyes. They work on all the muscles that contribute to the ability to do these things in every position they're in, and it's a culmination of strengths that work together to build each skill. *Do your best not to compare your baby to others and be aware that some inconsistencies in their skill presentation are normal as energy varies.* Progress might not be as fast as you anticipate. Your child may simply need to build more strength in certain muscles before their body is ready for more.

As you go, especially with a newborn, plan their positions and activities to be no more than about fifteen minutes in duration. Since baby is going to spend a lot of time sleeping, too, you'll want to spread out what energy they do have during wakeful times over a variety of experiences. Cycle or rotate positions and activities and repeat the cycles between naps and feedings. Tummy time, for example, might realistically be practiced five to ten times during the day, but only for three to five minutes at a time. And during these practice sessions, each attempted head lift may only be one or two bobbly seconds at first.

Paying attention to baby's responses in each position will help you develop the skill to recognize when their energy needs a break and ease them from one position to the next before any protests become worked-up meltdowns. For example, if your baby starts fussing while in tummy time, you might choose to calmly roll them into side-lying, safely prop them, and begin engaging them from this new position. Or your baby may do better if you allow them some solo time, within a different, safe position under supervision, to self-explore. After a little time on their side, you may choose to roll the baby to their back, and after some time there you may then move to their other side before reapproaching tummy time or switching to your arms, a carrier, or a bouncer seat for more upright time. Perhaps for the next round of tummy-time practice you make the activity subtly different by including a mirror prop to motivate your baby to look up. Returning to the previously challenging or upsetting position, you may find that they've warmed up, eased further into moving, and can now handle with gusto what was previously a challenge.

When your baby is bobbing, squirming, and wiggling, they're experiencing the framework of muscles, bones, and joints that make up their body, moving against gravity. With each movement attempt, the sensations and experiences of their efforts create input for their brain on how they interacted physically. This process of learning how to move with control and balance is referred to as "motor learning." It takes time and experience (said differently: *lots of practice*); and, it begins at birth when gravity is encountered. Over time, motor learning results in imprints of instructions in your baby's brain for how their nervous system is to execute movements within different muscles to result in coordinated movements. Baby also gains more understanding of where their body is in space (aka "proprioception").

Because every position and movement holds the potential to teach your baby what their body is, how to control it, and how to use it to interact with the world, there needs to be focus on helping babies physically in terms of positioning and—essentially—protecting them against gravity until their muscles gain the strength, endurance, coordination, and stability to do so on their own. This is why the guidance you'll be provided via the activities in Part II is so important. By facilitating age-appropriate physical challenges and using select hand placements to position and stabilize your little one's body, you'll be bolstering their proprioception and their ability to control their body to navigate their environment.

For those whose children were born prematurely or have special needs, almost regardless of the nature of those needs, this approach can be utilized *with appropriate care, caution, and guidance for any necessary adaptations from licensed medical professionals familiar with baby's unique needs.*

Be aware that as you go forward, your baby may do a few things that look curious to you, and you may question whether they are "normal" or "good" for them. Newborn reflexes, which disappear or "integrate" by later stages in their first year, are possibly to blame. We aren't going to discuss every reflex in this book (that would be information overload and there are plenty of videos on the internet that show and teach about these), but we do want to make sure that you aren't overlooking some of these acts or thinking you need to stop babies from doing them. In pages ahead, you'll gain understanding of the Moro or Startle Reflex, the Rooting Reflex, and the Asymmetric Tonic Neck Reflex (ATNR), to name a few. You'll get some insight into why babies bringing their hands to their mouth is actually a good thing. You'll learn how you can utilize baby's developing visual skills to help elicit more movement.

A QUICK NOTE ABOUT REFLEXES

Your child's reflexes are routinely assessed immediately after birth and should also be at all subsequent pediatrician well-visit appointments. Regardless, should you happen to notice that one of the few reflexes discussed in the upcoming pages is no longer present or that its presentation looks different from one side of their body to the other, this should be discussed with your child's pediatrician.

   Also, please be aware that your child has other reflexes that your docs should be assessing in addition to what is mentioned in this book. We've selected the more obvious and notable ones that we feel you'd do well to be privvy to.

Anticipated Progression of Strength and Skill Development

Every baby is unique in their genetic expression and structural foundation, their nutrition, their energy, their strengths, weaknesses, and exposures to movement within their natural environments (home, daycare, outdoors). They won't all reach expected milestones at the same time or with the same skills. What opportunities they are exposed to and how much practice time they get will absolutely impact their physical expression as they grow.

As you're likely aware, certain physical advancements are expected to occur within certain ranges commonly referred to as "milestones." For the purposes of this book, we are less concerned with milestones occurring "on time" and more keen to empower you to strengthen your child thoroughly so they are ultimately rising up with stability as they gain control of their body.

Read on for more understanding of what to expect in the natural progression of movement, strength building, and skill development, organized into three-month increments. Being aware of this will be helpful in choosing how to engage your tot. You don't want to overstrain them nor do you want to eliminate challenges that spur healthy growth and development. As you read the overview ahead, keep in mind that Part II will provide specific activities to help guide this growth process. Also keep in mind that there is *so* much more to growth and development than just what we touch on here. These are simply the big points we feel it's valuable to be aware of as you endeavor into this physical journey with your child.

MONTHS 1–3

During the first few months, one of your newborn's biggest challenges in every position is trying to lift their head. Their skills with this start incredibly small. In fact, first attempts at lifting the head may occur just moments after birth atop Mom's chest, thanks to an innate drive to "breast crawl" (they physically move to the nipple to nurse) and a reflex babies are born with called the Rooting Reflex. This might initially result in just the eyebrows and muscularly furrowed forehead rising. And the head might lift for just a fraction of a second. See the upcoming box for more on this natural reflex, which should disappear by baby's fourth month of life.

ROOTING REFLEX

Especially during their first several weeks, the baby is mostly sleeping and when they are awake, they are very motivated to eat. The **Rooting Reflex**, which enables baby to move head and neck in search of their mother's breast, can be stimulated by a light stroke from the corner of the mouth across the cheek. In response, a baby will lift and turn their head in the direction of the stimulus as they open their mouth, looking for their food source. This can be strategically utilized to encourage baby to actively turn their head and neck.

For example, when being held for nursing, Mom can gently brush her nipple, fingertip, or a bottle nipple (meaning Dad or another caregiver can do this too!) across the baby's cheek on the side toward which she wants the baby to turn. Eliciting the reflex should cause baby to rotate to face that direction. Doing this toward both sides can be an effective way to layer in subtle work on the baby's neck's range of motion, *hidden within the functional act of nursing.*

Providing support at the base of baby's skull may be helpful with directing their movement to be smooth and controlled, especially in the early weeks, though it should be noted that some children will respond to that support by pressing their head farther back toward the hand supporting them. It's truly a little bit of trial and tweak as you go.

Also important to note here, we wouldn't encourage stroking the cheeks to elicit a child's rooting response and NOT providing the nourishment that baby is seeking, as that is nature's intended purpose of this reflex and it might be very upsetting for your hungry baby.

Simply knowing that this is possible gives you one more easy, natural tool to make your time with your baby that much more fruitful.

As muscular endurance builds, the duration of sustained head lifting, in seconds, progressively increases: one to two seconds becomes three to five, then seven to ten, ten to fifteen, fifteen to thirty, and so on. Over the first few months, your baby will gradually build the skill to lift their head and hold it in neutral midline alignment. This means that the crown of their head points to the ceiling and their chin points to the center of their chest without their neck tilting or rotating to either side.

By roughly three months of age, we anticipate seeing that a baby has developed a fair degree of neck control and is beginning to engage muscles farther down their body, in their upper to midback and core as well as outward toward their limbs.

On their back we anticipate that the baby can visually track you or a small toy that you wave across their line of vision from their periphery to their midline and from their midline to either side, as well as slightly up and down. They should be able to turn their head and neck fully to either side (from resting one cheek upon the surface to the other). This rotation may result in another reflex called the ATNR (Asymmetric Tonic Neck Reflex) until approximately months four to six. And another reflex you're likely to see shifting your child's body is their Startle Reflex (aka Moro Reflex). This also goes away by months five to seven.

ASYMMETRIC TONIC NECK REFLEX (ATNR)

The **ATNR** occurs in response to the baby's neck rotating to one side, as seen exhibited by our daughter at nearly three months old. With this reflex, the baby appears to be ready to take you on in a fencing duel: with one arm extended in the direction they are facing and the opposite arm bent at the elbow with hand resting near the base of their skull.

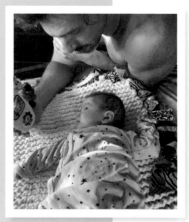

This reflex should integrate by the fifth to sixth month, sometimes sooner, and will result in asymmetrical posturing until then. *We point this out because this is one case where asymmetric posturing is NOT a negative, curious as it may appear.*

While this book will not go into detail about how you would approach treatment of reflexes that do not integrate on time, we want to make clear—it would absolutely be something to discuss with your child's pediatrician should you notice that the expected reflex response is (1) never present in the first place, (2) presents differently on one side of the body versus the other, or (3) continues to present beyond the seventh month.

At this stage your baby's hands should no longer rest in tight fists and should be beginning to open and close more at will. Over months to come (beyond these first three months), watch how different positions of the wrist and forearm will impact your baby's ability to functionally grip with the side of their hand that is closer to their thumb versus the side of their hand that is closer to their

MORO REFLEX AKA STARTLE REFLEX

This reflex, when triggered, causes the baby's arms and legs to move up and outward from their body in a quick manner, before then recoiling close to the body as if to self-protect. This generally happens in response to actual or perceived changes in their body position, such as when you transition them down into a crib or bassinet, or pick them up. It also happens in response to a loud, startling noise—hence this also being known as the **Startle Reflex**.

This reflex can be triggered just about anywhere, on any surface or in your arms, while awake or asleep; and it can be very upsetting for some babies who will cry out. It can wake a sleeping baby, so take care to monitor your own volume as well as that of your

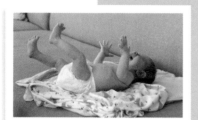

baby's environment. Also, it's important to be careful when transitioning your baby between surfaces because sometimes the reflex is accompanied by the head and neck extending back in a quick, jerky manner. This reflex is another reason it's so important to learn to support your baby's head, neck, and body well. Stability can help prevent it.

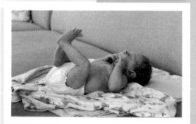

As babies grow older and acclimate to the sounds of the world they live in, the Startle Reflex will occur less frequently. It should integrate by months five to seven.

Many resources will encourage parents to swaddle the baby to attempt to calm and prevent this occurring during sleep so that the baby is not awoken by the reflex. Swaddling prevents the limbs from moving, plain and simple. Being supporters of movement and unfurling once the baby has exited the womb, allowing them to experience the various sensations that come with movement in various positions, we want to refrain from commenting on the practice of swaddling except to point out that every child is uniquely different and what is calming for one might not be for another.

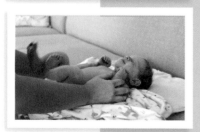

Here we see a three-week-old whose reflex was triggered. Baby responds by suddenly flinging her arms and legs up and out as she cries.

After the initial reaction, she brings her limbs back toward her body, as if trying to shield herself from whatever caused the disruption or to instinctually hug or hold on for safety.

When this occurs, you can help to calm your baby with a loving touch that brings stillness along with warm, calm, stable pressure. In the final image here we see baby lowering her limbs further and easing into a smile as her mom uses broad contact from her hands and forearms to encompass her.

pinky. This will differ from their early reflexive grasp. By the end of this first window of time, anticipate that your baby will exhibit more bending and straightening of their arms, alternately and together, and they will begin batting at and reaching for objects that you present to them, utilizing their hands to effectively hold something for several seconds. They should be able to grasp your fingers and even a small towel, cloth, blanket, or toy such as a rattle, with a tight grasp of their palm and all their fingers together. Also, by sometime between the end of this window and roughly month five, you can expect to see your baby bring their hands together in the front and center midline of their body when they are on their back.

Their legs should freely kick, bend, and straighten; and the force that generates, coupled with their ability to turn their head, should result in gaining the ability to roll from their back to either side. That's because at this early stage their spine moves all together as they reflexively "log" roll, as opposed to a more mature "segmental" roll in which we see their legs, hips, and lower portions of their spine lead the way followed by their arms reaching across the midline of their body, and then the upper body following.

In this early stage, the gains in your infant's neck and upper back strength, endurance, and range of motion are perhaps most apparent during tummy time. By the end of three months we anticipate seeing that a baby is now able to lift their head and neck in neutral alignment and maintain this hold to look up at least forty-five degrees from the surface. They should do so by pushing their limbs into the surface and propping their weight increasingly more through their bent elbows, forearms, wrists, and hands. Their hands may still be closed in fists, though likely more loosely, and are held less tightly to their body.

You may find your baby is accidentally rolling over from their tummy to their back during their first several weeks. This often makes parents feel their baby has an advanced skill of rolling over; but the truth is, this can happen as a result of the weight of your infant's head being a bit more than he or she has learned to handle. Meaning, they turn their head to one side and suddenly they reflexively logroll their whole spine and end up on their back. For some little ones this can be surprising and upsetting, especially if they have not yet coordinated the ability to then roll off their back to a side. This early reflexive type of rolling can lead to more coordinated skills over weeks to come, though, so you don't need to stop your baby from doing it. Just keep a careful eye on your infant and be mindful of where you place them. If rolling occurs, guard against any position that might impair breathing. Rolling will be a safety concern until your little one gains the strength and coordination to turn their head and neck to clear their airway independently.

While being held in upright positions (with the lower portions of their spine, hips, buttocks, and legs all well supported), they should begin using their arms and hands to push their weight into the chest of a person holding them, thereby adding control and stability to the base upon which their head and neck sit and align. By three to four months they should be able to maintain a neutral head alignment and exhibit the ability to turn their head and neck to both their right and left sides while maintaining this alignment.

If you support your baby in sitting, you should see that they hold their back in a rounded position, their trunk and arms not yet having developed the strength and stability to muscularly hold their body upright upon their seated base. Ideally, by three to four months, you will see that they can hold their head and neck up, neutrally aligned, with approximately forty-five degrees of an angle between their chin and their chest. Their chin should not be pressing into their chest, nor should their head be flopping toward their back or to either side, requiring the level of support it did when they were first born.

A FEW NOTES ON YOUR BABY'S HANDS

Fine motor skills are the coordinated movements of the arms, hands, and fingers. This includes reaching, opening and closing of hands, pinching, and poking. Though not the primary focus of this book, some mention of aspects of fine motor skill development has been woven throughout since they are, of course, developing at the same time. Fine motor skills are the focus of occupational therapists and there is a great deal of crossover and collaboration in pediatric physical and occupational therapy. Pediatric occupational therapists (OTs) are trained in the development of fine motor skills and sensory skills; with some having additional training in feeding and oral motor skills (latching, sucking, swallowing). *A brief discussion on the development of sensory and fine motor skills in the first year of life is provided at the end of this book.* But before we proceed, we want to make you aware of a couple of reflexes related to the hands that are important to keep in mind as you progress through this book. Please note that if you have questions or concerns about your baby's fine motor development, it is best to consult with your pediatrician to determine if you need a referral to an occupational therapist.

The **Grasp Reflex**, which lasts until month five or six, is when your infant's hand closes shut when pressure is applied to the palm. This is not actual strength or control, but a neurological response to input. It is important to be aware that anything you place in their hands will likely be dropped. Remember that they are not yet capable of holding up their own weight at this stage. You never want to hold your infant up with their grasp since it can easily damage the joints and ligaments of their shoulders and arms. There is a condition called Nursemaid's Elbow that is a direct result of such forces to young, developing arms. So, swinging your baby by their hands is something most pediatric PTs and OTs will advise you against.

The **hand-to-mouth movement** in infants is due to physiologic flexion and should be encouraged. When your baby brings their hand to their mouth in the early weeks of life, it provides pressure input to the face, lips, and inside/outside of the mouth. This promotes the skills of latch, suck, and swallowing. As your baby's grasp strengthens, continue to encourage this pattern by providing appropriate toys and teethers to help them explore and develop these oral motor skills.

If you support your baby in standing, you should see that, while they cannot self-support their weight upon their legs, they can put their feet on toes or flat to the surface with their knees slightly bent. You should also see them exhibit what is called the Stepping Reflex, which is characterized by lifting one foot and then the other as though they are walking. This reflex typically goes away around two months of age.

In terms of cephalocaudal development and spinal curves, this period of time has a dramatic impact on the development of a child's uppermost portions of their spine. The important relationship between how their head is held on their neck and back is being built daily.

MONTHS 4–6

In this next period of time, now that your baby can comfortably lift their neck and head to look up and to their sides, they are now working to strengthen and control muscles farther down their spine into their upper back, torso, and hips.

This is especially apparent when pushing into the floor during tummy time. Your baby should exhibit increased skills with lifting and rounding their upper back as they push their chest and upper abdomen away from the surface below them. To accomplish this, your baby is increasingly engaging the muscles in their upper back, chest, shoulders, and arms, while also engaging their abdominals with more control. In fact, expect during this time to witness your tot experimenting with these parts of their body from all angles, not just flat on the floor, but also in your arms, and while sitting too. This helps them to learn how much of their body weight they can support as they shift through these various positions. It's a perpetual learning process— doing, building strength, playing, and refining skills. This has a huge impact on building the kyphotic curve in the upper to midback.

With all the pushing and pivoting done, your baby's arms respond by becoming stronger and more controlled, with their hands loosening so that palms eventually lie flat against the ground. This helps them advance further as they gain the ability to press up higher through open palms, straighten their elbows, and better handle their body weight with more stability.

During this time, expect to see your baby experimenting with

lifting their hands from the ground, as opposed to keeping both elbows planted on the floor for balance. At first these motions may appear wild and disorganized, as if your child is batting at invisible bugs
and raking at toys like leaves. Over time, though, this will result in
your little one being able to reach out for and successfully scoop up
and grab objects using one or both hands. As the precision and dexter-
ity of the hands and fingers increase, your baby will develop the ability
to do such things as hold their bottle independently and finger feed.

Your baby's legs might appear to be on a slower development cycle,
though this certainly isn't the case. Anticipate that while the baby
is playing in tummy time, there is less flexion at the front of their
hips than in previous weeks, and their legs are likely to be positioned
widely behind their body, potentially in a froglike position. These wide
positions of the legs add balance and stability to the base of the baby's
body, making it easier for the energy of their movement efforts to go
into their upper body without them falling to a side or face-planting
into the surface as they coordinate pressing up and shifting their body
weight. Some babies may even begin scooting along the floor toward
the end of this stage, pulling themself along with their arms, as they
push with the inner aspect of their legs. And don't be surprised if you
see your baby scooting backward before they move forward.

You can also expect to see your kiddo's purposeful control of their
rolling skills improving. On their back they begin to establish the
skill of reaching for and grabbing their feet, rocking and rolling to
their side and beyond to their tummy. Not only are you likely to see
your baby grabbing their feet and rolling around month six, but you
are also quite likely to see them bringing their feet to their mouth.
Strange as this might appear, it's not a bad thing! It not only gives
your child more sensory stimulation to the learning center that is
their mouth, but this act also gives a great deal of movement to
their developing hip joints. This helps to lubricate joint surfaces and
enhance their range of motion, which will be beneficial as they experiment with moving and shifting their weight over their hips with
rolling, sitting, and crawling attempts. All of this helps prepare their

body for the bigger tasks ahead atop two limbs—kneeling, squatting, transitioning to standing, and walking.

Gradually, instead of relying on reflexive logrolling, babies begin coordinating their movement with greater strength, moving more segmentally through their spine. That is, they will eventually begin to coordinate separate upper body and lower body actions to more elegantly and efficiently perform a roll, with their legs, hips, and low spine rotating first, then their midback and upper back following as their arm reaches across the midline of their body to come to the floor and provide stability as they push up from the surface. Expect to see that baby is able to better control rolling from their back to their side as their ATNR integrates. You should now find them hanging out on their side, supporting themself with one arm while reaching for toys with the other. From their belly they have likely figured out that they can turn their head and neck to a side, and follow with their shoulder and arm and then the rest of their body, to purposefully control a roll to their back.

Keep a keen eye on how this skill is expressed in both directions, back to belly, belly to back, over right and left sides. It's crucial to speak with your child's pediatrician if you notice that your little is rolling one direction more than the other, because this skill builds up critical muscles in your child's core and hips essential for their sitting skills. Most babies will favor one direction at first, and you can give them guidance to go both ways.

Speaking of which, another huge leap for babies during this window of time is with their sitting skills. Your baby should be developing the strength and coordination to sit upright atop their bottom and legs, with their legs in a ring, such that their weight falls through the midline of their body and is supported by the outer portion of their legs with their feet very close or touching. Their trunk should be stronger and positioned increasingly more vertically above their legs as they exhibit greater skill with maintaining balance, even while turning their head. Around four months we expect to see that babies are developing the ability to prop themselves up with their arms out in front of them for balance. They should also be developing a natural Protective Extension Reflex to catch themselves should they experience a bump or startle that challenges their balance.

THE PROTECTIVE EXTENSION REFLEX

The **Protective Extension Reflex** develops over time as opposed to other reflexes mentioned thus far that are present at birth and integrate over time. This reflex enables the baby to self-protect and catch themselves if they lose their balance in sitting.

As this skill is developing, you are likely to see your child first catch their balance with their upper arm kept relatively close to their body and their weight falling more through their shoulder or the upper portion of their arm or elbow, basically still tumbling over with their reaction slow and ineffective. This is not abnormal, though; and they are learning through each effort. So don't block them from tumbling. Protect their safety by making the play zone safe, but allow those experiences.

As the skill becomes more finely tuned with strength and stability building, expect to see them responding more quickly and catching their balance farther down their limb with their forearm, wrist, hand, and eventually their open palm.

Over weeks and months to come, this will develop further, allotting your baby the ability to catch their balance to their sides on a single outstretched arm around month seven, and behind them around month ten.

Toward the latter end of this window of time, babies should be experimenting more with shifting their weight over their seated base (meaning up and over a leg) to reach for toys in a small arc around the front and sides of their body; and they may also begin to shift from sitting down to horizontal positions on the floor. Returning back upright from the floor to sitting, however, is not as easy to control and coordinate; and, babies may take more time to develop control with the skill.

All these acts—pushing up, rolling, sitting, and reaching—serve to help strengthen a baby's midsection through their trunk to their pelvis, hips, and arms.

MONTHS 7–9

As their core grows more stable, we anticipate seeing babies develop more control outward of their bodies into their limbs. These gains lead to more exploration of movement that includes greater ranges of motion in segments of their bodies farther distal still, in terms of cephalocaudal development, as babies prepare to come more upright from the floor onto all fours and also onto two limbs in the coming weeks and months.

In terms of rolling, your baby is likely now exhibiting a great deal more control. Placing them on their back for playtime is now likely to result in them immediately shifting out of this position, rolling to their side and beyond to their belly. And they don't likely just stop once they get there. Between the previous time window and now, anticipate seeing that your baby is developing the ability to roll over and over to effectively move about their space. This independence of movement is huge in terms of building their core strength in their back, belly, hips, and upper legs, which is all quite important as this muscular control provides what your baby needs to better control their upper trunk on their seated base when it comes to their sitting skills.

Your baby's arms are now stronger, able to press their torso off the ground during tummy time while providing support and stability. Your baby's legs, which were previously out to the sides of the torso, are now spending more time directly under it. With these gains, you are also likely to see your kiddo pressing up onto all fours and shifting their body weight in all directions, rocking back and forth and pushing from side to side. These moves strengthen the muscles, adding stability and preparing the joints for crawling.

With both arms and legs relatively powerful and coordinated, your child has probably started crawling by the early portion of this window of time. Crawling usually starts by pulling forward with arms low to the ground, and possibly dragging the belly. At the same time, your little one should exhibit pushing with their legs, which will typically begin externally rotated with their inner aspects in contact with the ground and knees out to the sides of their body, more than directly underneath them. This is a temporary phase until your child builds the strength and coordination to perform more sophisticated crawling, such as moving on hands and knees with the belly hovering over the ground.

Note: A small percentage of babies are *perceived* to "skip" the crawling stage. If your child appears to be among them, consult with your pediatrician and seek a referral to work with a pediatric physical or occupational therapist; and consider an assessment and treatment with a pediatric chiropractor. We say *perceived* because it is an inaccurate perception that they are "advanced" and need not spend time with this task if they seem to be showing interest in pulling upright on two limbs instead.

The act of crawling is important because it provides strengthening practice that will build more muscle stability and control, as well as improve communication between the two sides of the brain. More shoulder stability means better arm control, which means more opening of the palm. More pressure through the palm further wakes up the smaller hand muscles, priming them for further development of control. And the improved communication between the brain's hemispheres contributes to smoother control of reciprocal (alternating) arm and leg movement, which benefits not just crawling but also walking.

Your baby is developing the ability to sit with better balance, increasingly more motivated to play with toys and reaching all around them to grab things that would have previously been out of reach. This repeated act of reaching and recovering their upright seated balance, shifting from sitting to the floor and from the floor back up to sitting, provides a tremendous amount of core control for your baby. It is also within these months that babies develop their Protective Extension Reflex to their sides (typically month six or seven) and, later, behind them (typically month nine or ten), which adds better control and safety to their sitting skills as it takes their ability to reach and shift their weight even further.

Babies at this stage are also likely to be experimenting with pulling up to kneeling and standing, and probably while leaning into support surfaces (e.g., furniture, a wall, you). It's important to wait until this stage of the first year to start promoting standing practice because the anatomy (bones and growth plates) of babies' hips are simply not in a good place to hold their weight much earlier. Expect for kneeling to be low at first, with bottom close to feet versus more vertical with hips extended. As babies develop more strength and control between their abdominals, low back, gluteal muscles (bottom), and hamstrings (back of the upper thigh), they will achieve a more upright, strong kneeling position. In an upright stance your baby is likely to keep their legs very wide as this gives them a broader, balanced base of support for their upper body. Shifting their weight from one foot to the other and up and down in squatting are ways your baby is likely to experiment with movement; and you may notice them bending and rotating their torso, shifting their body weight in all directions over their hips, as they explore what their now better-developed lower body can do to move them about their environment. These acts all serve to further strengthen their core and legs, adding to their coordination.

As for spinal development, your baby is steadily gaining control farther down the cephalocaudal chain. Crawling and transitioning their body upright gives more shape to the developing lordotic curve in their lower back. At times your little one might look like a cowboy or cowgirl riding a bucking bronco. In reality they're actually building critical core muscle strength and coordination between their torso and lower limbs with their motion experiments, and this will help balance and align their spine as they grow more upright. This is all important prep work for walking.

MONTHS 10–12

In this window of time, babies exhibit much more control over their floor skills. They have likely mastered the ability to shift from sitting to horizontal and crawling positions on the floor and back to sitting with fluidity, control, and balance. Protective arm extension should now be intact in all directions. These solid gains in core strength provide babies a more stable base from which their limbs can more freely move with increasingly better control. Your baby's rolling skills have likely been traded for crawling on all fours as their preferred means for moving about; your little one is likely to be becoming quite the little speedster with their crawling. All this crawling works wonders for strengthening a baby's shoulder girdle (including their scapula on their rib cage and the mobility of their upper spine), arms, and hands.

With these gains in upper extremity strength and the Grasp Reflex a thing of the past, fine motor skills will also be flourishing. You can expect to see your baby picking things up with a variety of grips, holding and passing them between their hands with more smooth control of releasing objects. They should also be gaining more independence with their budding feeding skills, not only using two fingers to put small items in their mouth but also gaining the skills to manipulate utensils. Using the increased strength and control in their arms, hands, trunk, and hips, babies at this stage will exhibit more and more pushing and pulling to achieve more vertical "bipedal" positions, that is, on two feet.

At first kneeling and stance might not be totally upright or fully aligned and will probably require that your little one use some sort of surface for support. Expect to see most tots working to find their balance, teetering as they lean their chest, stomach, hips, arms, and hands to the surface in front of them. There's likely to be a lot of flexing of the hips and knees and sticking their bottom out behind them, alternated with rigidly locked-out, straight knees. Also, their ankles might plantar flex, shifting them up on their tiptoes (which is okay as long as it's for just a few moments at a time and not your kiddo's primary position). In other words, finding the sweet spot where they are upright and balanced over their flat feet is a gradual process.

As your baby practices kneeling, half kneeling (i.e., weight balanced between one flat foot and one bent knee), squatting, standing, and more advanced movements such as sidestepping to cruise along furniture, they begin to transform into a more independent little mover. Bipedal movement is a major leap in their relationship with gravity. This will require ongoing development of muscle strength, coordination, control, balance, and stability to further refine their skills. Of course this all requires practice and exposure, support and quality-controlled movement. It's not up for debate—babies will absolutely figure out a way to move, regardless if this quality control is offered. But their alignment and skill expression are, as previously talked about, not guaranteed and malleable in nature throughout the process.

Most babies will naturally transition back and forth between crawling and walking for as long as they need to in their strength-building process to build both confidence and stability. It's not something you want to rush; rather, support and thrill to observe. Stumbles and falls will happen. Ideally you've effectively babyproofed their environment for safety, and nothing beyond a few bumps will happen. It's worth saying, in short, that how you respond to those bumps can absolutely shape how your baby responds. Behavior and movement go hand in hand. Be sensitive to this as you go. Understand that some bumps are okay and will actually help to build bone density: so, try not to react quickly by scooping up your baby if they fall. Be aware of your observable responses (facial expressions and verbal reactions). Rather than wearing concern on your face or gasping, try to smile encouragingly and calmly allow your child the opportunity to self-correct and learn as they experiment with more movement. If they are upset or melting down, they may need you to comfort them and help them find their calm so they can return to action. Be their comfort and their cheerleader. Praise their efforts and encourage them to play more (e.g., "That was hard and you did great," or "Go, baby, you can do hard things," or "If you fall, get back up again"). Assess the situation for safety, meet baby's needs for security and

SHOES AND SURFACE CONSIDERATIONS

When your baby begins to walk, be picky about shoes. As adults, we typically consider our own shoes in terms of arch support (or comfort or fashion); but babies don't have an actual developed arch yet (and while comfort is certainly important, fashion really shouldn't be).

As your baby practices walking, the muscles of their lower legs will start to pull more across their ankles and feet and their arches will begin to form. This may have you wondering if there are pros and cons of shoes versus going barefoot. Time practicing both is beneficial. Barefoot walking challenges the muscles to learn to accommodate to various surfaces of the floor; and the main purpose of a shoe is to protect the feet. Both are important.

With or without shoes, some kids will end up overpronating their feet, which looks like their arch is collapsing inward with their weight rolling over the inner side of the feet and possibly giving the appearance of their knees leaning inward. To help combat this, we suggest alternating time spent barefoot with time moving about in more supportive shoes that are firm and fitted through the area where the arch will be, cup the heel adequately, and are not too wide or long in the toe box that it would lead to the foot slipping. And that would do well to be alternated with a shoe like a moccasin that will protect the skin but allow the child to feel the shape and contours of the environment below them. If finding shoes with the right support is difficult, there is also the option to purchase small inserts ("orthotics") that cup the heel and support the arch to prevent overpronation. These can help train your baby's muscles to eventually support the foot naturally. If you choose to go this route, we strongly encourage having a PT or chiropractor check your child's alignment while still and while moving.

A word of caution about all shoes: Avoid built-up heels. This goes for boots, sneakers, and sandals. If the heel is built up, it positions the child's foot and ankle into plantar flexion (toes pointed downward, heel raised). This will alter the mechanics of how your baby moves their leg from the ground upward to their hip; and this can have impacts on positioning all the way through the pelvis, spine, and head. So while it may look adorable, it does the body no favors.

Generally speaking, "low top" shoes are less supportive, whereas the early walker may benefit from a "high top" shoe that crosses the ankle joint. These give a little more support to the joints of the low leg and feet, which may be beneficial until baby's muscles develop and take over that role.

When it comes to the surfaces your child is moving upon, the terrain and texture of the ground are important sensory (and safety) considerations. Watch your child closely and see how they respond posturally and behaviorally to the various challenges that come. Be close enough to lend supportive hands, especially in new environments. Consider what the support below their feet offers them. For example, carpet is more cushioned and may be tickly or scratchy on the feet, whereas tile/wood/cement are firmer and possibly cold, slick, scratchy, or gritty. Outdoors, grass is different from sand (wet and hard-packed versus dry and loose), leaves, and mulch (which can be slippery and unstable).

Also consider whether the terrain is flat or has an incline or decline. Flat surfaces are more supportive and reliable whereas inclines/declines present balance challenges. Little ones may require more support as they learn how to negotiate these challenges, even if they exhibit decent balance on flat terrain. And, of course, as with all other movement skills, their abilities may wax and wane with energy and disposition.

comfort, and shift the activity if needed to introduce a new activity to spur them on.

Toward the end of this first year, your baby should be ready to start walking with the help of your support or possibly a walking toy. Independent walking requires strength and balance and some babies will be ready toward the end of their first year. Some won't be ready until months thirteen to fifteen, or even later in some cases. Note: If your child reaches fifteen to eighteen months and is not yet taking steps, ask your pediatrician for a referral for PT evaluation and consider also seeing a chiropractor skilled in pediatrics. *Whenever a baby officially starts walking, it's a milestone to rejoice, marking a massive leap in their remarkable journey from horizontal to vertical. Even though their journey is far from over, it took a LOT to get here, and a whole new world is accessible to them with this leap of independence.* Hope you've babyproofed!

Your child's center of gravity is going to shift as they become more solid and stable over the top of their feet. More activation of their posterior chain farther toward their tail and beyond down their legs will give them more balance and control as they spend more time upright. Walking may begin with arms held somewhat rigidly in the air, in what we call a "high guard," "mid guard," or "low guard" position. In these positions the arms are held up as a means of adding stability to the upper portions of the baby's spine, as opposed to a more mature pattern of being kept low and swung reciprocally in alternation with the legs. You will know your baby is gaining strength and control, their walking skills maturing, as you see their arms drop lower. In fact, you may note this first by their willingness to carry a toy around with them. Pay attention to how they hold and carry it.

You can anticipate seeing more control of legs with walking forward and backward, increasing speed with walking becoming running, more control of single limb balance while the opposite leg is swinging and kicking a ball, and also with jumping, beyond the first year. More control of hands for self-feeding and toy manipulation as well as more use of arms for swinging, throwing, and catching are also anticipated. And, of course, more dancing and lots of silly wiggling.

As you go through this year, we encourage you to model movement and encourage your kids to explore their world via movement. They truly are little sponges, soaking in all they observe and learning from your words and actions. Your facial expressions and sounds have the power to help your child create positive mental correlations with movement. As cheesy as it might sound, there's no reason not to give your child positive affirmations like "I move because it makes my body feel good! When I feel good, I feel happy!" After all, you want them to be happy movers for a multitude of reasons, not the least of which is because lack of movement will slow down their digestion. If that slows down and the body is consitpated, or full of poop, it will likely feel like poop . . . which can turn behavior to poop. And that's not what you want for your baby.

Now, with all this said, let's charge forward positively and go over some key ways to help your baby in their journey of building their movement skills.

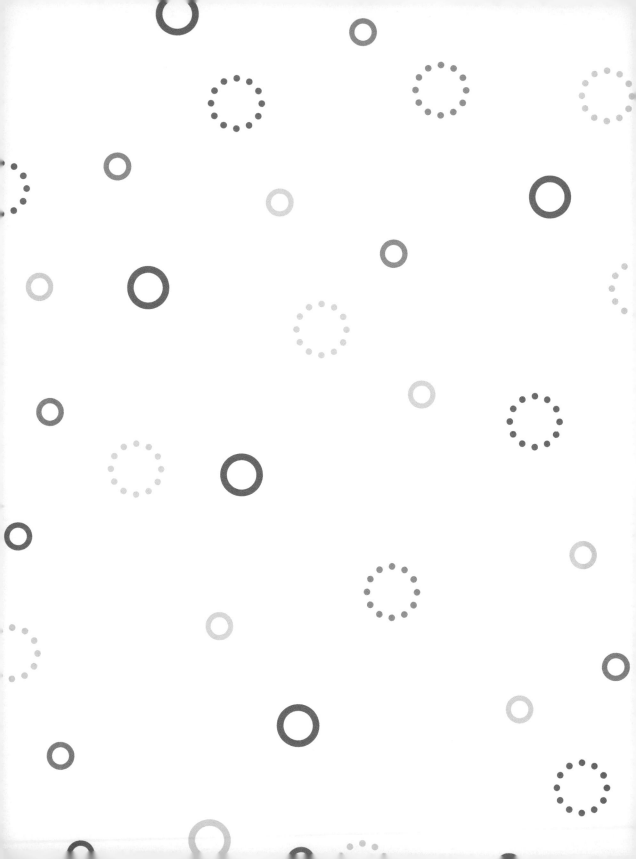

GUIDING YOUR BABY FROM HORIZONTAL TO VERTICAL: ACTIVITIES TO OPTIMIZE DEVELOPMENT

This part includes dozens of concepts and activities that help guide your baby toward optimal physical development. Many of these are presented as activities, created by photo journaling real babies in real play sessions. You should find these to be both engaging and fun (though sometimes challenging and frustrating) for your little one, and they will help to steer your baby toward steadily strengthening and enhancing their physical development. The activities are visually represented by hundreds of photos with several different babies, including our own. Some of the images might appear less polished because they were unstaged and captured in the moment with the intent of helping by sharing from our own experiences.

Accompanying every photo is a description highlighting its most important details, making it easier for you to understand each step of an activity as you work to replicate it with your own baby.

Generally speaking, these activities are organized in a chronological manner, working from the newborn stage to the end of the first year, culminating in the skill of walking.

We encourage you to aim to introduce each activity to your baby in its order and at your little one's pace. Your child will typically need the strength and skills gained from practice of earlier activities to prepare them to tackle each new one. The introductory paragraph of most activities identifies the age at which your baby is likely to be ready for it,

expressed as a range of months within the first year.

If you aren't sure whether your baby is advanced enough for an activity, try introducing it during a time when they are awake, alert, and likely to be more receptive. This should help as you gently guide them through the movements to see how they respond. If they can't manage the challenges, working backward in the activities may help you to determine problematic, weaker areas. *Meet your baby right where they are with support and love and gradually work on any lagging areas using earlier activities.* As strength is built and opportunities to explore movement are provided, don't be surprised to find your baby experimenting with some of the skills you've introduced as well as some you may be planning to try next.

Be sure to constantly supervise your child during these activities. They're designed for at least one caregiver to be participating or overseeing, and ready to step in if needed. If a second caregiver is available, it only benefits the baby to have another set of eyes and hands participating—even if that's just presenting toys and "bringing the excitement" to entice the baby to participate. This can help to free the hands of the parent implementing the activity so they can assist the child with two hands versus just one (presuming the other hand is busy trying to engage and motivate the baby with a toy).

As you go, if something appears unusual to you—such as your child consistently favoring one side or avoiding one limb during certain movements—don't hesitate to bring this up with your pediatrician *before your next scheduled visit*. If there's a genuine issue, it's best to identify it and treat it early. With the overview of physical skill building (at the end of Part I) in mind, if you find that your baby is passing age ranges without the described skills developing or trending late, a call to their pediatrician for a checkup is a good idea.

Psychology, emotion, and movement have intimate connections, and while that's not the subject of this book, it's worth keeping in mind as you go. The activities and concepts presented will be most effective for your baby's development if you implement them with playfulness, positivity, and encouragement. The more your baby enjoys their movement experiences, the more willing a participant and happy an explorer they will be. And similarly for you, the more joy and confidence you feel guiding your baby through these exercises, the better a job you're likely to do.

Among so many other roles, as parent, you are their first coach and biggest cheerleader. Share your support and love as you encourage them and build a trusting bond. Try your best not to compare them to other kids or get anxious about doing well. *We've created this resource to help take any guessing or worry out of the mix so you can enjoy the magic of your little one growing and becoming a physically connected MOVER.*

Building Baby's Baseline by Holding, Positioning, and Their Earliest Physical Challenges

Two of the most invaluable things you can do to positively shape your baby's physical development are *hold and position them effectively*. This takes some initial learning and steady mindfulness. Previous sections gave you some of the important anatomy background to understand *WHY* this is important, and ahead you'll find images to show you *HOW* to provide the support your child's body needs. This is your physical guidance for how to encourage the engagement of their muscles in ways that will benefit continued healthy development *and* prevent a myriad of issues.

When your baby is brand-new, you should aim to hold them with 100 percent support because a newborn has virtually no control over their delicate body.

This can be done in several ways, and you and baby will both want and need a variety of strategies throughout the day. Keep in mind that it's important to keep switching their position, whether in your arms or on a flat surface like their crib, so that they experience their body differently against gravity. And do your best to protect your newborn against the harsher effects of gravity. You can accomplish this by positioning your baby, while awake or asleep, in your arms or elsewhere, in postures as close as possible to neutral alignment. Utilize your hands or props, like rolled blankets, towels, or burp cloths, to help position the baby. Because of physiologic flexion, what this looks like will change throughout the year.

When moving your baby in and out of their crib, car seat, or bath, passing them between caregivers, or simply bringing them up for close face-to-face time, you want to do so with careful attention to their spine and both hands fully supporting their body. Use one hand to broadly support their head, neck, and shoulder to upper back region, and use your other hand to support their lower back, bottom, and upper thighs, as in the photo below.

Spread your fingers widely to provide as much support as possible and allow the baby's body weight to be more evenly dispersed.

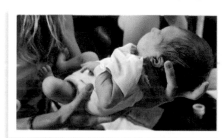

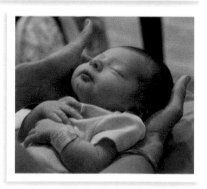

Another comforting way you can hold your baby on their back, which allows for great eye contact, is on your lap. These first two pictures show a five-day-old, and the picture that follows is a one-month-old.

Here the five-day-old is held in the caregiver's lap. Her head is supported at the base of her skull and the side of her skull in such a way that her chin is guided to neutral alignment. Her relaxed face speaks to the calm, stable, and comforting support she is receiving.

The image of the one-month-old shows the mother with legs elevated so that the baby is both flat on her back and resting with her head elevated approximately forty-five degrees, a position that aids in the natural digestive flow (making this a great position for after a feeding). As for the baby's arm position, Mom is simply allowing the baby to move and accommodating her support in response. Baby is seen here resting with one arm down at her side, her hand in contact with her mother's leg, palm open as she is exploring

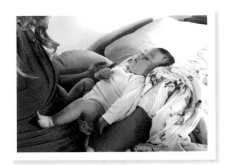

what she feels with her fingers. Her mother's hand is providing a base of support below her opposite elbow as she bends the arm and pushes it back, her hand in contact with her own chest, exploring. We also see that the baby has her feet in contact with the mother's abdomen. This allows the baby to feel where her body is in space with each push of her legs meeting resistance; and this provides great feedback that helps her brain develop further muscle control and body awareness.

Generally speaking, when you cradle your baby close to you, focus on neutral alignment. Take care to not wedge your hand under an armpit, knee, or hip, as this can push one side of the body too far upward or forward. This comes with the risks of contorting or compressing nerves, muscles, and joints.

If you see your baby's shoulders rising up to their ears, their neck tilting or turning to one side, or their chin pressing down into their neck, shoulder, or chest, there is a good chance that there is too much pressure somewhere. Be watchful to correct such happenings right away as they don't help your baby learn to support their own head well.

This image shows a baby with a small hand towel rolled and positioned under his head and around the underneath and sides of his neck, creating a bumper roll to protect and support the area where his lordosis will be developing. The image beautifully captures a mother doing her best to prevent her child's chin from

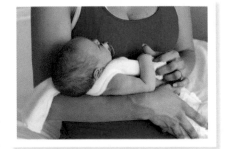

compressing down into his neck as she cradled him during a guided session. This position provides a great option for how you can support your baby while feeding, or after, when you would want to avoid them being flat on their back or stomach. More holding for feeding images are coming next.

Holding for Feeding

Countless hours will be spent feeding your baby, and a little mindfulness can go a long way when it comes to both the caregiver's and the baby's posture.

Breastfeeding a Newborn, Seated with Props

This image shows a mother using props to keep her nursing posture aligned: a pillow between her knees, a nursing pillow below the baby, and a pillow below the nursing pillow to ensure that the baby is propped in line with her breast. We consider this to be an active "reset" posture. We recognize that assuming such a position for every nursing session isn't realistic, but if you study this image, it highlights the exact reason you should incorporate the ideas presented here and in the next several activities. It may not jump out at you right away but if not addressed, it can wreak havoc on the nursing mother's body.

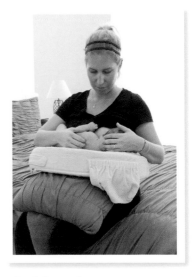

At first glance you may simply note that this mom is doing what comes naturally by leaning her neck forward and looking down to ensure that her baby has successfully latched and is feeding well. The problem with this? Too much time spent in that position can stress and strain the cervical spine, nerves, and muscles, and compromise blood flow to the brain. When you consider all the hours in the day that are cumulatively spent nursing, it really adds up fast.

Our advice to nursing parents: aim to incorporate a few minutes of this active feeding posture a few times throughout the day. Even just five minutes, three to five times a day is a good start. More would certainly be better!

In this next image, you see a profile view of how she repositioned her head and neck into a stronger alignment, bringing her chin back as she raises her head upward to keep her neck tall over her torso.

To set this up well, do the following:

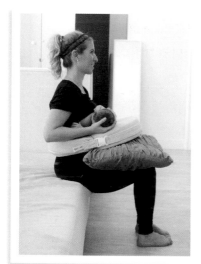

- Come toward the edge of your seat with your feet flat on the floor and your big toes pointing slightly toward each other, with the outside edges of your feet parallel.
- Place a pillow, a small ball, a folded blanket or towel, a stuffed toy, or a water bottle between your knees to squeeze to activate your inner thighs.
- Elevate the position of your baby using pillow and nursing props to *bring the baby to you rather than bringing your body to the baby.*
- Focus on taking slow, big "decompression" breaths (more on this in Part III) as you work to elongate your torso and expand your rib cage.
- Bring your chin back, chest up, and work to allow your eyes to look straight ahead, versus downward, once you've ensured that your baby has latched.

Keep in mind that there are many ways to support your baby. You need not buy a fancy pillow to do so, but use of a prop is encouraged

as this will reduce the likelihood of the baby's spine contorting atop
your own arm or your own body rounding down to reach baby and
experiencing compression in the process.

Now that we've discussed Mom's posture, let's zoom in on the baby.

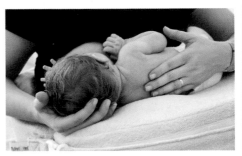

The goal here is to keep the baby's
spine in as close to a neutral alignment
as possible. No leaning, bending, or kink-
ing the neck to reach the breast. One
hand is cradling the infant's head to
help keep the base of the skull stable and
well aligned (this will become less necessary as your baby grows and
gains more control). The other hand should also be in contact with
the baby's body facilitating neutral alignment. This is a great time
for gentle loving touch and light massage. The bonding potential is
truly exponential here.

The number one concern when it comes to feeding should be for
the baby to successfully latch and effectively coordinate their suck
and swallow to receive ample nutrition. Specifics of the latch with regard to nipple depth and baby's lip and mouth placement are things
we encourage you to educate yourself on as soon as possible, ideally
before the baby arrives. Resources exist online and there are also
professionals who can help you, such as a certified lactation consul-
tant or a therapist (speech, occupational, or physical) proficient in
oral motor work. To the best of your ability, learn the basics and try
to apply them.

Breastfeeding an Older, Larger Baby

The next four images give helpful cues for breastfeeding a larger,
heavier baby. They specifically target considerations for posture if
nursing your baby in the standing position.

Full disclosure: In these images, I hadn't slept much and, despite the best of intentions, I was nursing our six-month-old in a weak posture. Thankfully a call to awareness and some gentle guidance from my well-meaning husband went a long way. This is real-life nursing and I was caught in the act. Let's be honest—we don't always sit still for a multitude of reasons. Perhaps you are home alone, tending to another child or pet, or some other chore. Or perhaps you're exhausted and worried you might fall asleep with your baby if you

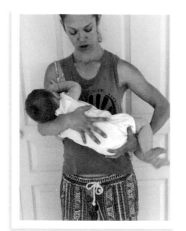

sit but you just aren't comfortable nursing in a lying-down position. Maybe you just feel better moving and, like us, have a baby who enjoys nursing while walking outside in the fresh air.

In these images, I am working to make nursing physically beneficial for myself and prevent irritation from poor neck alignment while holding the weight of our child in my arms. Note how my arms support our baby's head and neck, torso, bottom, and legs while keeping her spine neutral.

While holding your baby's weight, expand and elevate your rib cage as you breathe. Use their weight as a counterpressure to help you leverage this 360-degree expansion of your torso. I found it helpful to think of the baby in my arms as a platform that was strongly coming outward from my expansive torso. It's a workout for sure, but the best and most natural kind.

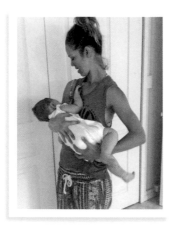
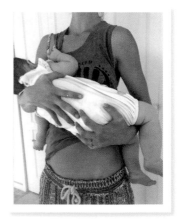

You'll notice my right elbow and forearm support her head, neck, shoulder, and upper back, wrapping my hand around and broadly placing it across the whole of her back and upper pelvis. My left arm comes between her legs, my palm broadly cupping her bottom, supporting her pelvis and low spine. In the images on the left on the previous page, I'm looking down at my baby to double-check her spinal alignment—this puts my own neck into poor forward head alignment that must be corrected before I get moving. You'll see me do that in the next shots. This is a completely natural occurence and not terrible as long as one recovers from it with smart maneuvers.

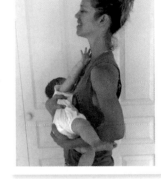

In these photos, I'm keeping Sunny's spine neutral by keeping my hands spread broadly toward the center of her body's frame. At this stage, she was around fifteen pounds and it was growing increasingly more challenging to hold her well supported while nursing on the move and still maintain my own posture.

In this profile view you see that my head and neck have been pulled back. I'm working to align my own spine neutrally, with the crown of my head pointing toward the ceiling and ears stacked over shoulders, stacked over hips. Her little hand exploring my chest and neck speak to her comfort and stability here.

Bottle-Feeding a Newborn with Props

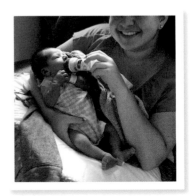

Here we see a mom utilizing a nursing pillow to elevate her baby high enough to cradle her close as she gives her a bottle. Mom is doing a phenomenal job of supporting her tiny bundle's body, keeping her whole spine in line while also keeping her elevated and turned so she can face both the bottle and Mom. Supportive, comforting, and functional.

Note how Mom is using her upper arm and elbow

behind her baby's head and neck, while her forearm and wrist support along the length of the baby's torso, and her hand is securely

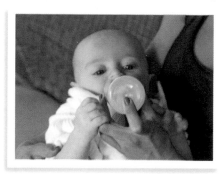

holding the baby's low spine and pelvis stable by wrapping around her hip and bottom. Lots of points of supportive contact offer great feedback for baby.

Bottle-Feeding an Older Baby Without Props

This image shows a nearly five-month-old baby having his bottle, and the caregiver utilizing a simple technique to help the baby learn to bring his own hands to his bottle. While he wasn't willing to put his hand to the bottle itself, he was willing to hold on to one finger very near the bottle. Over time a caregiver can gradually bring the child's hands in closer contact with the bottle, until they are ultimately holding it themself.

The caregiver's other arm is wrapped around the baby's upper back, neck, and shoulders, with hand cupping around the baby's arm and giving gentle pressure to encourage him to keep his hand toward the bottle. The pressure is light but gives a sense of stability; and, you can see him beginning to explore the caregiver's thumb with his hand that was between the torso of the caregiver and his own body. By the later half of the first year, most babies will have developed a fair degree of neck control and will no longer need direct support from your hands to control their head and neck alignment. Instead, a rolled receiving blanket can be draped in the region to offer a gentle, supportive cue to help the baby maintain well-aligned posture.

Even though this baby had taken his bottle, he was making effort to bring his arm back close to his body, pulling away from the bottle. In response, the caregiver provided more support at the base of his skull, neck, and upper back and engaged the baby by talking to him and keeping eye contact. With his body feeling stable and supported and his attention to the caregiver, he brought his hands back toward the bottle.

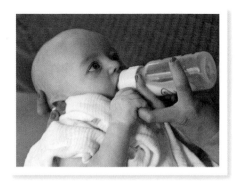

Let's consider for a moment what happened here. This particular baby had great neck control in other positions, *but* he was tired by this point in our session. When the physical demands of coordinating his suck and swallow were added on, which requires more core engagement for stability, his neck control suddenly became a little more challenging, and the effort to coordinate his hands holding the bottle was too much. So instead of holding the bottle with his hands, he tried to bring his arms back close to his body for more stability. When the stabilization of his upper spine was added, he more freely moved his arms to attempt hands to bottle.

Attention to posture and stability can make a huge difference in a baby's feeding skills. You can find more advanced feeding posture info within the upcoming chapter "Container Considerations."

A FEW IMPORTANT NOTES ON BOTTLE-FEEDING ERGONOMICS

The baby should be reclined about forty-five degrees. This is important to help the flow of milk from the mouth through the digestive tract. You never want to place the baby flat on their back with a bottle as this allows too many muscles necessary for swallowing to relax. It isn't good for your baby's skill development and it makes them more prone to gag or choke on the fluid. The bottle should also be tilted forty-five degrees so that any bubbles float to the surface instead of down the hatch. Bubbles can cause gas, tummy upset, burps, and spit-up.

We do not encourage propping a baby in any device or propping their bottle during bottle-feedings. We strongly encourage a caregiver being an integral part of the process until the little one is big enough to sit independently (in a proper high chair or flat on the floor) and hold their own cup. Of course, at that point, you'll have other things to consider like whether a sippy-cup can have negative impacts on the alignment of the mouth, or whether to use a cup with a straw or an open cup. These things are outside the scope of our practice, but we hope you will explore this further.

Holding Your Baby Upright in Your Arms, Facing You

This position, while upright, can also be considered like a partial tummy-time experience for a baby. It puts significantly less pressure on the stomach than when lying fully on top of it and is therefore

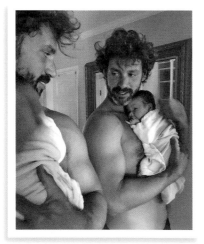

a great position for after feeding or just to help calm those babies who get upset being directly on their tummies.

Here we see that newborn Sunny's hand is pressing between daddy Eric's chest and her mouth, and even starting to open, all of which gives her body great sensory feedback (pressure, warmth, heartbeat, breath) that she can use to help self-regulate some of her own physiology. We see Dad using mirrors for more than just his own visual feedback of his posture and his daughter's. He is also using the mirror to entice the baby's

VISUAL AND AUDITORY TRACKING

Moving a toy in baby's line of sight to get their attention provides a visual stimulus. If they proceed to lock their eyes on the toy and follow it (with their eyes) when you move it, we refer to this as "visual tracking." Tracking can be used as a tool to help engage and motivate movement; and it will be mentioned again in activities to come.

In the same way that a baby can be enticed using their sense of vision, they can also be encouraged to move by the things they hear (auditory stimulus). Calling their name or making a silly sound that piques their curiosity are examples of ways to motivate your little one to turn their head to see from where a curious sound is coming. Using the sense of hearing in this way is called "auditory tracking."

It may seem unrelated to movement, but we want to caution you to be mindful of both the volume and tone of your voice. Sensory system input can easily overwhelm and impact energy and behavior. And behavior can impact movement. Loud talk can "rev" a child's engine, so to speak; and softer, slower speaking where baby can observe your mouth forming words can be more calming. A "revved up" or overstimulated baby is likely to be anxious, tense, and unlikely to be your most willing participant.

Your child is learning from the sounds you make, the movements of your mouth, and the movements you impart. It's dynamic and we hope you enjoy the process. As you go about engaging movement, also consider engaging your baby to be an active participant in communication with you. Focused eye contact and cooing count before language is established. Speech therapists refer to this as "joint attention" and they encourage it because it can enhance the baby's participation, learning, and foster bonding at the same time.

Newborns lack interest in toys for their first several weeks. You—your face, your voice, your smell—are baby's first favorite toy. This makes the first month extra sweet because the very sight or sound of you can be a wonderful motivator to entice your baby to look up while on their belly, to look left and right while on their back or on their side. At this early stage, in every position, look for moments of eye contact with your baby. In time you will focus more on where they are looking and how they track with their eyes.

It's helpful to understand what visual capabilities your child has so you use toys at the right distance. A newborn can see approximately eight to twelve inches in front of their face, and it's easiest for them to fix their eyes on an object if they are on their back with their head supported.

Another important consideration is that we have six tiny muscles around our eyeballs that control the path that each eye holds. A shift in the angle of the neck and head during play can impact how muscles are used. Imbalanced muscles and tilts in the neck can begin with visual issues as your child attempts to accommodate their position to better take in their environment. This is not always the case; in fact, a neck muscle imbalance can occur first, but due to habitual poor posture, the eye muscles may end up also developing imbalances. Such imbalances can have a negative impact on a little one's developing movement skills. *Please note that if your child does have known visual difficulties, this exercise program is most certainly still for them*; and, it would be a great idea to work with an eye doctor to determine what your child's unique needs are, as well as an occupational or physical therapist who has training in implementing and teaching visual exercise programs.

visual engagement. He moved slightly and looked for her eyes to follow, or "track" him. This is one way to work the tiny muscles that
control the direction of the eyes, or the visual path. As neck muscle
strength develops, the head and neck will also turn to visually track
objects, making this an even more dynamic way to hide work (neck
exercises!) in a lovingly held position.

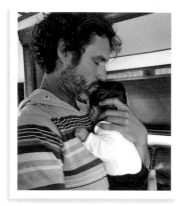

This image shows them a few weeks later, with
Sunny at one month. Eric's hands beautifully encompass both ends of her spine, with exceptional support
of her head and neck, and he is bringing his face in
close contact with her head. The breath from his
nose, kiss of his lips, warmth of his body, and feeling of his heartbeat all give her comforting sensations
that not only help regulate her own heart and respiration rates, but also contribute to a beautiful bond of
connection.

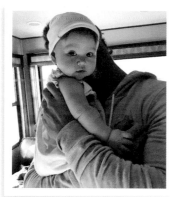

Here we see the progression. Sunny is now four
months old and exhibiting increases in neck strength
and range of motion. Her head is upright and she is
able to turn her neck fully to her side, looking over
her shoulder. Dad is supporting her spine with one
arm under her bottom and upper thighs and his other
hand at her midtorso and back. We see Sunny's hand
is no longer in a fist and is now open and holding
Dad's, which speaks to her increased core control and
decreasing physiologic flexion.

VISUAL SKILLS AS THEY RELATE TO MOVEMENT

For the first three months or so, children observe what they are seeing by moving their whole head, not just their eyes.

In the first month you should see your baby track an object from the sides, or periphery, of their vision to the midline of their body.

By two to three months they should be able to track from side to side, across the midline of the body, as well as downward and upward slightly.

By three to four months your baby should be able to visually track while in a supported sitting position (such as on your lap or semireclined in their bathtub). They should also be able to maintain their head in the midline of their body by this time, which in turn helps vision as the head and eyes are not leaning off-kilter.

By four to six months they should begin exhibiting the ability to visually track with just the eyes moving and no head movement.

By five to six months they should begin to notice distant objects and have the control to turn their head, neck, and upper torso to take in their environment around them.

It will take months before these skills are refined in all the positions babies find themselves in throughout the day. Coordinating the ability to turn the head to a certain degree and visually track up and down and side to side, while holding a well-balanced seated position or a more dynamic posture like all-fours crawling, kneeling, or standing, are more advanced skills that develop throughout the first year (and beyond into the second).

If you're at the stage of introducing toys, start by choosing toys that are black and white with a few pops of bright color as this is easiest for a baby's eyes to focus on during their first several weeks and months. Toys that light up and make sounds offer more stimulation, so if used, pay close attention to your baby's reactions and avoid overloading or overstimulating their sensory system.

Watch how your baby's eyes, face, and posture react when you bring a toy closer to them versus farther away. How do their eyes accommodate those changes? And how do their posture, balance, and movement respond?

These are important considerations when planning your child's play activities and setting up their environment for success.

Holding Your Baby Upright in Your Arms, Facing Outward to Their Environment

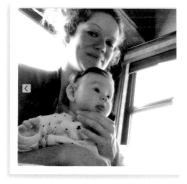

This is one dynamic way to help a baby at two to three months (seen here is our ten-week-old) to strengthen their neck and eyes. Here Sunny is sitting upright on my lap with a Boppy pillow around the front of her body and a toy suspended in front of her at eye level. She is receiving several gentle cues for her body position. Her chin is stabilized, pointing to the center of her chest, with light pressure on both sides of her jaw. My chin is in contact with the top of her head, and my other arm is around her torso with my hand on her abdominal muscles. We see Sunny respond to this by opening her eyes widely and raising her eyebrows, showing she is intrigued by what is in front of her line of sight.

The hanging toy was about twelve to fourteen inches in front of us. A newborn can see approximately eight to twelve inches in front of them, so at this age (two and a half months) we would anticipate this baby can see farther.

Without knowing a baby's exact visual skills, the point is to make sure that they are motivated by what they can see ahead of them. For the caregiver, utilizing mirrors in front of you and to your side (for a profile view) will allow you to observe your baby's responses and better gauge their participation.

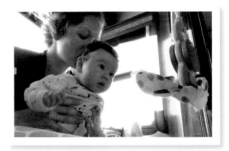

Once Sunny's eyes were locked and she was intrigued, I removed the facial support and moved both hands to broadly support her trunk, with fingers wrapping to her chest and abdomen as I leaned her toward the Boppy pillow in front of her. With her trunk supported and her eyes locked, we see that Sunny not only maintains neutral head alignment, but she also begins to bring her hands down to the pillow. This is fantastic all around. I maintain gentle contact to the back of Sunny's head throughout the activity, hiding a subtle cue that helps her budding proprioceptive skills of knowing where her body is in space within a loving kiss.

Playtime meets work meets bonding, all wrapped in one.

This can also be done with the caregiver standing, using the wonder of the world around as the motivation to get the baby looking; thereby hiding the work of neck strengthening within life's activities.

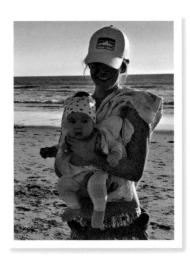

This shows a great way to hold a baby upright with their trunk and lower body well supported. Here you can see my upper arm and hand is broad around Sunny's torso and under her arm, with my hand across her chest and my thumb and fingers coming up toward her shoulders. My other arm is creating a shelf for her to be seated upon, with my hand holding gently but firmly around her inner thigh. Sunny's bottom is supported, leaning into my abdomen.

This provides a fantastic option that allows your baby to view their environment, which creates endless opportunities to motivate them to turn their head and neck. This benefits their range of motion and strengthens their upper spine.

In the frontal view on the previous page, we see Sunny is holding her head in a strong midline alignment (chin in center of her chest and not tilting either ear downward), as she is also rotating her neck slightly to one side to see the caregiver attracting her attention with the camera.

In this profile view by the sea, you see me progress the challenge, leaning Sunny forward so she is biased further toward a tummy-time

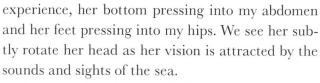

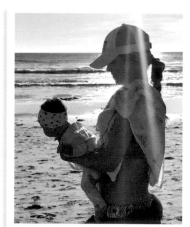

experience, her bottom pressing into my abdomen and her feet pressing into my hips. We see her subtly rotate her head as her vision is attracted by the sounds and sights of the sea.

Last, another image of the same supportive, forward-facing hold with a larger baby of almost five months. This baby is significantly heavier and is therefore more work to hold. To that end, I want to humbly direct your attention to my neck position and encourage that once your arms and hands are in place supporting your baby, correct any downward gaze and neck alignment to a more upright, strong posture. Note that this baby's hands are not only relaxing open, as compared to eleven-week-old Sunny's hands being in fists, but they are also exploring his own legs. Subtle shifts like this in your child's posture are like little clues that speak to how they are doing and if they're progressing.

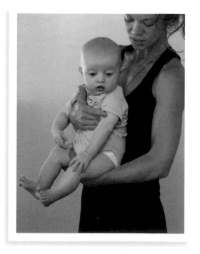

One very common mistake we have observed from parents and caregivers out in the world: carrying a baby on one's side or hip too early.

If baby has not yet developed enough trunk strength to sit independently and is not yet actively engaging the muscles of their inner thighs to "hug" your side with their legs, they can end up with their trunk slumping and legs widely positioned. This risks overstretching your infant's hips, tilting their pelvis, and tightening up areas of their body in attempts to find a sense of stability as they basically are left hanging by your support arm. It also puts asymmetrical weight and forces on *your* body as you move and carry them. So in short, not helpful for either of your bodies.

One thing you can do to help your baby build strength in their trunk and inner thighs is carry them forward facing, like in these images. Taking care to switch the arm you use under their bottom is important, not only for balancing the forces your body experiences, but also because this will switch which of their inner thighs your hand is wrapping around. Holding the leg in this way puts pressure to the inner thigh's muscles (the "adductors"), encouraging them to contract. You can pair words to the actions by telling your baby, "hug me with your legs" to help their learning process. Over time this can help contribute to strengthening those muscles, enabling baby to hold on tighter with their legs.

Remember to frequently switch which hip they are on when you do finally carry your baby on your side. This not only alternates the stresses to your body, but it switches up the visual perception they have of the world (feeding their eyes' muscles and brain with more input) while also giving their neck and core postural muscles slightly different challenges.

Babywearing is another solution to combat the potential problem of asymmetrical force distribution that occurs with holding your baby on your side. Using a wrap, carrier, or sling to carry your baby close to your body can provide a beautiful bonding experience that helps protect both the caregiver's and baby's bodies.

Babywearing: Wraps, Carriers, and Slings—a Few Do's and Don'ts

Wearing your baby provides another option to mix into the array of how you hold and position them throughout the day. This practice has beautiful benefits in terms of forming a loving bond of connection and also giving your baby different views of the world around them. They will be close enough to feel your heartbeat, your breath, and the resonance of your voice in your chest. *And their tiny body will be at the mercy of gravity and the support they receive from both the carrier and the caregiver's body.*

This chapter includes some key tips to make the experience as ergonomically safe as possible for both baby and the wearer of the baby. You can find more images that show how to incorporate babywearing into a few Foundation Training exercises at the end of Part III.

When it comes to wearing a baby, there are many choices of make, model, and material. These next several images are showing what we chose to use with our own daughter, and how that looked over the course of her first year. We have no brand affiliations and are simply sharing what we found to be safe and supportive for both parent and baby.

We'd like to encourage you not to think of carriers as "hands-free" devices for carrying your baby. We encourage that you always keep at least one hand on your baby and, instead, think of carriers as another set of hands to help support them.

As you view the coming images, note where the wearer's hands provide postural support and read the details for helpful ways to make the experiences beneficial for your baby's physical learning and growth. All the images we've included show baby carried in front of or on the side of the caregiver. We did not include wearing a baby on one's back. We aren't fans of this practice for the simple reason that it is physically impossible for the wearer to adequately observe the baby's position or make necessary hands-on adaptations moment by moment.

Wearing a One-Month-Old Baby in a Carrier, Facing Their Caregiver

We chose to wait until our daughter was a full five weeks old to start utilizing a carrier. We trialed many and ended up going with an Ergo (360 Cool Air Mesh) for its structure, which we felt offered more stability to our baby's tiny frame. We also liked the mesh material as it allowed us more control over temperature, since it was more breathable than the canvas and, of course, we could layer in receiving blankets to keep baby warmer if necessary. Remember, your baby does not yet have the same thermoregulation that you do AND your body heat will certainly impact them. Starting between one and two weeks of age we had begun trialing different wraps and shirts with pouches designed to hold a baby, but we didn't love how they positioned her legs, flexed underneath her similarly to how they were in the womb. This is because, once a baby is outside the womb, though their tendency will be to pull their limbs under them, they are truly meant to be "unfurling" (refer back to discussion on physiologic flexion in "Baby Fundamentals" in Part I). While it is certainly possible to wrap a tiny baby in such a way that their legs are out and, essentially, dangling, it may require too much unnecessary force to their little hips to do so. Furthermore, we must consider the situation more than surface appearance. Science tells us that our muscles learn in many ways, one of which is through vibrational input. Alignment of the joints and limbs while receiving this input is important because within our joints are receptors that take this information and register it within the brain. This input reinforces our body's understanding of where it is in space, and also teaches our muscles how to hold our body. *So the concern from a developmental perspective really ought to be: If the body is in a less-than-ideal position and baby is feeling the impact of every step the wearing caregiver takes, what are we teaching them?*

By five weeks of age Sunny was within the designated weight range to use Ergo's "infant insert" (meant for newborns seven to twelve pounds) to help with positioning in her carrier, which was a game changer for her alignment and comfort. To add clarity here—she was born at seven pounds and four ounces, and steadily gained weight. However, before adding additional weight, size, some ability to control her head and neck, and having practiced tummy time enough for her hips to no longer flex so closely toward her tummy, she simply didn't appear comfortable nor did we like her posture.

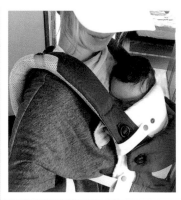

Comfy and asleep snuggled up close to me, Sunny exemplifies what is likely to happen when positioning is optimal. A baby's head should be close enough for the caregiver to lean down and kiss the top of it. They should not be down low on the wearer's chest or abdomen.

Baby's arms and hands should be between their body and the caregiver's chest. This allows for pressure and feedback to their tiny joints that will help in building their body awareness and control. This is superior to having an arm hanging down or possibly rotating into a poor position that can be potentially harmful.

Their legs should not be bent up underneath or beside their body into positions reminiscent of physiologic flexion.

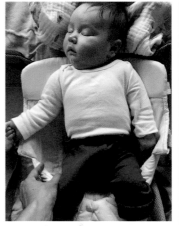

Seen here is our sleeping Sunny atop the infant insert, positioned horizontally to assess her fit. She is centered atop the seat cushion, with her hips and knees both at close to ninety degrees of flexion, which is ideal; but look at the gap of space between the side of her legs and the edge of this insert. For a body this tiny, that leaves a lot of space on both sides of her that she can slump into; we point this out because a baby at this stage simply lacks the body control to prevent that slip. At this stage, a baby is still dominated by physiologic flexion; so, if you're going to carry them in something like this, do your best to pad and protect their body from contorting into a poor alignment. Baby should be seated with their trunk atop a tall pelvis with the bottom, hips, and upper thighs well supported within the carrier or wrap. If you pay attention to the materials that Ergo provides with their carriers, they do a good job of showing you that your baby's hips and legs should be positioned to resemble an M, where the baby's hips and legs are supported such that both are flexed and their knees are slightly above their hips. This is to help prevent developmental hip dysplasia. If you have a child with this condition, we strongly advise working with a licensed professional who can help you to understand best practices for your unique child.

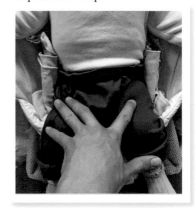

Note: Sunny is horizontal here, so you cannot appreciate this in the same way, but once vertical against gravity, the weight of her body changes her alignment.

This second image atop the infant insert shows pink burp cloths rolled and tucked on each side of her lower trunk, hips, and upper legs. These pieces of fabric provide a bumper to take up the space between her body and the insert so that when the carrier is fastened around her and the caregiver, it will pull taut and help prevent her body slumping into the space. Any fabric will do for this. Just be aware of the baby's body temperature as you go, steadily checking in with gentle touch.

Wearing a Nearly Six-Month-Old Baby in a Carrier, Facing Their Caregiver

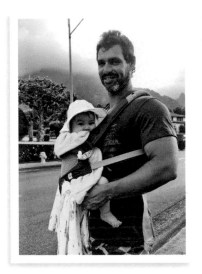

Here's an image of our sweet girl progressing, weighing somewhere around fifteen pounds and comfortably forward facing on her dad's chest. Due to a warmer, balmy environment, she was in just a diaper and the carrier was lined with one blanket around the upper portion (light blue) and another rolled and running across her low back (white with print) as additional low back and hip support. This served to gently cue her body away from rounding her pelvis under her and to instead find a more neutral alignment. Both Eric's hands are under her bottom, in a broad carry, providing support for her bottom and upper leg, all the way to her knee joints.

We see that Sunny has gained the strength and mobility to turn her head and neck over her shoulder to look at me as I call her name. Her hands and arms are between her chest and her dad's. At this age and stage, she enjoyed holding on to small teething toys, which you can see clipped to the outer edge of the carrier. This convenience meant she could play with these toys between caregiver's chest and her own body without us having to worry about them being thrown or dropped.

Note that Eric's shoulders are not rounding forward. His elbows are out wide and his chest is broad as he consciously keeps his head and neck tall and his torso expanding with each breath. As you wear your baby, you may do well to consider their weight as a healthy counterpressure to your own breath-led rib cage expansion. Lovingly support your baby and don't be so rigid that their body can't comfortably conform to yours. This should be a rhythmic flow that becomes a natural part of your wearing experiences. Think of it as exercise. You just happen to have the cutest "baby-weight" attached to you.

Wearing a Nearly Nine-Month-Old Baby in a Carrier, Facing Outward with Their Feet Supported

As babies gain more trunk strength and control, they will become more ready to face outward and view the world around them (we began alternating around five to six months once the neck was strong enough to keep the head up, neutral, and look all around without flopping against gravity). This offers your baby a great deal of visual stimuli as well as social engagement potential (which has very real perks for their developing social-emotional well-being and language skills).

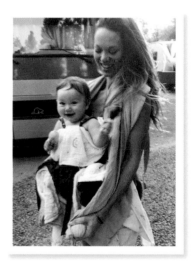

We do not advise that a sleeping baby be held forward facing as the lack of neck control that naturally comes could be potentially harmful. However, if awake and in good spirits, this can be tremendous fun for baby.

Taking care to adjust straps well is important for the baby's body as much as the wearer's body, especially if the baby is energetic and moving about like you see our daughter here. She was holding maracas in both hands, shaking them and rocking her body side to side in the cutest little happy dance. This layered in some great fine motor and core "work," weaving it seamlessly into a delightful evening walk.

As far as the baby's position in the carrier: the seat in this image had been adjusted so that the portion between her legs was made narrow as opposed to the alternate wider option, which provides more coverage for a seated bottom and thighs if the baby is facing the caregiver. My hands provide a supportive base or platform below Sunny's feet, maintaining them flat and her ankles at approximately ninety-degree angles to her lower legs. As such, this gives her a "closed-chain" experience. Her feet can push into my hands, giving her body cues as to where she is in space as well as potential force translated all the way up her legs and into her pelvis and low back. This helps her to gain more control of her body in sitting, to push and make adjustments to where her body is within the carrier; thereby making this activity more fruitful than if she were just hanging out with legs suspended. Even if the wearer needs to utilize a hand within their environment while wearing their baby, keeping one hand in contact and alternating their support can be highly beneficial.

Wearing a Nearly Twelve-Month-Old Baby in a Carrier, Facing Outward with Their Bottom Supported

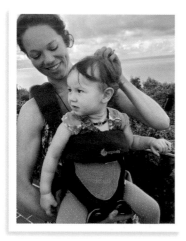

And here we are at just over a year old, forward facing. Since Sunny was heavier and had more control of her trunk, my hands were not below her feet. Instead I was providing support with one forearm, wrist, and hand to create a shelf under her bottom. Here you see my left hand playing with her hair. Loving touch and kisses to the top of the head can provide a nonverbal cue to your baby for where their body is in space and, in so doing, help them to align further upright.

Wearing a Baby in a Side Carry Using a Ring Sling While Nursing

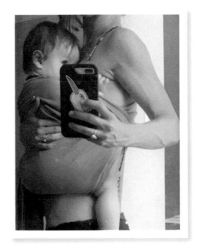

Seen here is our daughter, at somewhere between ten and eleven months of age, positioned within a ring sling and biased to one side of my front so that she can nurse. Her legs are wrapped around my side and front. A ring sling is simply a long piece of fabric sewn at the shoulder with rings to weave the fabric through and create a sling for the baby. Once your baby has gained the trunk control to sit independently and is beginning to move their upper body with strength and control over the top of their lower body (e.g., shifting from sitting to horizontal or from sitting to all fours), you can safely consider using a ring sling to hold your baby on your side hip. We advise against starting this sooner, though, because this style of carrier lacks structure and stability.

While the fabric is broadly covering Sunny's body from shoulders to knees, creating a full coverage seat for her, you can also see how I use one arm around her torso to create added stability. My baby is responding to this with visible curves in her back, including a thoracic kyphosis and lumbar lordosis. She is not rounding her back or tucking her bottom under her. This provides a healthy option for how a mom can remain active while nursing her baby. Note: Because nursing took her head and neck forward, I refrained from lots of movement that would jostle her about and give her body input of this alignment. This is very helpful while trying to do small chores about the home or working at a standing desk, but not ideal for a hike if baby is going to nurse.

Perhaps the most important consideration when using this style of carrier is the asymmetric forces that it distributes across the wearer's body. Looking at this image of the first time I tried a ring sling with

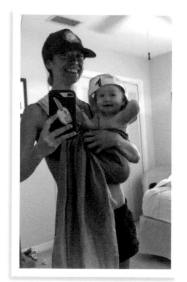

my daughter, you can see that my whole torso and pelvis shifted to one side in my attempts to safely hold her weight. It is important to be mindful of this very natural tendency to shift the body and to remember to switch sides, with effort made to spend equivalent time with the baby on both sides. This is important not only for the wearer's symmetrical muscle usage, but also for providing the baby some variety in their own muscle usage and visual input.

The attention you pay to positioning while holding, day after day, can add up to profound results.

Attentiveness to your baby's posture is equally important whether they are in your arms, in a container, or on the ground. Ahead you will find images and guidance for healthy postural alignment in some of the most common containers that babies are likely to be spending time in throughout their days.

Container
Considerations

Guarding Against Harm from Baby "Containers"

There's a buzzword in the world of kiddo movement for the devices we hold and position them in: "containers." And since they're quite common nowadays, we are going to touch on this before we dive into how to position your baby on the floor and other activities to build their physical structure. You want to consider the upcoming info carefully because, most simply put, containers can hinder your baby's development. Have you ever accidentally slept at a bad angle? When you woke up, zingers of pain in your neck informed you that muscles got squished, bones got jammed, and nerves got pinched. Stretching out of that damage might have taken several painful hours or days, or you may find yourself with a tendency to repeatedly tweak the same areas and end up with nagging irritation.

When an infant's neck is maintained in a poor alignment, that same damage can occur and it isn't so easily fixed. A baby lacks the strength and control that we adults have to actively stretch out a tight muscle and realign their bones. And they certainly don't have the cognitive ability to understand this needs to occur, or how to prevent this from happening in the first place.

Further, a baby's muscles and bones are so small that a subtle malalignment might not even be noticed at the time it happens. It can nonetheless lead to problems over time.

Posing special challenges to your baby's body are products marketed as convenient for hands-free parenting, like wraps, carriers, slings, bouncers, and other styles of seats, and other items considered common baby necessities, like car seats, high chairs, standers, and walkers. These can scrunch your child into positions that compromise their posture, or that they simply aren't ready for, allowing gravity to drag your little one's body parts into misalignment. Some of these things are okay for small windows of time, with adequate attention to baby's alignment, but attention is key. *And inattention can lead to a lot of damage. It's best to alternate baby's position and location throughout the day, between your arms, the floor, and containers.* We urge you to consider a rotation. More on this to come.

How to best handle some of the most common container-like devices is discussed, one device at a time, in the pages ahead, starting with the most universally used and necessary one, the car seat.

Positioning Baby in a Car Seat

This might be the only truly necessary baby "container" since it protects your baby for car and airplane travel. Also, some strollers and wagons are outfitted to tote your tot in their car seat. When you need to place your kiddo in a car seat, aim to do so only for the duration of the ride. Once you arrive at your destination, don't let your child hang out in their seat, because it doesn't offer them any benefit beyond transport. This is NOT a place to let them nap.

When you place your infant in the car seat, do your best to ensure their neck, spine, shoulders, and hip joints are protected, stable, and well aligned. Simple landmarks to look for are that their head is back in the seat, their chin points to the center of their chest, and there is an even amount of space between the bottoms of their ears and the tops of their shoulders when comparing right and left sides. Looking at their torso, you want to see level shoulders with an even amount of space between the shoulders and the hips. They should not be cinching, leaning, or twisting to either side (this can look like one leg or side of the pelvis hiking up higher than the other). You want to see their bottom as far back as possible with their legs as symmetrically aligned in the seat as possible. For the first several months this will likely mean knees point to the sides of the seat, whereas an older baby will have their knees pointing more ahead of them.

You can help your child achieve improved alignment by using the car seat's straps in combination with small props you create by strategically rolling and tucking receiving blankets, burp cloths, or small hand towels beside their head, under or along the sides of their neck, along the sides of their torso, and/or along the outside of their hips and legs.

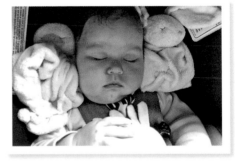

Here you see our daughter with a soft "lovey" (a tiny blanket with a plush animal head) rolled and tucked on either side of her head and neck, effectively creating bumpers to keep her from tilting as much as she was in the previous photo. While you can still see a subtle degree of tilting toward the pink bunny on her left (note that her chin is pointing subtly to her right shoulder), this is a marked improvement from her previous position, seen on the next page.

Please note: Any modification you make to a car seat can void its warranty. However, we personally feel that the extra protection is worth strong consideration if you can commit to monitoring your child's responses for the duration of their time in the seat.

Most infant car seats come with a soft, rounded halo of a cushion that cradles the baby's head. It has a worthy goal, which is to protect the head and neck. However, these can position a child's head too far forward, causing the chin to press down toward the chest, which can compromise blood flow or respiration. These cushions do nothing to prevent the head from tilting or rotating into uneven positions. In place of these standard one-size-fits-all prefabricated positioning devices, I like to suggest something I was introduced to during a course I attended specific to the assessment and treatment of neck muscle imbalances in infants: a simple rolled-up receiving blanket. As a clinician and a mother, this has proven to be my preferred cushion for protecting a little one's alignment, regardless of position or container type.

Placement under and/or along the sides of a child's neck, essentially filling in the space where the lordotic curve will eventually exist, provides a cushion and stability, and prevents the heavy head from causing the neck to tilt or turn into an asymmetric position.

THE REAL-DEAL RISKS OF THE CAR SEAT

Letting baby nap in a car seat is extremely unsafe as they can overheat in their sleep or their airway can be compromised. Read: Suffocation and SIDS risk! Instead, consider wearing them on your chest in a carrier if you aren't in a safe place to allow them to be flat on the floor, in a crib or some other form of safe bed.

One of the most common mistakes I see well-meaning parents make with regard to the car seat (and the stroller) has to do with how their baby's body slumps over because of the weight of their head against gravity and their lack of of muscle strength and control. The next time you are out and about in your community, have a peep at the kiddos you pass. All too often what you are going to see is a head and neck in some wonky,

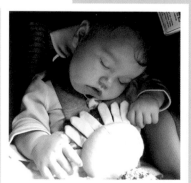

non-neutral position flexed forward and rotated or bent to one side with an ear resting on or very near a shoulder and their chin compressing their chest. This is concerning for their blood flow and breathing, as well as muscle and joint health.

Seen here is our daughter at two months old. We placed her in her car seat and she fell asleep before the car was fully packed. The posture she shows is terrible for a little body to remain in for any period of time, but this is a completely typical response given her body and the seat. This is what can easily happen to a heavy head when a baby falls asleep and gravity dominates.

More specifically, this alignment, with her left ear all the way to her left shoulder, her left arm elevated, and her chin pointing to her right shoulder, is a recipe for painful irritation.

You likely don't think about the impact this has on the nervous system and what it may be teaching a tiny body, but it can be profound over time.

Time spent in a poor alignment, especially in a seat that is likely to have their body jostling about and experiencing vibrational sensations, which gives them subconscious feedback about their position, can lead to pain and imbalances in the muscles. It brings with it the risk for asphyxia or nerve irritation and, at minimum, is a recipe for a fussy baby. It's also a recipe for confusion of caretakers who are unable to pinpoint just why their babe is waking fussy.

Other places to utilize bumper rolls in the car seat are tucked along the sides of the torso from below the armpit to the hip bone, and also along the sides of the legs from the hips to the knees. The blankets, if effectively placed, can take up the extra space around the baby's body to prevent sliding into a poor position in the seat.

When creating a prop for the baby's neck, take extra care to support the lordotic curve below the head and above the shoulders. Protect it from flexing forward, tilting sideways, or rotating too much to either side. A sign of such an issue is if one of your baby's ears is notably closer to a shoulder than the other, or their chin is either compressing downward or out of alignment and not pointing to the middle of their chest.

It's extremely important to take care to tuck the fabric around your baby's head and neck in a way that doesn't pose any risk of impairing breathing. Don't run the risk of hands with their Grasp Reflex still intact moving a blanket over their face and then the baby being unable to self-help with a roll or turn to free themself. One option is to weave the end tails of the bumper roll under the shoulder portion of the car seat's chest straps as seen in the next photo. Another is to roll or fold the ends of the fabric between the sides of your baby's neck/head and the sides of the car seat (like pillows on either side of a head, similar to the photo shared earlier of our daughter positioned with rolled-up loveys).

New babies have yet to build any trunk strength and being small in their car seat means that they might shift and could easily twist into poor positions. If you notice your baby holding an arm and leg closer together on one side of their body when compared to the other, they may be subtly putting asymmetrical pressure into their spine or elsewhere in their body. That pressure shouldn't be there while baby is sitting in their car seat, and it could result in painful irritation or muscle imbalances within their trunk. To aid alignment of the torso, you can use rolled blankets or other fabrics (burp cloths, hand towels, washcloths, lovey-type blankies) tucked along the baby's sides between their armpits and their hips in a snug, sandwiching cushion that prevents side-bending the trunk.

A blanket roll along the outer edge of the hips, bottom, and thighs can be utilized to prevent the legs from rolling outwardly. This helps a baby sit their weight taller over their pelvis and, coupled with other strategies, helps to prevent them from slumping down in their seat. Bear in mind that younger babies are prone to physiologic flexion. Their spine will round, which naturally presses their back into their seat but not flatly, tucks their pelvis under them, and flexes their thighs with their legs rolled outward.

Anytime you place your baby in their car seat, gently guide their body toward neutral, taking care not to rush them with tense hands that may startle them or create tension in their body. Do not force them to bring their back flat or their legs down; their body may simply be unable yet. Then utilize strategies to support your baby in the healthiest position they can reach without getting upset or overheated. Constant supervision and being within a hand's reach are

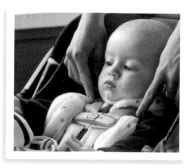

important for safety because a blanket can be a suffocation risk and car seats can get hot fast.

Side note: These blanket bumper roll strategies can also be applied beyond the car seat, to just about any other type of "container" that modern kids are spending time in during their days.

Seen here is a nearly five-month-old baby boy, with his head and neck well centered in his car seat.

A receiving blanket is positioned under the base of his skull, taking up the space between his ears and his shoulders and supporting his developing cervical lordosis with a safety cushion.

To replicate this safe positioning with your baby: Once you've protected your baby's neck, secure the chest plate (connecting the two chest belt straps) at roughly nipple to armpit level. The straps that suspend the plate should be tight enough that you're unable pull any slack up in a pinch between two fingers.

For the hip/leg straps, place them on top of the baby's thighs, near the hip crease, but not so high that they put pressure on the baby's abdomen. In the event of an accident, you want the force distributed through the strong leg bones as opposed to your baby's delicate organs.

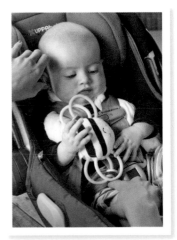

Here is another view of the same baby. The caregiver's right hand is pointing to the positioning of the lap belt atop his leg. Note that the baby is well seated deep in his car seat.

As you make sure your baby's bottom is sitting deep in their seat, ideally their torso is stacking well toward an upright position. Due to physiologic flexion, expect that this is a challenging position for your infant. They might naturally slide their pelvis forward, with it tucked slightly under them (causing them in essence to sit atop their low back) as opposed to being upright atop their "sitz bones" (the underside of the pelvis and bottom muscles).

If tucking the pelvis occurs, use your hands on the sides of the baby's low trunk-hips-upper thighs to slowly and gently ease them backward into their seat. Move with patience, allowing your little one to wiggle with you as you make each shift, feeling the support and guidance you're providing.

Be mindful that your guidance is calm and gentle versus moving quickly and forcing their position. Your speed and pressure can make a difference in how their body responds; and, silly as it may sound, the last thing you want to do is to create a negative sensation or association with car seat experiences.

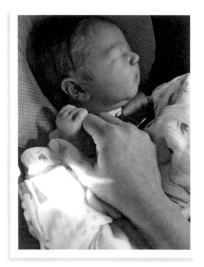

Seen here is our newborn daughter's first car seat adventure, leaving the hospital after her birth. You can see her head is centered and well aligned within the infant halo (her chin is up and her nose is pointing straight ahead). No bumpers are being utilized beside her head or under her neck, as I was right there with my fingers ready beside her neck to prevent any tilting during bumps and turns.

As your car is on the move, ideally you or another caretaker can sit with your baby in the back seat. If not, hopefully, at minimum, you have a mirror in the back seat that allows you to view your baby in the rearview mirror. Keep an eye to their body for anything slipping into a poor, compressive alignment as a result of a big bump, a sudden swerve or stop, or your baby falling asleep.

Between the cushioning you've created and the adult supervision you provide, your child's body—and especially their delicate head, neck, and spine—are likely to be extremely well protected.

The next few images capture some big leaps in our daughter's first-year car seat posture progression.

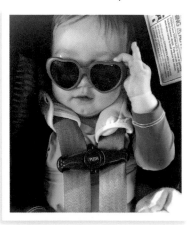

Here is our daughter at approximately nine months old, pinky up and stylish in her shades. No blankets were necessary around her neck as she had developed great neck stability and spinal alignment by this age. Instead, we utilized cushioned wraps for the top of the belt straps. These worked great as a temporary bumper to prevent side-bending of her neck if she fell asleep, buying us a few moments to pull over and create more effective props.

Beside her left hip you see a yellow lovey rolled

CAR SEAT POSITION: REAR FACING OR FORWARD FACING, WHAT'S THE DEAL?

The standard safety recommendation that car seat safety technicians give parents (which I learned while I was working within a hospital system and went through the National Child Passenger Safety Certification, a program of Safe Kids Worldwide) is: a child should remain rear facing until they are at least two years old or weigh forty pounds.

This has to do with the risk for whiplash being substantially higher in the event of an accident with a forward-facing car seat configuration. Severe whiplash can be fatal for a little body. This is horrible and not meant as a scare tactic. It's extremely important to consider your child's muscle strength and stability in their seat so they're optimally protected should unexpected forces suddenly jolt their ride.

and folded. We kept these handy in case she fell asleep, to protect her posture if necessary.

A few months later, at thirteen months, showing off her long and strongly centered neck. No bumpers here as this gal was wide awake and sitting well.

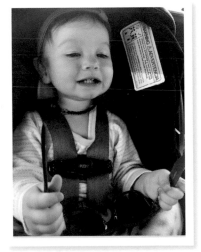

You can see that her head is now at the top of her car seat. It was right around this time that we upgraded from an infant seat to a convertible seat so we could continue to help her toward healthy posture and sit her more upright.

While this discussion has been about a car seat, you can apply a similar approach to other baby "containers" such as bouncer seats, swings (please see the following box with a word of caution about these), and standers, if you should choose to use them. In general, our advice for all containers is this: use rolled receiving blankets to protectively position and cushion your baby as close to neutral as possible. Steadily monitor for airway safety and temperature. Think of containers as part of the rotation of positions your child is alternated through during the day. As much as possible, minimize the amount of time your child spends in each device and opt for firm, flat floor space.

SWINGS, STROLLERS, AND WAGONS

A word of caution about swings: We are not fans of these for the simple reason that they are not flat. They put your baby in a concave position that does them no favors in terms of coming out of physiologic flexion, instead allowing a rounded or asymmetrically aligned spine and tucked pelvis. And because they are moving your baby, they come with the risk of shifting them into compressive alignments that can be detrimental.

A flat surface is always preferable as it simply gives your baby more feedback about where their body is, leaving it up to gravity and the baby's muscles to generate the forces they are experiencing.

A word of caution about strollers and wagons: Similar to the swing, these put the young body, which has yet to develop muscular control of their head, neck, and torso, at the mercy of gravity. We don't love these for a newborn, and personally chose to wait until our daughter was able to sit up with fair trunk control (in her case at four months) before we began to use a stroller (with bumper rolls at her neck, along the sides of her torso, and between the sides of her hips/upper thighs and the edges of the seat). Our rationale here is that the vibrational input that comes with the stroller's wheels moving over the ground will, on some level, be translated to the baby's body. Unless your baby is perfectly positioned in a healthy alignment and you're able to watch them as you stroll, jog, or run, they run the risk of their little body and brain receiving feedback about a less-than-ideal alignment. While many of these devices allow you to attach your car seat to them and others offer the ability to simply lay your baby flat, we would instead recommend carrying your baby in your arms or wearing them in a supportive carrier once they've reached about two months (refer back to the previous chapter on babywearing). Once your baby has developed the ability to sit independently and transition out of sitting to all fours, you can safely presume they have more trunk control and will likely slump and slide less in these devices. We still caution you to watch them closely and implement bumper rolls if they should fall asleep before the ride ends.

Positioning Baby in a Bouncer Seat

Seen in these images is a style of bouncer seat made by BabyBjörn (no affiliation or advertisement; this is simply what we chose for our own daughter because it's made of organic cotton and is simple yet support- ive). Its flat back and shelf seat allows the child to be positioned upright, against a reclined back, in a way that allows them to take in their environment. This particular make of bouncer seat has an adjustable amount of recline, which allows caregivers to control how much pressure their child experiences through- out their body and their visual perspective.

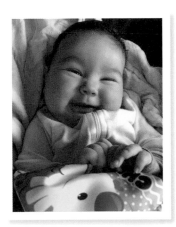

   This gives another variety for positioning that can be woven into the day's activities. Something like this is far superior to the option of propping your baby upright on your couch or bed pillows, two options we cringe at because they lack steady support and your baby can easily shift. This puts baby at risk of falling victim to gravity, recruiting any muscles they can to try to self-stabilize, and potentially compromising future alignment and growth.

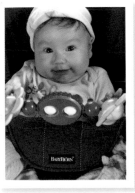

   In the first two images you see our daughter at three months old during her first experiences in her seat. In one shot she is tilting her head one way, and in the next shot it's the other. This might seem subtle, and her squinty little smile is certainly ador- able, but this could compromise her alignment in the long run if not corrected. What you see here is why we waited until we were beyond her third month, embarking into her fourth, to start using this seat in our rotation of positions for wakeful periods. It boils down to neck strength and the budding skills of holding the head aligned in neu- tral. We encourage you to spend a solid two months, at minimum, focusing more on time spent initiating head control skills with your baby on flat surfaces (in tummy time, lying on their back and lying on their sides before you consider using something like this seat. Until they develop adequate strength to tolerate a seat like this with fair head control, your baby can and should still experience time with their head upright in other ways, such as in your arms and, as necessary for travel, in their car seat.

See the next several images for how we improved Sunny's posture by utilizing a neck bumper roll. In these images we see her chin lifting to look up, her head extending on her neck, as she reaches her hands to contact the toy in front of her (which is a bar with spinning toys on it, attached to the seat's two sides and placed in front of her at eye level). This very clearly shows the effectiveness of adding the bumper roll—she is no longer tilting either ear toward a shoulder. Her neck is cued to be tall and well aligned. She can both lock her eyes on the toy and focus her energy on manipulating it.

Using this sort of seat needs to be done with care and caution because babies can easily have unplanned reflexive movements, or simply move more than you might have intended them to move, as they explore and experiment with what they can do. Which means *they can potentially fall out of this type of seat. Parents need to exercise diligence with fastening the front portion of the seat to secure baby in place, especially once they start developing rolling skills.*

Also keep a watchful eye on your baby's trunk. While a seat like

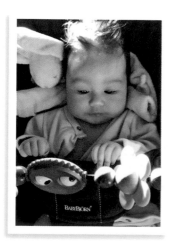 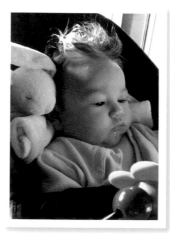 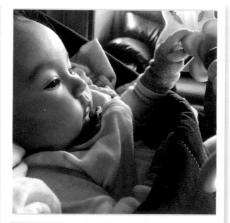

this is nicely supportive behind and in front of the baby, the sides of the baby's body are lacking substantial alignment support. Your baby won't fall out as long as the seat is fastened, but they can slump to their sides with gravity, putting their spine into less-than-beneficial positions and potentially compressing their tummy and other organs. Much like the car seat, this can be controlled (to a degree) with rolled receiving blankets tucked along the side of your baby's torso, between their armpits, hips, and even along the sides of their thighs.

Another part of the difficulty for a baby in this seat is the fact that it leaves their feet, in a sense, dangling. Because the baby's feet are not able to sit flat on the floor, they cannot experience pushing their weight into the surface below them. This is considered "open-chain" sitting versus "closed-chain" sitting, which would be the feet down upon a surface. This is an important consideration anytime you put your child into a seated posture. Without the pressure and feed-back that having the feet flat gives the baby's body, they have more difficulty pushing and effectively positioning their body in a strong, upright seated posture. And not just at the feet, but all the way up their legs and into their pelvis, low back, and up their spine. This is why it's also important that your child experience time practicing sitting with you (starting at about five months) when you can ensure that their feet are flat on the ground and that they are well aligned up their legs. More specifics on this to come.

This type of seat provides your child an opportunity to sit upright without the direct help of a caregiver (beyond initial positioning and steady observation to ensure that positioning isn't lost with movements explored, of course) and without the risk of totally falling over. *If well aligned and supported within the seat,* this can allow for excellent visual stimulus and motivation to turn the head to look around the environment. This promotes visual tracking and neck strengthening, as well as fine motor practice with reaching, activating toys, and bringing hands together in their midline. For all these reasons, we feel this is a decent option to add to your baby's growing repertoire of daily positional possibilities.

Positioning Baby in a Sit-Me-Up Floor Seat

The seat pictured is by Fisher-Price; *again, no affiliation, this is simply what we trialed with our daughter and a commonly found style of baby seat.*

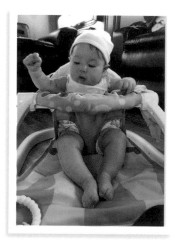

This type of seat has a wide and balanced plastic base and upper back with a tray around the top at approximately the armpit level, and a fabric sling-style seat that creates a bucketlike saddle. The fabric attaches to the tray, with holes for the legs to come through and toys at the top.

Despite the hard plastic behind the back, the fabric seat means there is a less solid, less stable surface below the baby. The structure will grossly support your baby's trunk more upright atop their bottom than the bouncer seat (because the bouncer seat is more re-clined). Like the bouncer seat, it's also going to put your baby into an open-chain sitting position. Baby's feet are not going to rest flat on the surface with their soles to the ground and, as a result of the lack of support, their pelvis may tilt and tuck under, their side may cinch if their spine bends or rotates, and their legs will likely roll outward (as you can see Sunny's doing here, notable by her knees pointing out to her sides versus up to the sky).

Poor postures within a chair like this might easily be subtle and undetected. The concern with this is: if muscles are continuing to be worked by reaching for toys, grasping, shaking, banging them to the tray atop the seat, this is generating force and giving feedback to your baby's brain from a potentially poor position. This could essentially reinforce their poor posture and lead to further issues.

Until babies have solid trunk strength to sit up atop their bottom without falling, utilizing a seat like this means that your baby could easily end up slumping. Do not initiate using this type of container until your baby's neck is strong and stable with the mobility to turn fully to look over both shoulders. And even then, we encourage waiting until they have established some degree of trunk strength and control, such as pushing up from the surface while on their tummy, rolling over their sides, and prop sitting using their arms as a tripod (around months four to five).

You can assist poor postural alignment by using blankets or towels around your baby's torso and hips within the sling, essentially taking up excess space and giving them a protective girdle for alignment as well as a greater sense of stability.

These final two images show our daughter at three months. She was teething and motivated by her toy teething ring, so I placed the ring up her arm and created an opportunity for her to explore and manipulate it. These images capture her pushing her back into the backrest of the seat with a solidly neutral head and neck alignment (note the chin tuck and rise while maintaining neutral). We encourage waiting for upper spine control like this before utilizing this type of chair so that it doesn't cause preventable issues. Like all containers, we recommend limiting and supervising time spent inside it.

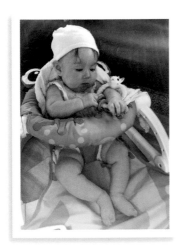
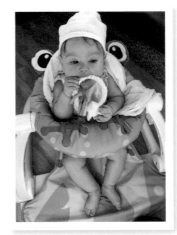

Positioning Baby in a Bumbo Floor Seat

This chair is being included as it is a fairly popular one, and every pediatric therapy clinic I've worked in has had at least one.

The Bumbo seat is advertised to support babies three months and older to sit on their own. The seat design itself is deep and sloped with elevated leg openings at its front and a high rounded back. This causes a child's body to lean backward toward the backrest and does not allow for their feet to be flat on the floor, making this another open-chain sitting situation (meaning their feet cannot sit flat on the floor). It has a three-point safety strap for the child's lap, which came about a decade ago after the US Consumer Product Safety Commission issued a voluntary recall on the product because babies were suffering injuries from falling out of these seats. It now comes with warnings not to place the seat on elevated surfaces because there is a risk that baby and seat can topple over.

Most pediatric physical therapists are not fans of this seat for a child's development for a few very legitimate reasons that you would do well to consider.

In a nutshell, this chair positions a body that is not yet ready to sit independently into sitting. At three months of age a baby has barely built control of its neck. There is no trunk support or muscular stability yet at play for the average baby at this stage. To put a child lacking that muscular control into sitting will typically cause their spine to accommodate to these forces in directions that not only lack symmetry but also can put the child at a developmental disadvantage, especially if their tiny structures sustain injury from time in a poor position. You might see their neck tilt and/or rotate sideways, their neck may crane forward, their torso may side-bend, their hip might hike up, their pelvis will probably tilt under them causing baby to sit with more pressure into their back than into their bottom, and their legs will be elevated somehow without their feet touching the floor. The last thing you want is for strength to be developed within a poor alignment or for a nerve to become irritated and end up perpetuating a poor alignment outside the seat too.

In short, all this can interfere with a young baby's natural progression of strength and skill development. You must consider what this is teaching your baby and what it is, more or less, robbing them of. In this seat babies can't experience actively bearing their own weight as they can on the floor. Without propping and pushing through their hands, arms, and legs, their bodies miss valuable feedback that teaches them where they are in space and helps build muscle strength and control.

We did have a Bumbo in our home, which was basically for our own research purposes with our daughter since this book project was underway at the time. For the above-stated rationale, we did not even give this seat its first attempt with our own daughter until she was eight months old and able to transition in and out of sitting independently. By that point we knew she had solid neck and trunk control and enough hip mobility to shift her own pelvis to a strong degree. She was already capable of sitting upright atop her bottom in her high chair, without tucking her pelvis and sitting on her low back. These next two images show how that went and we'll explain how and why we came to our own opinions of the seat.

This image of Sunny at eight months shows her arms flailing wildly as her trunk rotates toward her right in her attempt to find stability (notice the asymmetrical creases in her tummy muscles). You can see that there is a good inch to inch and a half on either side of her trunk, which means she could end up leaning or slumping her body in either of those directions in her attempt to find balanced stability. You can't see her feet, but they were not flat on the floor. From this position she lacked the ability to push her lower body into the surface for feedback and assistance to find a more stable alignment. She's smiling and adorable, but this position and

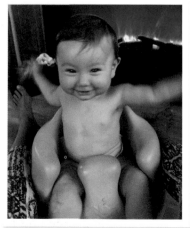

movement do her body no favors. In fact, this could predispose her to irritation or injury.

In this next image you see an attempt by her dad to use this seat in place of her high chair. Variety is important, so a novel effort was made to trial the seat as an option for snack-time.

Note in this image how Sunny's arms are lower, resting atop her

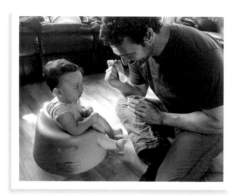

chair with her hands closed in fists. These are signs of more stability than what she exhibited in the last image; however, her feet were still unable to rest flat upon the surface and the alignment this puts her spine and pelvis into is questionable (note one leg is higher than the other and toes are clawing for more stability). As your baby is eating, you want them to be as safely stable as possible to prevent choking.

In short, we were not fans of this seat and did not end up using or keeping it. We simply don't love that this chair is advertised by the company "to support small babies who cannot sit up unaided."

Side note: This company also has a product called the "Multi Seat," which they advertise as being "for babies and toddlers who already sit up unaided." We did not bother assessing this one personally as it's another seat that promotes open-chain sitting; and, even though they advertise it as not having the rounded backrest or sloped seat, this just didn't make biomechanical sense to us as being an ideal choice for a developing body.

Our advice with regard to sitting is to keep the activity to floor time as much as possible; and for feeding your baby in the first year and later fine motor activities with your toddler, utilize a high chair that has a platform for their feet. More on this to come.

In the activities ahead you will come upon guided ways to help your child build their trunk strength and their trunk-over-hip mobility (i.e., sitting and reaching for a toy and then recovering to upright seated balance). This will naturally improve their sitting skills. You will also come upon guidance on how to align your child's body well when sitting upon your lap to practice a sitting to standing activity. This will further improve their seated skills, hip mobility, and hip strength as you naturally prepare them for the developmental progression toward more advanced upright movement skills.

Positioning Baby in a High Chair

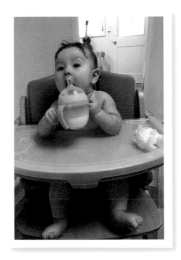

This photo shows Sunny at six months old, right around the time we started introducing solids. What's great about this image is that it captures that our tiny baby could sit with her feet in a closed-chain position (meaning, feet on a surface versus dangling). This is superior to utilizing something like a bouncer seat because a bouncer (1) is open-chain sitting (feet are not planted) and (2) could potentially allow too much movement. When eating you want your child as still and stable as possible to prevent choking. In this closed-chain position, she is capable of pushing her feet into the platform and using the force generated to press her body against the backrest. We see she kept her arms stabilized atop the tray as she worked to get the bottle to her mouth. With all that going on, her head and neck were still fairly neutrally aligned, which is fantastic for a six-month-old who was building independent sitting skills at the time. At this stage we used the five-point harness in the seat to help cue her trunk upright. While this seat was an excellent option, we ended up switching to one with a more contoured high back and a small pommel between her legs for a little more support. You'll see that in the next images, in which she's nine months old.

While you cannot see her feet, which were flat atop a platform, what you can see is her taking a strawberry and turning it around between both her hands as she curiously inspected it and brought it to her mouth for a taste. This speaks to her core stability as she can now more freely move her limbs to manipulate and control things with her hands. Her alignment from her head to her bottom is neutral in the midline, with her spine strongly stacked.

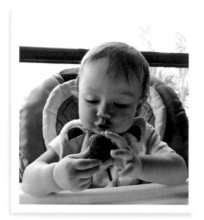 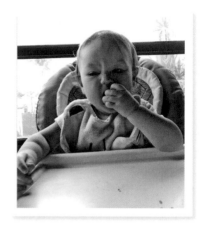

In these next four images, less than a month later, we see her exhibiting more upper extremity movement and control, thanks to her steadily increasing trunk strength, mobility, and control. She was happy to explore food using either hand, seen on the next page using grip variations (known to pediatric OTs as the "three jaw chuck" and the "pincer grasp") and exhibiting more freedom of arm motion—turning them up and down (supination and pronation) as she manipulated a spoon between both hands. An important note to make here is that babies at this stage should not yet be showing hand dominance or preference.

In these pictures, her tray was still positioned fairly high. We did this because when it was lower we noticed she tended to flex her body forward more with less control of her spinal alignment over her seated base. With it elevated, her trunk could remain more extended and upright. Around month eleven or twelve with more trunk strength established, we were able to drop the tray lower without her losing alignment. By this stage she was able to reach either arm in any direction about her tray to grasp food and was self-feeding fairly well with both hands.

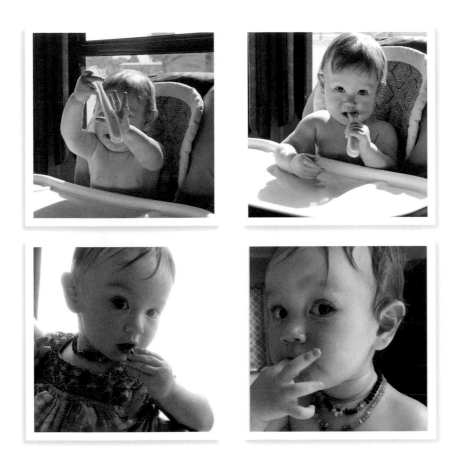

At around month fifteen we went back to using the first seat you saw her in at six months old, which offered fewer contours in the seated and backrest surfaces. In fact, she still uses that chair today at three years old because the seat height and foot platform are both adjustable and the tray removable to sit at the dining table, allowing for great mealtime ergonomics.

AMBIDEXTERITY AND HAND DOMINANCE

Ambidexterity is the ability to use either hand, functionally, in the same way. It seems from reviews of past scholarly articles that there is not an exact age determined for dominant hand selection, which falls in the realm of fine motor skill development; however, I can share from my experience working alongside pediatric occupational therapists that most agree that this is not something that should develop until roughly age five years! This has to do with development of a strong and stable core being the base from which the upper extremities, the arms and hands, extend. This also has to do with the cross-lateral control from the brain's two hemispheres, which, simply put, means that the right side of the brain controls the left hand and vice versa. Fascinating indeed, and *that information should prompt you to watch your child for early hand selection.* The cause, of course, is not yours to determine; but this is mentioned as it should instead direct you to a conversation with your pediatrician and a referral for evaluation by a pediatric occupational therapist.

To give you more understanding, here are some words from pediatric occupational therapist Allison Cost:

"Hand dominance is established only after the fine motor skills have been learned and practiced equally on both sides. The longer children utilize both sides of the body equally, the more opportunity they get for sensory input, cognitive problem solving, and integrated motor patterns. Once the fundamental fine motor skills of the hand become a stabilized pattern, children tend to pick hand dominance for complex motor skills like scissoring more out of repetition than necessity.

"If hand dominance is observed before age three, this often indicates a deficiency in coordination or strength on one side. But this is not always indicative of a medical condition. Often it is brought on by loving caregivers unintentionally in the setup of play and eating tasks. For example, parents who are right-handed typically place items in their baby's left hand when they are facing the child. To avoid this, make sure that you provide utensils, toys, and even take the time to place yourself on both right and left sides of the baby. And when you demonstrate, check in that you are alternating between hands yourself. If you find this challenging, I promise you that your baby is working just as hard and grateful for the empathy."

More from Cost on fine motor development can be found in the supplement at the back of this book.

Positioning Baby in a Stander with Supportive Sling Seat

Another common container that people love to utilize with babies is a stander. These come in an array of designs and sizes and their use needs a brief discussion.

There's a school of thought that a baby should not be introduced to any position that they cannot get into on their own; but we are including this to show how you would make this safe, since this is something many people are likely to include in their mix of daily positioning options. A word of caution with standing: Wait until your baby is at least seven months old, as the joint surfaces in their hips are simply not ready for much pressure before then.

Very simply put, it all comes down to padding them in, supporting your baby's trunk to be well aligned and stable, and ensuring that their feet can be flat on the floor (this may mean you raise the level of the floor up to meet your baby with something firm and stable like a weighted box or a book).

In these first images, our daughter (who was between six and seven months old here) has receiving blankets tucked around her torso to gently pack her in like a little girdle, adding stability to her

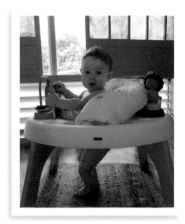 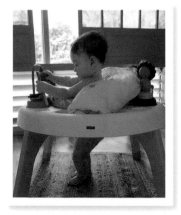

tiny frame and preventing back-bends, side-bends, or excessive rotation of her spine or her trunk over top of her little pelvis. This is
helpful to protect her developing body because she is sitting in a loose
sling atop legs that are just learning how to support her—that's a lot
of instability. You can see that her legs are flexed at every joint and
her feet are flat on the floor with her trunk upright over the top of
her pelvis and hips.

The main point we want to make with regard to using such a container is this: the container itself is essentially out of your control, but
how your child is positioned within it can and should be optimized
because too many points of instability can lead to your baby leaning
into off-kilter positions that potentially compress and compromise
nerves and joints, amongst other anatomy. Of course, that would be
no fault of your baby's, rather, a scenario of them falling victim to
gravity, their environment, and their body position. They simply lack
sufficient strength at this stage to self-support without external help
(which, in this example, is the blankets around her torso padding her
in). See in the next image what happened to her trunk alignment
when those blankets were not in place.

We see her left foot is flat and her right is up. Her head and neck
are leaning to her left, with an obvious asymmetric alignment. Moments of asymmetry are not necessarily an issue so long as the body
can right itself back to symmetry. In this case, though, this could
become problematic if it were habitual and the baby were spending a
lot of time in such a position. Her grandpa, on the other hand, is exemplifying a strong hinge (thanks to regularly practicing Foundation

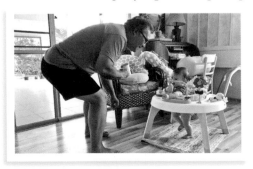

Training exercises; see Part III for more
details) to come down to her level and engage her with eye contact and face-to-face
joint attention. Here is another image of
Sunny standing while engaging with her
grandma, who was able to comfortably
squat with ease (thanks to her own regular FT practice). Physically modeling

healthy movements while holding engaged attention are valuable gifts for
the little ones in your care that promote
more than just bonding.

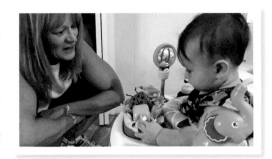

All this said, we'd like to emphasize
that what you are seeing here is nothing more than an introduction to being
upright in a manner that allows a child
to explore the sensation somewhat independently, albeit under the
watchful eye and hand of her caregivers. It was only one of several
positions Sunny was spending time in throughout the day at that
stage, as her core strength was building and her legs were moving
more, beginning to plant and pivot off the ground as they also built
strength and endurance. We felt she was ready for the inherent challenges of such a container because, at that stage, she was pushing to
stand when held with support at her low torso, and she also exhibited
pushing with her legs to try to stand when supported in sitting.

As you learned earlier in this book, gravity is a powerful force in
teaching muscle activation. Little bits of being upright with support
are not negative for a child at this stage if done so with care. This
is no different, perhaps better in some cases, than a parent holding
their child in an upright position with their feet on the ground.

Standing builds bone density while eliciting muscle activation
and activating joint receptors that help to teach where the body is in
space (proprioception). Standing brings another option for the positional play of babies who are physically ready.

We wouldn't advise this activity for a child this age who has not
yet developed adequate neck and upper thoracic control, or the ability to roll and sit independently. This is not an activity for a three- or
four-month-old; rather, it is suited to a child who has developed a fair
degree of trunk control and is actively seeking leg movement.

It could be argued that a child will rise, stand, and walk when they
are ready, and we don't disagree. However, that doesn't mean upright
postures should be avoided until then as opportunities could be lost.

For the integrity of their anatomy and based on what science tells us about bone growth and a baby's hips, wait until at least the latter half of their first year.

What we saw during this practice was our daughter experiment with shifting her body weight. She would alternate between moments of being flat-footed and then push up and off the ball of her big toes as she pivoted around within the stander. She was motivated to look around her environment, engage with caregivers, play with the toys on the tray of the stander around her. All of these moves created stimulus of the joints, tendons, and muscles in her feet and legs, giving her brain feedback that helped to further engage her muscles, and teaching her more about movement, positioning her body weight, and balancing. With this practice, she was further learning how to hold her weight upright over her pelvis, using her feet, legs, and pelvic girdle muscles—the same as a child who has pulled to stand at a support surface, minus the leg work of the actual transition. (In truth, it could probably be debated that she even may have had better control capabilities since she was packed in the container with blankets helping to align her trunk and she was able to keep her feet flat on the floor with legs in healthy alignment.)

So why does all this matter? If you don't pay attention to this, what are you teaching your baby physically? It's a bit of a rhetorical question at this point.

You wouldn't want your baby to be in a stander that only allows them to be on their toes. Nor would you want their spine leaning, twisting, curving asymmetrically. However, if a child can push up and come down flat-footed under their own control, and without their trunk alignment being compromised, that's a different story; and, a device like this can provide another positioning option for the day.

Another similar container is the wheeled walker variety that holds the child within a sling seat (which is not the same as a stand-behind push toy walker that you will see in activities ahead). While this is not pictured, it deserves a quick mention. We are *not* fans. We simply don't encourage having them move in a walking manner in a device. Their muscles and joints just aren't ready and all the potential movement without control could result in harmful forces through your baby's legs, hips, and trunk. (For clarity, we are not speaking about assistive walking devices, which can be extremely helpful for those with limiting disabilities.)

And since it's been asked of myself and nearly every PT with whom I've worked, I'm going to go ahead and bring up the jumper type of toys that bungee the baby suspended in the doorway in a saddle. In one word—NO. These simply allow too many forces to go through your baby's spine, hips, and legs that are potentially detrimental to their little joints, muscles, and ligaments.

So far you've learned about a variety of diverse topics related to your baby's positioning within your arms and in common devices or containers they may encounter during their first year. Now let's shift our focus back to the newborn stage and talk in more detail about how to best position and challenge.

The pages ahead cover positioning your baby outside of containers on other surfaces in their environment, and include cues and tips for how you can both support and challenge them in these early basic positions: supine, prone, and side-lying. These strategies can be used from your child's first day of life onward, and are what we consider to be the "activities" to do with a newborn, barring any special needs that require a licensed medical professional to provide education on adaptations suited to your child's unique situation. It's through these challenges that they will slowly and steadily increase their baseline of muscular endurance and strength, body awareness, purposeful control, and muscular stability of their joints, as their balance and movement skills blossom. Images will be included to aid in your understanding of how to progress through the challenges.

Positioning Baby for Tummy Time

One of the most helpful activities for encouraging your baby to engage with gravity is tummy time—that is, spending time "prone" on their stomach. This activity helps develop strength of the body's posterior chain of muscles as the baby first learns to lift their head, neck, and upper back, giving rise to the spine's natural curvature. At the same time, this encourages elongation of the body's anterior chain of muscles (meaning it helps your baby come out of physiologic flexion). As the natural progression goes and your baby begins to push against the ground with arms and legs, eventually pushing up on flat palms and extended arms and then back into an all-fours position in prep for the stage of crawling, further strength is established down the body, a stronger core is built, and the limbs coming off the core are also strengthened. These progressions provide important baseline strength-building opportunities that you don't want your baby to skip because skipping robs them of necessary strengths upon which other skills will be built.

Tummy time is so helpful throughout the course of this foundation-forming first year, it's typically good practice to start it the very day your baby is born so it becomes a regular position within your baby's day to day. A tummy-time session lasting just a few minutes, approached several times throughout the day, can end up being of tremendous benefit. And if you feel your little one is initially too frail for tummy time, or simply not keen on it, rest easy, we have multiple approaches for you.

Tummy time is more than just a floor activity; in fact, the most gentle and comforting place to start is on your own body—atop your chest, abdomen, and even your arm.

Atop your chest, your baby can feel and hear your heartbeat and breath; and this helps them to physiologically regulate their own body temperature, especially if given the opportunity to be skin to skin (a practice that is especially beneficial for those born prematurely). Atop your chest and abdomen, especially if you're fully reclined on your back, your baby has more of a flat surface, which means they will experience more pressure to their stomach than if you were seated upright and they were more vertical on your chest. Atop your arm is a similar experience depending on how you position yourself.

A baby will experience different degrees of pressure on their stomach and digestive organs based on how upright or reclined their caregiver is sitting, so it's important to consider how recently your baby has eaten.

Waiting at least forty-five minutes after the baby has eaten is a good rule of thumb to follow as this gives time for the contents of their stomach to move farther along the digestive tract so that it's less likely to come back up. Pressure experienced in tummy time can actually be highly beneficial to your child's digestive process as this helps bring blood to the area, positively impacting the function of the digestive organs and aiding motility (meaning it helps things—food and gas bubbles—to move along) toward elimination. As always, observe how their body is responding. Try holding them more upright if the pressure of being directly horizontal is upsetting or causes reflux.

When it comes to tummy-time practice, babies can be very sensitive. There's a bit of a psychology to it that's important to consider. And it's really rather simple. If practiced when the baby is energetic and in a good mood, and not immediately after a meal, it is very likely that your baby will enjoy the activity, or at the very least can be coaxed to have fun with it if you bring the right flavor of excitement for them. Gently calling their name, singing, making different noises, eye contact, and different silly faces are pretty much the best play to engage them in the newborn phase before they'll have the interest to visually attend to a toy around their second month and participate in more "tracking" types of work beyond that age. This has been my experience time and again, even with some of the fussiest of babies.

GUT HEALTH AND TUMMY TIME

If your baby is majorly fussy during tummy time, consider their stomach status. Are they spitting up? Is their stomach tender to pressure? What's the root of this issue? Are they breast fed or formula fed? If breastfed, is there something in Mom's diet, causing shifts in her milk supply, that is irritating the baby's tummy? Are they sensitive or possibly even allergic to something in their formula? Is their digestion backed up . . . or the opposite? A tender tummy will absolutely result in a baby putting up a fuss with attempts at lying prone. This goes beyond the scope of physical therapy, but, again, everything is intimately related and issues of this nature can hinder a child's physical progression. They can even lend to behavioral resistance to what the baby will begin to associate as being an uncomfortable experience. Be in tune with your baby. Consider that agitation may go beyond simple behavior or being tired. If you find it occurs every time your child is atop their tummy, this is definitely worth discussing with their pediatrician.

Little bodies are wondrous, miraculous, and sometimes mysterious, and also similar to our adult bodies in many ways. They truly need to be looked at as a whole because issues bigger than muscles, nerves, and bones can impact your child's willingness to move.

Because the term "colic" is so common, yet so poorly understood, I encourage you to consider what colic truly is, especially if your baby is resistant to tummy time. In short, it's a catchall term for kiddos whose crying persists and can't seem to be explained. This irks me. Why are we using a term like that instead of making it common practice to consider the baby's physical alignment, considering if a nerve is being compressed and irritating things from digestion to muscles and, truly, vice versa? Why is it not common practice to consider your child's gut flora? Or how they are digesting what they are ingesting? What is their elimination like? And why is it not common practice to explore Mom's health, too, if the baby is breastfed?

While this absolutely goes beyond the scope of PT, I hope it stimulates you to look deeper and to think bigger picture when it comes to your child's health.

So What Does a Newborn on Their Tummy Usually Look Like?

Expect that the baby will rest with their neck rotated so that a cheek is resting on the surface below them. While the neck rests to one side, they should have the ability to lift and turn their head and neck. Expect to see the arms bent at the elbows with hands kept close to the shoulders or under the body. The hips aren't likely to rest flat on the surface and the knees will be bent and likely "froggied" out to the sides of the body. All these positions are visible remnants of physiologic flexion and will gradually change with experience working against gravity.

In the tummy-time position, a baby learns so much about their body's movements with each little shift of their weight transferring their body's center of gravity and shifting how they bear that weight through their body's core and limbs. If you watch your baby's early attempts to move, you will see that as their head lifts, their weight shifts backward. As their head turns, it shifts to the side of their trunk. If their arms are close to their body and their pelvis is elevated (because of their flexed hips), then their weight shifts forward toward their head and shoulders.

Over the weeks and months to come, their shoulders, elbows, and hands will more comfortably support their weight, extending more from the body and pushing their body upward from the surface with their palms gradually opening. They begin to coordinate propping higher in prone. This means further posterior/inferior (meaning farther down their back and lower down their body) weight shifting, which in itself requires more muscle activation and recruitment farther down the spine and body as a whole (recall that whole cephalocaudal piece of development described earlier)—so this means it's no longer just the head and neck muscles being summoned to action, but also the muscles of the arms, shoulders, shoulder blades, upper and midback, chest, abdominals, pelvic girdle, and hips.

Over weeks and months to come as baby presses up and backward toward hands and knees, the neck, core, and limbs all progress in their coordination. This teeter-totter over time gives challenge and stimulus to the muscles, an engagement that typically causes them to build in their strength. As they do, they increase in their ability to give stability to the spine in the neck; that is, of course, if their pull is relatively even around the neck and the alignment is not being pulled off-kilter and irritating nerves. Seeing and understanding this relationship of subtle moves in the head and neck affecting overall weight transfer should hopefully help you to make sense of why subtle guidance is important and how it can have a big impact on your baby's movement and strength building.

Actively guiding early tummy time is as simple as being hands-on to feel your baby's natural strength increasing. Your hands are ensuring that they spend time with their head rotated to either side, attempting to lift their head, and encouraging acceptance of weight into their hands. In the first few weeks this is time spent on you, and then gradually on firmer surfaces like the bed, couch, or a table or the floor with a yoga mat or blanket that won't slip or be too cushy, engaging in eye contact and visually tracking your face and using their hearing to track your voice. This begins with the tiniest movements of the head and neck, with zero muscle endurance at first. Then it progresses to one to three seconds of holding a position; and, over time, your guidance is weaned as your baby grows in strength, endurance, and body control.

Ahead you'll find several images showing great options for ways to achieve tummy time when your baby is awake and alert or restful and napping. Side note: Taking care that this is atop an awake caregiver is key. We don't advise falling asleep with your child unless you are both under close watch of another adult, for the obvious risks of compromising a baby's airway, dropping them, or rolling over on top of them.

Tummy Time on Your Chest

Baby elevated on Mom's chest like this is a nice way to assist the natural digestive flow of milk after nursing. Gravity helps every-thing go where it should and the elevation prevents excessive pressure to the tummy, which helps prevent reflux.

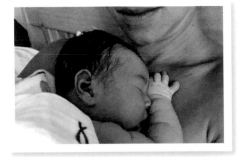

Tummy time on Dad's chest looks a lit-tle different. Here we see his fingers gen-tly caressing the baby's head in a way that prevents her neck from side-bending under its own weight when met by gravity and the contour of his body. She is also close enough to hear and feel his breathing rhythm and heartbeat, in addition to the warmth of his skin. All this sensory information helps her to regulate her own body temperature and to feel where her little body physically is in space, and it promotes soothing and bonding.

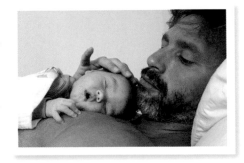

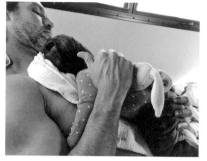

Here is another view on Dad's chest as the baby got a little bigger. She has a blanket under her head and neck helping to keep her spine in one long neutral line from head to tailbone. Dad's fingers are gently lying along her spine with his right hand while his left hand cups her bottom, providing both security and feedback as to where her body is in space.

As your baby ages and the strength and range of motion of their upper spine, arms, and core advance, you can add some challenge to their being on your chest by letting them prop as you sit reclined. This offers wonderful face time for bonding and social-emotional development.

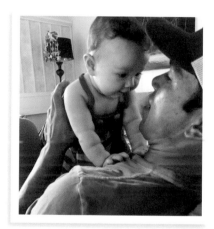
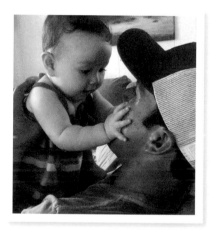

Here we see Sunny making wonderful eye contact with her uncle Jessie, while exploring his face with her open palms. Note: His supporting hold around her rib cage (front, back, and sides) gives stability to her thoracic spine that allows her to keep her neck alignment strong and neutral as she explores with her hands. He is careful not to cause her shoulders to elevate with his hold, remaining stable under her armpits. In short, his stability allows her mobility and all of this is hidden in loving, bonding playtime.

Tummy Time on Your Abdomen

This is a great position for more restful tummy time for a baby with Mom's hands cupping her bottom. From here the mom can lengthen her own legs and perform a Supine Decompression or an Internal Leg Trace exercise quite nicely (see Part III for details). If your baby is napping like this, be sure to rotate their head and neck the other direction partway through the nap so that they experience different ranges of motion instead of resting in one steady position.

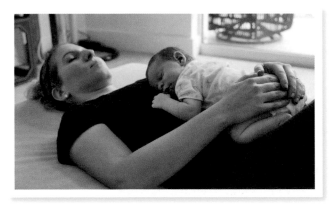

Move the head/neck with gentle hands to the skull, spreading support between the base of the skull and the sides of the forehead but taking care not to press on the temples where delicate blood vessels run.

Baby woke up? Here's how Mom lovingly supported her little one's arms and upper back, while lifting her up for some eye contact and affection. Baby responded by lifting her head and neck and keeping them in line with her upper back. This is actually work for baby but it's hidden in a loving moment.

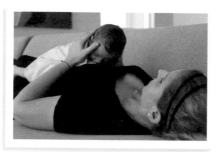 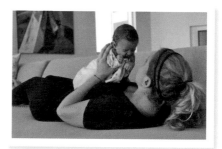

Tummy Time on Your Arm

These photos show how you can fully support a baby who is mere weeks old by laying them over your arm. This variation of tummy time can be utilized from the start of life until the baby is simply too big to comfortably hold this way while also keeping a strong posture yourself.

Dad places his baby daughter over his arm in such a way that her spine is fully supported, from her pelvis to her neck, in a solid neutral alignment. At the same time, his hand is broadly supporting her shoulder, jaw, chin, and head.

Meanwhile, Dad himself is implementing Foundation Training principles, with his other arm in a broad, open position at the shoulder (called a Long Wing position; see Part III for more details). With his spine and rib cage expanding and elevating with each breath, he is exemplifying the ability to "decompress" while also freeing one hand to utilize in other ways.

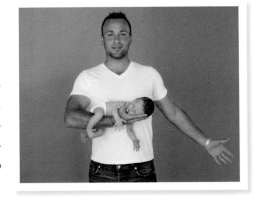

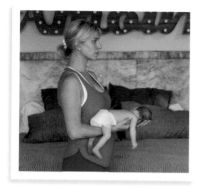

In this second example, a mom uses two arms and hands to support her son in tummy time. You may simply feel more strongly balanced using two versus one.

Meanwhile, the mom herself demonstrates excellent efforts at strong posture. Her head and neck are elevated, allowing her to expand her rib cage with each full inhalation, as she makes a conscious effort to lift her upper body to create ample space atop her digestive organs and the space that quite recently housed her growing and developing baby. This promotes better blood flow and nervous system communication, which will absolutely be beneficial as her body realigns and heals following pregnancy and childbirth.

There's no specific period when you must stop holding your baby this way. However, after around three months of age or so, you'll need both arms to sustain your larger and more actively moving baby, as in these next examples.

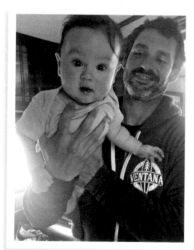

This image shows a visible progression of skills. Sunny is now able to hold her head in neutral midline alignment (notice how her chin points to the center of her chest and her head stays up in line with her spine versus dropping her chin toward her chest). Eric is modifying the previously used "prone on arm" position to one that is more supportive and challenging for a baby who has developed this neck strength. He has one arm extending the length of her body with that palm broad across her chest, and his other hand is broad across her abdomen, which serves as a cue to her tummy muscles to engage (because, very simply put, gentle but firm pressure to a muscle encourages its contraction). This allows you to "fly" your baby about their environment to visually experience what is around them. You can see how this baby has her eyebrows lifted and her eyes wide open as she thrills to see the world around her. This is a great way to hide the work of lifting the head and neck in some joyful play. It also serves as an arm workout for the caregiver, who will want to take care to stand with their spine strong, tall, and decompressed.

Similar to the previous image, this photo shows an older baby being supported slightly differently. The caregiver has one arm under his bottom and pelvis, with the palm broad on his low abdomen, and the other forearm and hand broad across his chest with fingers encompassing his shoulder and upper arm. These images better show how the weight of the baby is a workout for the caregiver. It might be helpful to think of your arms as a platform for the weight of the baby. As you stand tall, think of breathing big into your upper back and chest as your arms create a counterbalance of leverage to your efforts. This baby is doing a great job of keeping his whole spine in line; and, he is not dropping his head down as he turns to look over his shoulder. Again, this position is a fantastic one to utilize to entice babies to work on their visual tracking and neck mobility skills. At this stage they are incorporating more trunk muscles to self-stabilize as they lift, which means the caregiver no longer needs to support the baby's head and neck and can space their support more broadly, as seen here.

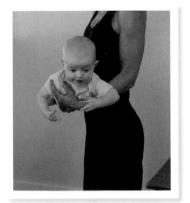

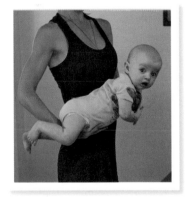

Tummy Time on a Flat Surface . . . and the Progression of Prone Skills

Generally speaking, it's best to initiate tummy time when your baby is awake, active, and alert. This increases the chances that they will be in an agreeable mood for the challenge, have the most energy for healthy practice attempts, and that motor skills your baby practices will have the best carryover. It's also safest because your baby, being facedown, risks impairing their breathing if they have a hard time lifting and turning their head to clear their airway (which all newborns do).

It is for that reason that you should avoid your baby sleeping on their stomach in their early weeks and months. Once your baby has developed sufficient strength to roll on their own and change position, there's less risk for compromised breathing.

The main activities to practice in tummy time during your baby's first three months of life are centered around visually tracking and propping increasingly higher from the surface. At first the baby will barely be able to look up,

IMPORTANT TO KEEP IN MIND AS
YOU APPROACH TUMMY TIME

A word of caution about the surfaces you choose for tummy-time practice: A soft and cushy surface, like a plush blanket atop your bed, can make it harder for your baby to push into the surface and receive the physical feedback they count on to help them grade their force as they learn to lift their head and, eventually, push up. Since it instead acts as more of a shock absorber, babies may end up working harder with less ability to control their body. This also poses a suffocation risk if the baby is sinking into the surface and has difficulty clearing their airway.

Another word of caution: some babies will protest tummy time if it's not done well, which may simply boil down to timing and energy. Unfortunately it can seriously put a monkey wrench in their development if tummy time is done with poor alignment that is painful or irritating for the baby, or if it's not done at all (often parents will avoid it altogether because they think their child simply hates it and it's not worth the battle).

so focus your energy on helping them to make eye contact with you. Don't be surprised if at first you simply see their eyebrows lift or forehead furrow. The head is heavy and gravity is powerful; they are using some muscles but not yet enough to get the job done. Helping your baby to feel stable in their core and guiding their head to lift with your own hands can be wonderfully beneficial, if done with careful hand placement and slow, gentle moves. Giving them this experience begins to teach their systems how to take their body in that direction on their own.

Once a baby can lift their head, they will likely be looking at the level of the floor and then slightly to both sides. This gradually increases as the baby gains strength in their neck, and next you should find that your baby is able to look a little higher, like at the level of the horizon; and they can also look to both sides at that horizon level. Looking upward, above horizon level (and to both sides), takes even more work. You should begin to notice your baby pushing their arms into the surface as their attempts increase in endurance, strength, and control.

WHAT DOES TUMMY TIME DO FOR FINE MOTOR AND VISUAL SKILL DEVELOPMENT?

"Tummy time provides invaluable setup for arm movements and visual skills. The work of pushing up and staying up establishes the role of the bigger muscles of the midsection as the leader. This opens the way for the smaller muscles of the arms and hands to focus on specializing to their designated roles (building muscles that will later be used for such skills as grasping, holding, and beyond to manipulating utensils feeding, cutting with scissors, and writing). The sensory input provided as the forearms and hands start pressing down is a catalyst for body awareness to create these isolated movements. Visually, tummy time also provides a unique opportunity to build the muscles of the eyes that being upright or lying down simply cannot in the same way. The prone position can limit the visual field so a baby is not overwhelmed with a lot of visual input. Practice of focusing on single objects becomes easier with less distraction. As items move, eye muscles and neck stability are established, and this becomes a motivating factor of reaching, increasing arm and hand skills. Everything is working together to build into a web of adaptability and future growth."

—Allison Cost, pediatric occupational therapist

By about three months of age we expect to see babies pushing higher from the surface (about forty-five degrees) and be able to turn their heads to visually track a toy, such as a rattle, or turn toward the sound of parents calling them. As your baby is coming up farther from the surface and bearing weight farther down their arm, increasingly closer to their palm, you can add new layers of supportive challenge by placing a rolled towel or blanket under their upper chest with their arms over top of and in front of the roll. Depending on the thickness of the roll, this will challenge your little one to prop higher. Placing toys to reach toward in front of the roll will keep them enticed to play longer as well as enhance their visual tracking and reaching skills. This "play" equates to a workout for baby!

Over weeks and months, your assistance should be gradually weaned. Your hands may still cup the shoulder joints, but now with less contact, that is, two fingers to the very front of the shoulder versus the whole hand. In time two fingers will become just one, then none at all. If you work with your baby often, you should come to feel the difference in their energy and capabilities as they gain strength; and this will help you to challenge them by reducing your assistance level. In time, you may challenge them further by only assisting one side of the body at a time; of course, taking care to alternate sides.

It isn't until later months that you can expect your baby to push up on both palms with their elbows straight, and later still before you'll see them self-support on just one palm while the other reaches for a toy (approximately month six-plus).

This valuable "work" time prepares them for not just bearing weight through one arm, but alternating sides in reciprocal fashion, which is an essential foundation for building crawling skills to come.

As this progresses, be on the lookout for imbalances by checking in:

- Is the chin in the center of the chest?
- Is there an equivalent amount of space between ears and shoulders on both sides of the body?
- What's going on with the arms? Is one advanced forward of the other, or do the hands rest in line with each other on the ground? Do the elbows straighten the same amount on both sides?
- What's going on with the legs? Like the arms, is one advanced forward of the other, or do the knees rest in line with each other? Do the legs rest in the same position much of the time?

Generally speaking, subtle differences are okay at first, but if there is a habitual asymmetry from one side of the body to the other, there is the possibility that a muscle imbalance is occurring. In this situation it is best to have your pediatrician refer you to a pediatric PT who can evaluate your child's unique strengths and weaknesses and help guide you as to how to best address them. Another excellent referral would be to a pediatric chiropractor. We encourage you to trust your instincts if you think you're seeing something slightly off, and make an appointment with your pediatrician to assess. Early intervention can prevent later work. And sometimes very minor gentle guidance can make all the difference. Exercises performed with proper posture and without overexertion lead to better-quality outcomes when it comes to guiding your baby toward developing their motor milestones.

Depending on the space you have, you can create an exercise-play setup for your baby on a bed or changing table at a height that will allow you to stand as you do this, aiming for your body to be in a subtle hinge as in the Founder exercise in Part III of this book. Another option is to place your baby on the floor or a lower piece of furniture such as a couch, as seen here, and work in a kneeling position (see the Kneeling Founder exercise). Either position can help you to strengthen and protect your body as you focus on theirs.

Here we see a newborn (ten-day-old) baby lying prone without

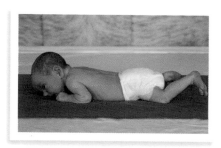

any guidance. His arms are flexed at his elbows and his shoulders are flexed and rolled inward, bringing his fist close to his mouth. This is normal, natural, and absolutely okay; but we want to draw your attention to the proximity of the baby's jawline to his shoulder.

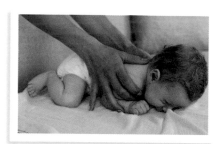

This posture holds all the structures close and tight, which is to be expected; but now that baby is expected to be uncurling and unfurling, we can guide them to engage their muscles to begin to find positions that create more space and avoid compression of the delicate structures in the area.

The next images will show you how to guide your baby.

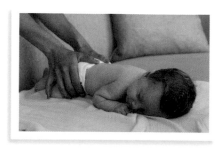

Gently place your baby on their belly with their arms slightly underneath them, hands under their shoulders. Using both hands to contour your baby's body gives them more tactile feedback to feel where they are in space.

Tracing your hands down from their shoulders/arms/upper back to their lower trunk/

pelvis/buttocks before moving into activities gives the baby even more feedback about their body position. This also allows you to align their body—upper then middle then lower—to prevent any postural asymmetries. You are setting a template for their body by guiding their posture. They will naturally recoil to some degree because of physiologic flexion, so don't get hung up on them maintaining the ideal positions; just go slow and steady.

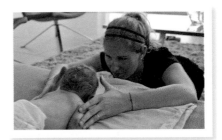

Using a few fingers to gently provide support and stabilization at baby's arms, you see her mother gently compress toward her torso. Notice in this first image that Mom's hands are not yet in contact with her baby's head. She is strongly kneeling and bringing her face down to baby's level to encourage eye contact as she lovingly calls her baby's name.

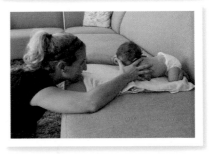

Mom's thumbs are now gently providing support at the forehead, her pointer fingers resting at the base of her baby's skull. She is not forcing this position, she gently rests her fingers there and allows the baby to move her head upward as she continues to verbally engage her.

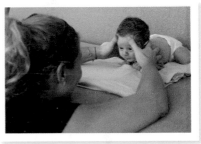

Beautiful eye contact! Motivation, connection, and bonding all in one.

This image gives another variation for how you can position yourself in relation to your baby, behind them versus in front of them. This allows for them to engage with another caregiver, view a toy, or even a mirror (which will be more interesting and motivating for a baby around three-plus months of age as their visual skills further develop). Your fingers can cup

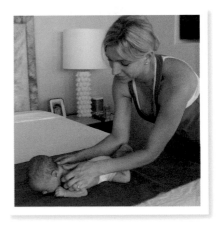

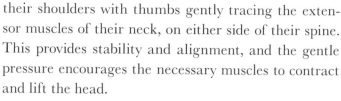

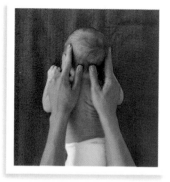

their shoulders with thumbs gently tracing the extensor muscles of their neck, on either side of their spine. This provides stability and alignment, and the gentle pressure encourages the necessary muscles to contract and lift the head.

If more support and assistance is needed, you can place your fingers higher up on your baby's skull to give them more of a cue for where to lift from, stabilizing them in a neutral alignment as they go, seen here in

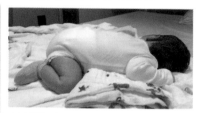

an overhead view. The thumbs trace baby's neck muscles; the index fingers are positioned on the bones at the base of the skull behind the ears, in such a way that you can help with a little pressure through the flat pads of your fingers to lift; and the remaining three fingers of each hand cup the shoulder and upper arm. The palms and forearms can drape and contour your baby's back, providing weight and pressure that give stillness and stability to the lower portion of their body, allowing your baby to better direct their energy into lifting the uppermost part of their body as they press down with their arms.

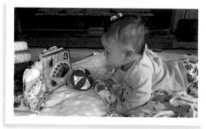

Note: If your baby is having a hard time making the transition from tummy time atop you to on top of a flat surface, you can try folding or loosely rolling a blanket and taking up the space under their abdomen and chest, essentially building the floor up to softly meet them, as seen in the second image.

The progression of bringing your baby up from the floor as they build arm strength, to encourage them to prop higher from the surface, looks quite similar.

Seen next is our three-month-old Sunny girl,

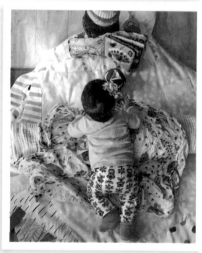

propping over top of a rolled blanket, with colorful, textured books and a small ball in front of her. You can see she is pushing through her palms with her fists loosely opened and her elbows are extending, but still show some degree of bend to them. From a bird's-eye view you can see that her left knee and hip are flexing and coming forward as compared to her right. Don't be surprised to see your baby playing with shifting their body weight at this stage to explore what they can do on the surface. Such play translates well to crawling skills to come; and caregivers can even explore helping their baby to find these subtle differences. That said, it is important to allow ample time for a baby to play and explore on their own, both with and without a prop like this in place. These photos show a great setup for your baby to self-explore, whereas the next two show how a caregiver can get involved.

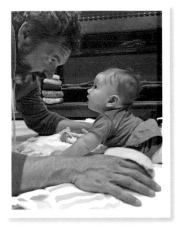

In these two images, Sunny, still three months old, is propped over a roll that is not as thick as in the previous two images. She has a toy in her hand that she had been banging on the floor, which is excellent arm-strengthening work as well as a challenge to the baby to keep her head, neck, and upper spine neutral as she plays. Eric is joining her in a plank (which could also be alternated with an 8-Point Plank; see Part III), and this naturally challenged her to look up (versus down at the floor) to make eye contact. Next I called her to look over her shoulder. Both these actions hid the work of using her neck muscles to control where she turned her head and directed her vision.

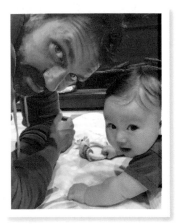

As visual skills develop further and your baby can see more than a mere foot in front of them, this sort of play can become even more fun by propping a long mirror on the floor in front of them. Most babies will be enticed to look up at their own reflections, so the motivation to work the muscles is beautifully hidden. And you can lie beside the baby so they see your reflection too. This is a great time to play with visual recognition, pointing to and labeling body parts (i.e., "Here are Mommy's eyes, here are baby's eyes. I see you with my eyes. Do you see me with your eyes?"). This allows you to provide limitless stimulating play ideas. In months to come as the baby is reaching more, you can even consider putting fun fabrics and textures, stickers, and toys on the mirror for the baby to be motivated to reach to touch and feel. Be sure the mirror is stabilized so it can't be pulled down; also, make sure it is vertical, not leaning, so that their visual feedback is not skewed.

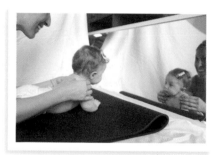 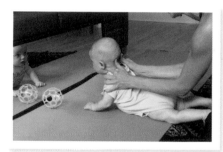

These images give you two different ways to provide stability to help your baby find neutral head and neck alignment as they work to prop and focus their eyes level on the mirror. If you remove the torso prop and your baby is looking low to the ground or habitually postures asymmetrically in their arms or neck alignment, you can use more hands-on supportive propping variations and layer in visually tracking a toy.

Notice how the child below has his right ear and cheek leaning very close to his right shoulder, and his left arm and hand are positioned

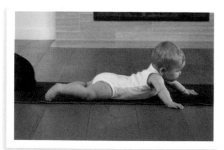 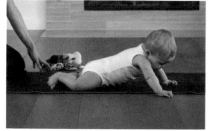

forward compared to his right. These shifts
could signify imbalance that could grow with
a little body if they are not addressed early. If
your baby consistently exhibits an asymmetry
like this after a solid two weeks of dedicated
daily practice, then we'd encourage evaluation by a pediatric PT to help direct your care
to your child's specific weaknesses *before faulty
movement patterns become habits.*

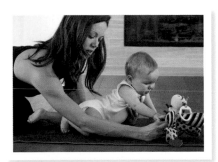

One arm under the trunk was not enough to
help prevent the neck from tilting. We see that
he brought his knee forward, which is great in
terms of precrawling skill practice; however, his
neck alignment isn't addressed with this assistance. The second image shows more support
provided to the trunk.

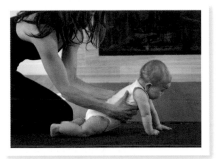

With two hands to the abdomen and
midtrunk, the child shows much more neutral
neck alignment and the ability to hold himself
higher over outstretched arms with elbows fully
extended and his hands closer under his body.
From here, seen in the third image, I switch
arms and maintain broad torso support with my
right hand and forearm. At the same time, I'm
using my left hand to hold a toy up at the level
that encourages baby to hold his head such that
his eyes are looking outward at horizon level.
From here I move the toy in an arc from his left
side toward his right, maintaining this level to
encourage him to follow it with his eyes. The
goal is to strengthen the neck (and core supporting) muscles from this improved position.

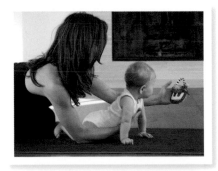

The final image in this series shows how I
have switched my right hand to provide support

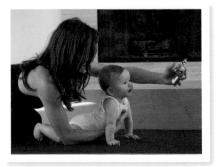

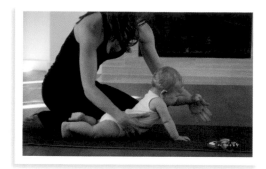

from a lower segment of his body, near the hip. As I make the shift, baby loses his tall arm alignment and begins to get upset, but he manages to reach his left arm up toward my hand as I drop the toy to the floor. This might not be the same tall press-up from ground as the previous image, but there are notable gains here. While his vision is lower, his neck is still more neutral than where we began (his right ear not dipping to his shoulder quite as much). His left hip and knee have flexed forward

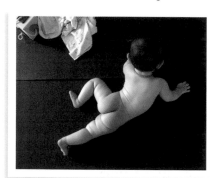

(as noted by his foot being off the ground), advancing his leg slightly on his own. Both of these things need to be able to happen to crawl; so, this sort of play can be beneficial to help your baby as they start to progress their tummy-time skill practice toward precrawling work.

Around six months of age, a little one in tummy time should comfortably exhibit flexing their "froggied" legs along the surface while also cinching their sides, as they hike their hips and side-bend their spine. You'll notice their elbows coming closer to their knees as in this next image. And this is hugely helpful maneuvering as your baby begins to crawl by pushing and pulling themselves along the surface.

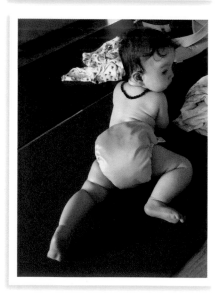

You can actually see the crease in this baby's low back, above her hip. This mobility helps to define the curve of the low back and is indicative of the mobility in the lower spine and hips that your baby will need to develop crawling skills. This mobility will also help your baby with more advanced skills like transitioning to standing and walking.

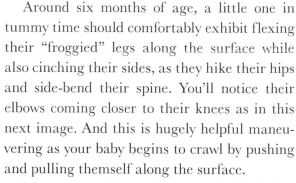

Look to see that your baby can not only prop higher on their arms by six months, but also that they can flex either leg at their hips and knees and push off their toes as seen here.

And as for reaching, they should exhibit reaching for items with either hand, typically whichever is closest, as well as reaching across the midline of their body, as seen in these next two images. No preference for a dominant hand should yet be shown; so, if this is occurring, speak with your pediatrician and seek a referral to a pediatric PT, OT, and/or DC (doctor of chiropractic).

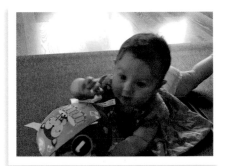 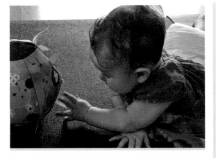

A quick reminder with these next three images—take tummy time to nature. Sensory play on various different surfaces (grass, sand, carpet, wood, tile) provides your child different levels of pressure and feedback as they are learning and exploring their movements. When able, bring a four-legged buddy to catch your baby's attention and motivate them to wiggle, stretch, and look up. Sometimes nature itself

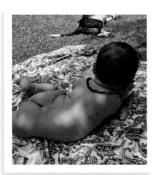 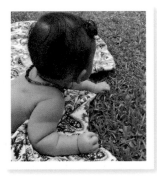 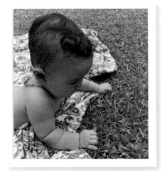

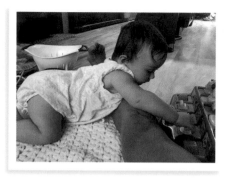

will be the very best toy to stimulate reaching and grasping. Grass under a blanket feels curiously different than carpet or tile.

Around nine months of age, good luck keeping your mobile baby in tummy time. Expect to see them shifting onto all fours as they press up and push back. On all fours you can expect to see them testing how their arms can hold their weight via rocking forward and backward as well as side to side as they reach for everything around them. These movements are excellent preparation for crawling, helping to strengthen their muscles while also building more core control, range of motion, and lubricating joint surfaces. Expect to see your child progress from tummy time to all fours (hands and knees) to pushing back to sitting, and then pulling up to kneeling and standing during this latter part of their first year.

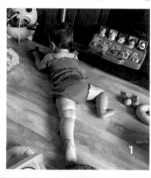

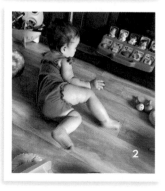

Over the top of your leg is an easy way to take floor playtime challenges up a notch. With baby on hands and knees, Mom can place a toy of interest (in this case a great cause-and-effect toy that appeals to baby's advancing cognitive development) on the other side of her leg to stimulate baby's reaching and propping. Encourage baby to alternate which hand is reaching for the toy and which is propping; working both sides is important. Same-side play and crossing midline are possibilities that can be easily directed by the caregiver simply placing one hand atop the baby's downward (weight-bearing) hand and enticing them to reach with their other hand. From this position the caregiver can also bring additional challenges by rolling their leg inward and outward, which will cause forward-backward rocking (more on this later). This movement challenges baby's neck and arm strength and core stability.

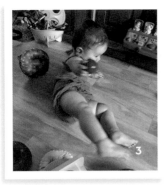 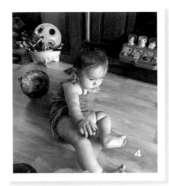 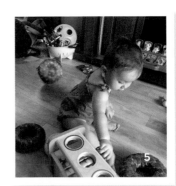

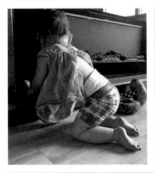

The next five-shot series shows how eight-month-old Sunny, placed in tummy time, rolled to her side and shifted her weight back to her buttocks, propping on one arm, and then reaching with the other for her toy. Activities ahead will guide you in more detail through ways you can help your baby to build abdominal strength as well as arm-propping strength, which are necessary to execute the moves you see here. This is being shown to help illustrate how, by this age, direct tummy-time practice is unlikely as it will naturally be leveled up for more advanced movement skills.

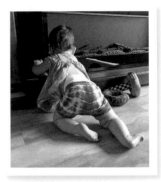

In the next three-shot series, we see the same child one month later, shifting comfortably from tummy time to hands and knees, coming farther upright with her trunk over her hips as she presses up on furniture. She is even beginning to extend her hips into more of a kneeling position, and extending her knees so she is nearly standing at this low furniture. The work of her muscle-challenging movement exploration is hidden in the game of reaching for toys. And all this began by being placed in tummy time with toys scattered ahead of her at eye level.

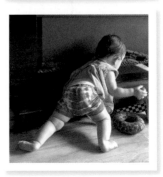

At close to a year tummy time is a thing of the past. Next, image left, we see Sunny at nine months old coming up farther still on the armrest of the couch. As she reaches for the magazine ahead of her, she is approximating a half-kneeling position (one foot, one knee), showing a natural progression in her skills toward a more upright bi-pedal posture. In the middle and right images we see practice taken outside to add more playful challenges in a sensory-rich environ-ment. Loose-packed sand offers more challenge than hard-packed, wet sand and this baby is charging forth with gusto.

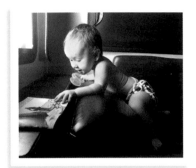
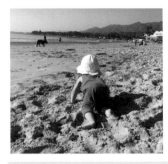
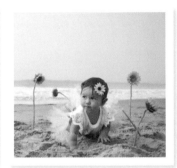

Positioning Baby on Their Back . . . and the Progression of Supine Skills

Lying on the back, aka supine or belly up, is just as important for your baby as lying on their stomach and sides; so be sure you actually dedicate time for the baby to just *be* in this position several times throughout the day, *without* swings or rockers or any other container device. It's important for them to have *still* time to observe their surroundings and experimentally engage with them, however they are capable, as well as for there to be time that you *engage and challenge* them. The former is best when the baby is both asleep and calmly awake, alert but still; the latter is best when the baby is alert and actively moving.

There is so much more to it than the phrase parents will read and hear everywhere: "back to sleep." For one, this position promotes eye contact and offers primo connection time that is so important for bonding. Visual tracking and "midline orientation" are other important baseline skills that will develop in this position. And being on the back also offers a variation in how your child's skull receives pressure; which, as discussed earlier, is important because it is that pressure that will help to determine the shape of their head, impacting their neck muscle activation and future skill building.

Please appreciate that lying on a plush, cushioned comforter atop a bed is not the same as other firm, flat surfaces. The concern is that "cushy" surfaces allow the baby's body weight to shift with gravity, causing joints to roll and shift into positions that are less than ideal. These shifts pose a risk where head shape is concerned because they can subtly bias your baby's head into an off-kilter position that can lead to a flat spot and/or other preventable shifts in facial features.

SUPINE AND DIGESTION

Providing a subtle angle of elevation for your baby's body while they lie on their back is another important consideration for time spent in supine. This can be done on your lap with your legs elevated (as previously shown in "Building Baby's Baseline") or in a crib with a positioning wedge that props them with their head, neck, and upper body inclined (with head higher than feet) about thirty degrees from the horizontal surface below them. These can be found online through medical supply companies and would be superior to using a pillow to try to prop your baby's head higher.

Using a wedge can help with the prevention of reflux (spitting up) since gravity helps the natural flow of food through the digestive tract. Should you need to utilize one, remain diligent in monitoring your child's neck position, especially if the baby is sleeping since it can easily slide with gravity into a poor position. You can utilize props such as rolled-up blankets to increase body awareness and help control their position.

So What Does a Newborn on Their Back Usually Look Like and How Does This Progress?

While it's important to understand what neutral positioning in supine should look like and how to diligently promote this, it's also important to recognize that your baby will move and shift and can't really be expected to remain in the positions in which you place them. This is due to a combination of lack of strength and the ever-present force of gravity.

The newborns seen on this page are between three and ten days old.

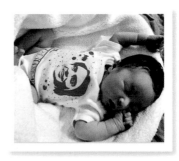

A newborn baby does not yet have much of a lordotic curve in their cervical spine (to picture a lordosis, think of a backward C with the rounded part facing the front of the body and the concave part facing the back). As such, their neck will typically be flat to the surface with their chin tucked toward their chest. Their head will typically rest in a slightly rotated position (meaning their nose isn't likely to stay pointing straight up at the ceiling) due to lack of muscle control and strength to keep it in the midline of their body.

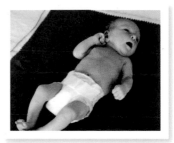

Their arms will be kept close to the sides of their body with their elbows bent (there's that physiologic flexion again), and their hands, which will typically rest in closed fists, will be near their chest, shoulders, or face. Over weeks and months to come their shoulders will naturally open into a more outwardly rotated position, their elbows will be less flexed, and their fists will gradually open. The seemingly uncontrolled wild batting

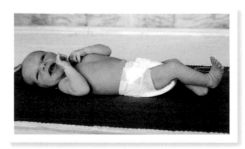

and swinging arm maneuvers they will exhibit are your baby's way of exploring their possibilities, and an important part of how your little one learns to control their joints. Because control will continue to develop from the core outwardly, their shoulders, elbows, wrists, and then, finally, their hands will gradually be held less closely to their body and will be less erratic and more refined in their movement attempts. In the weeks and months to come, your baby will begin to reach their hands for people and toys that are presented. Their hands will be more open and are likely beginning to explore surfaces, people, and textures.

Their visual skills of tracking, midline orientation, and eye-hand coordination are also developing at the same time. "Midline orientation," that is, having their focus to their body's central line, will begin with their eyes being able to see straight ahead with focus, and then beyond. This is an important skill as it will later translate to the ability to bring their hands together in the midline of their body, which is an important precursor of things like being able to reach across their midline, catch a ball, and self-feeding skills. Early on your baby's attempts will be uncontrolled and they may miss a toy that is right in front of them or smack themself or you right in the face. This fine-tunes over time, and around three months of age you can expect to see your baby bringing their hands together at the midline of their body and to their mouth with much more accurate control.

As for your baby's hips, they are generally flexed and rolled outward, meaning knees will typically point toward the outsides of their body. Knees and ankles are also flexed to some degree at rest (again, this is a remnant of physiologic flexion). At restful/quiet times, your baby's heels might sit on the surface below them, but their legs will typically still remain flexed to some degree. If their legs are gently pulled straight, held by the ankles and feet, they will naturally resist and pull back upward. At active times expect to see kicking, individually or both legs together, with movement generated mostly at the hip. Over time, like the arms, control will be developed from their core outwardly toward their hips, legs, ankles, and feet.

If the bottom of your baby's foot is stroked, they will reflexively bend their hip and knee to recoil away from that stimulus. This integrates over time so that, later in the year, your baby can accept pressure and eventually stand up and hold their own weight. Before then you'll notice little feet splaying toes, touching and exploring their environment or their opposite leg.

Around months four, five, or six you may see tiny hands successfully grabbing feet, opening a whole new phase of movement and
exploration as their body weight shifts, rocks, and rolls. Around six
months or so, with increased core control and hip mobility, you may
even see your baby playing with the amazing skill of putting their
feet all the way up to their mouth. Before you leap to stop them in
the act, consider that it is the exploration of all these ranges of movement that adds more control to how your baby moves. These acts
naturally stretch and strengthen muscles and add joint mobility to
their tiny structure.

Seen here is a nearly five-month-old baby,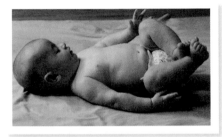
showing a strong neck in neutral alignment,
tucking his chin to look down as his hands explore his legs, and his feet explore each other.
This show of neck strength is a good indicator
that the neck bumper roll is no longer necessary. It's okay to continue to use one though,
for comfort, almost like a pillow (in fact this is what our daughter,
now age three, still prefers and uses).

As your baby gains more control of their core, which comes in large
part from their rolling skills, don't expect to see them remaining on
their back when placed there. Between months four and seven, these
skills are really booming in most babies, so much so that placing them
on their back is likely to result in them rolling over from their side to
their tummy, and then trying to figure out how to move farther from
there, be it to crawl or to press upward to sit. Like all other budding
movement skills, you'll want to observe that they perform these skills
symmetrically over both left and right sides of their body.

In the pages ahead you will learn more about how to help position your baby, introduce their joints to movement through range-
of-motion activities, as well as how to challenge their muscles in ways
that build endurance and strength. For the most part, these activities
are presented in a chronology that will be beneficial to follow as you

guide your child toward building a baseline foundation of strength and joint mobility that will, in turn, help them toward achieving their expected "motor milestones."

How to Physically Guide and Challenge Your Newborn in the Supine Position

For head and neck alignment you can implement the cervical bumper roll that we previously discussed using in the car seat for a soft and supportive positioning aid. This helps to cradle your baby's head and support their spine in the area where they will eventually be developing their "cervical lordosis." It also helps to ensure that pressure is evenly dispersed across the skull, not resting in one area, thereby helping to prevent plagiocephaly and torticollis.

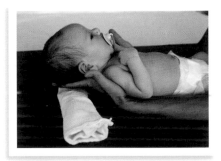 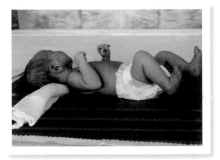

Note the caregiver support of the head and neck during placement and the space that is supported by the bumper roll, completely changing the child's head and neck alignment from the previous images of him with no bumper roll in place just a few pages back (page 145).

Be sure that the blanket is thick enough to take up the region behind and around your baby's neck, below the base of their skull, below their ears, and above their shoulders. Also be sure that the blanket isn't so thick that it lifts or flexes their neck or head forward from the surface. *You'll want to observe your baby's profile and make sure their spine is relatively parallel to the surface.* Use your baby's ears, shoulders, and chin to assess this as previously described in the car seat positioning discussion. The roll should not limit the baby's ability to move their head. They should be able to raise and lower their chin, as well as turn their head to either side.

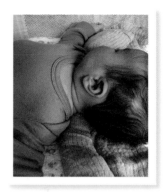

Here's another view of an effective neck roll with a two-month-old baby. You can see she fell asleep with her right hand exploring the bumper roll.

Throughout the day, you'll want to spend periods of time with this blanket in place, allowing your baby to view their environment and also engaging with your baby in ways to entice their active movement. And you'll want to do these same things without the blanket in place. The alignment you facilitate with the roll should start to become second nature for your child as their muscle strength, head and neck control develop.

Aim to lay your baby in a straight position with their shoulders in line with their hips, in line with their legs straight down to their feet. Knowing they will surely wiggle and move, try your best to make sure there is no bend in the side of their body that results in pulling a hip closer to a shoulder. From there you will have a better setup from which to practice neck, arm, and leg movements. You're also subtly teaching their body.

Gently Traction the Legs: Seen here is a newborn, ten days old, with his legs being ***gently*** pulled outward from his body, to help elongate his muscles from their previous state of physiologic flexion. Take note that the caregiver's hands hold the contours of the baby's legs as opposed to directly holding over top of a joint. Hands are loosely cupped around the tiny heel bones. 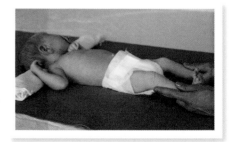 Doing this slowly helps your baby to get a sense for the new position, but expect them to retract their legs back into some degree of a flexed state when you release your hands. Don't expect your newborn's knees to reach or remain on the surface.

From here, since your hands are already on their low legs, we encourage you to try to flow into these next activities.

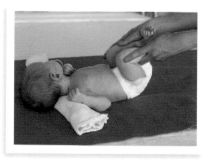

Leg Flexion and Extension: Gently flex both hips and knees toward the tummy. This not only teaches the legs movement but also provides abdominal pressure, which is a big helper of natural digestive flow. As the knees move toward the belly, they should be guided to point upward, versus outward, so that the baby's body receives input that ultimately will teach them this more neutral alignment. Keep in mind that the natural tendency (because of their in-womb positioning) will be to move toward a more "froggied" outward position. Also, because their pelvis and low back move together as a unit, you're going to see their bottom raise off the surface as you go. Take care that your hands are not compressing over top of any of the baby's joints. Keep a watchful eye on the diaper; make sure it's not too tight or abrasively rubbing the inner thigh or

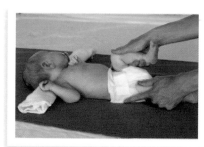

stomach during these activities. A few repetitions of this, flexing upward and extending downward, can flow right into either alternating the legs in a bicycle-like pattern or keeping the legs up and rotating the baby onto their side, as seen in the following two images.

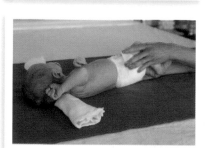

Baby Bicycle: Move one leg up, one leg down in slow, steady, rhythmic fashion. This teaches their joints and muscles a great deal and also gets blood flowing like an exercise warm-up. Hands gently contour legs, no squeezing over the knee joints. This is gentle guidance. Baby should enjoy this. Smile as you give eye contact. Pair action words of "up" and "down" to engage your baby. This activity flows nicely into the next.

Lower Trunk Rotation: Begin by flexing your baby's legs up as seen two images back. Keeping in mind that your baby's spine will naturally logroll as one unit, guide their knees to lead the way. You should see their legs, hips, pelvis, and spine rotate toward side-lying (note in the bottom image on the previous page how the baby's whole body is turning toward their left side, including their right arm lifting and moving with them). Go slowly, pausing when you reach the side to allow your baby to visually accommodate and feel their body in this new position. Be sure to practice both directions.

With these activities, don't be surprised to hear your baby's tummy contents shifting or passing gas as these moves put pressure on their abdominal contents and can aid digestion. They are paired well after a warm bath, but not directly after feeding/nursing (you'd do well to wait at least forty-five minutes to allow your baby's digestive process to move along on its own before you add pressure).

Keep in mind that the biggest thing a baby is trying to do at the newborn stage, regardless of position, is to control their head and neck movement. The previously introduced activity of ***visual tracking*** *is the primary means of neck-strengthening and range-of-motion-building work you will do with your baby in the supine position during their newborn stage.* Your job, as their movement coach, is to make sure that your baby can actively track and move their head and neck equivalently in both directions, left and right.

While on their back you can guide your baby to practice visually tracking you or a toy with their eyes. Over the course of the next several weeks/months, they should be able to look in a full arc around them, from over one shoulder to over the other. In time, your child will begin to shift their body weight and rotate more than just their neck, which can, and often does, result in rolling to their side or to their stomach if the movement is strong enough.

As you go, it's important to consider that if there are items of interest in their crib or the room, your baby might just keep their head turned in that direction because it's visually stimulating and gets their attention. Something as simple as a piece of furniture or a tree outside a window or even the recognition that their caregivers walk in through a door on one side of the room can lend to holding and using the neck muscles in asymmetric fashion. It can be helpful to switch where your baby is positioned in their crib and where their crib is in the room.

Along the same lines, be sure to present interesting items to your child from various directions. As you do, watch your baby's reactions to your pace and recognize that even the little muscles around their eyes, which help with focusing and depth perception, have a learning curve ahead of them.

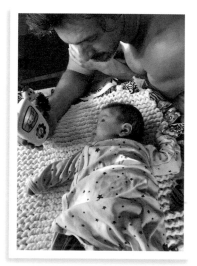

By three months of age, your baby should be able to visually track you or a small toy from their periphery to their midline and from midline to either side, as well as up and slightly down. (To clarify, "midline" is an imaginary line down the middle of their body from their head to their feet. More on this to come.) Your child should also be able to turn their head and neck with or without the neck bumper roll in place, rotating fully so that their cheek rests flat on the surface. At this age, as you see in the photo to the left (showing Eric coaxing two-and-a-half-month-old Sunny to track), the ATNR (reflex) may still be present.

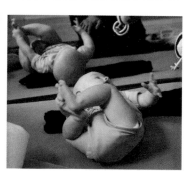

In this next photo of an almost five-month-old, we see just how much the baby's movement skills have advanced. He is looking and reaching to his left while his right hand is down exploring his feet (not up to his head), with his lower trunk rotating away from where he is looking. No ATNR dominating his position and his trunk is moving segmentally versus log rolling in the same direction he looks.

Midline Orientation Work: You can also dedicate time to working on your baby's midline orientation during this

early stage, while they are positioned on their back, by centrally placing mobiles above their bed or play area. This provides great visual
stimulus to get them first focusing their eyes and working their neck, and then reaching and shifting their body
weight. To clarify, this need not wait until three months.
If you recall back to the previous chapters on holding
your baby, you were shown another way to do this while
holding your baby forward facing, first stabilizing their
chin to help them focus their visual path. In short, midline orientation work is something to give your attention
because of what it progresses to over time: the ability to
reach across their midline with either hand. When they do
this, it means that the two sides of their brain are working
together to coordinate and control more advanced movements (in an
older kid this includes skills beyond just reaching, such as writing,
reading, and tying shoes).

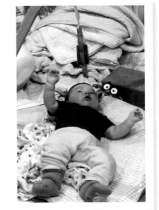

Seen here is our nearly two-month-old baby, reaching up toward
a mobile with her right arm and side of her body coming off the surface. At this young stage, as previously discussed, the spine moves as
a whole unit instead of segment by segment, so this actually translates to early rolling practice for her body. If you look closely you can
see what we did when we noted she was rocking up with her right
side. We bunched up her blanket to create a cushion under the right
side of her torso and pelvis to lift her to encourage more reaching
and lifting. Putting her just that little bit closer to the toy worked well
to motivate her to continue trying to make contact with it (not visible
is the bell in the center of the toy that gave her great auditory feedback when she successfully bopped it). If you choose to try something
like this, just make it gentle (i.e., not too thick as that could be too
forceful) and be sure to spend time practicing with it on both sides to
encourage symmetrical muscle usage.

Typically, a baby will begin reaching for an item with the hand
on the same side that the item is located or presented from. Between
roughly three and six months or so, babies will begin reaching across

their midline; that is, their left hand will reach across to the right side of their body to grab something and vice versa.

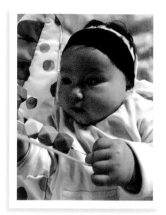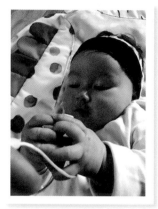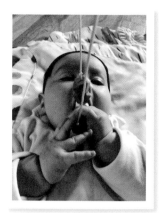

Here we see the progression of reaching with the same baby at three months old as she reaches for a string of beads, clasps them with her hands, and pulls them to her. This is great because it promotes the two hemispheres of the brain communicating to work together to accomplish tasks as the baby works on visual tracking, neck movement, reaching their arms, and the fine motor work of grasping and bringing hands together. Of course, this resulted in Sunny trying to bring these teething-safe beads to her mouth.

Note: Always be careful with what you choose as toys. Be sure it's a safe material for teething or touching as baby's movements are not necessarily predictable during these early stages of learning to grade their force while still lacking body control. Also be sure to check the cleanliness factor as potentially harmful germs can easily make it from little hands to mouths. Keys and cell phones will interest a baby because they see you playing with them all the time, but these are not the right "toys" for baby. And beware of any toy with a hole in it, like the popular Sophie giraffe and just about any other bathtub toy. A hole allows water or spit to get inside and when moisture is trapped, mold can grow.

The work you do with your baby to help them gain control of their head and neck movement, particularly lifting their head and bringing their chin toward their chest, sets the stage for their strength building farther down the front of their body (aka their "anterior chain" of muscles), into their trunk and core. And the more stable their core becomes, the more mobility you can expect to see your baby bolster in their limbs.

Up next are more strategies that you can begin with your baby while they are on their back to help them in the process of gaining strength and control.

Range of Motion

A more passive way to direct your child in their mobility work is via guiding them with your own two hands through the various ranges of motion they should be developing, providing a gentle way to show them what they can do. Not only will you be introducing their nervous system and brain to early patterning of movements, but you'll be enhancing their blood flow and joint lubrication as you assist their muscles and joints through their arcs of movement potential. This body input enhances your baby's awareness of their position in space and can be very guiding as they come out of their womb-primed positions. These activities also make for very nice calming prep for doing other activities like tummy time or side-lying play, for example.

We encourage you to consider the sensory experience and bonding potential as you approach this. Begin with eye contact between parent/caretaker and baby. Using a soft, soothing tone of voice, take the time to explain to your baby what is about to happen. Let them know where you are going to touch them and what you are going to do. While cognitive processing may not be 100 percent at this stage, this still prepares them for the activity, slows you down, and it may help them to make the connections between the description of what you will do and the part of their body sensing your touch. Other great options are to sing to your baby during the activity or simply express your love for them. Helping to create a sense of calmness and happiness can help your baby to correlate the activity with a sense of pleasure, which will likely have positive carryover effects to future practice attempts. This can help them to be more willing to engage again.

Another sensory aspect to be mindful of is how you are physically touching and applying pressure to your baby's body. Use the flat pads of your fingers versus flexing your fingers and pressing with their tips. Try it on yourself; it can make a huge difference in the sensations you impart. Babies are sensitive and your attention to these details can make all the difference.

Range-of-motion maneuvers are safe to begin right away with your newborn, though you must keep in mind that what you see may differ based on the amount of physiologic flexion your child is still exhibiting. The older your child, the less physiologic flexion will dominate and the less tightness or muscular resistance you are likely to encounter. As you go through these moves, it should be noted that you do not want to move too quickly nor do you want to forcefully stretch your baby's tiny muscles. Your smooth, controlled guidance provides valuable motor learning opportunities for your baby. Go slowly and expect your little one to gradually begin participating with you, attempting to lift and move their own body more and more as they develop more strength and control.

Range-of-Motion Warm-Ups: Guided Movements of the Neck, Arms, Trunk, and Legs

Seen in upcoming pages are two- to four-month-old babies participating in guided range-of-motion activities. The older your baby gets and the more they move around on their own, the less necessary or realistic it will be to hold their attention and participation with activities like these.

Most babies will be willing participants in this if you catch them in the right alert, calm, or even active state. Use a steady, gentle touch and slow, rhythmic movements for the best results. These activities are well paired with diaper changes since your baby is already on their back. They can also be interwoven as part of bathtime if you are using a seat that props your baby on a reclined surface (just recognize that a less-than-flat surface may be more challenging for your baby as it may create subtle changes to the alignment of your baby's bones and muscles). Following a warm bath is another opportunity for practicing these activities since your baby's muscles will be naturally warmed up.

RANGE-OF-MOTION ACTIVITIES ARE NOT THE SAME AS INFANT MASSAGE

Because so many wonderful resources are already in existence for the centuries-old practice of massage, we are not covering the topic directly in this book. We do want to encourage massage being part of your day to day with your baby. It can be a wonderful complement at any age, especially at this early stage of life. Gentle, loving touch can be extremely powerful in helping to develop your baby's body awareness. From nervous system stimulus, to blood and lymphatic circulation, to muscular relaxation or excitement, to sinus pressure and headache relief, to tummy massage aiding the flow of the digestive system during a time when natural motility simply lacks (we as adults get this as a benefit of more movement via walking, jumping, repeatedly flexing our hips as we move), there are just so many uses and benefits of massage that can impact how a baby feels and moves.

Facial massage, for example, can provide excellent stimulus to the region that needs to learn to function with muscular control for the purposes of latching, sucking, feeding, and eventually making sounds to communicate. These skills are crucial for taking in the nourishment that's essential for continued growth, strength gains, and the health of the body as a whole.

Massage can also be very helpful in terms of bonding, communication, and providing a calming aid in times of stress for your baby, such as right before and after a visit to the doctor's office.

We highly encourage massage being a part of your hands-on approach to caring for your baby.

As you approach these activities, go through the motions slowly and pause when you reach the end of the movement. Pairing words that teach your baby about the direction you are moving them and which part of their body you are touching can be helpful. Your baby is processing more than you may realize and you are likely to find that pairing the actions you impose with the words is helpful in not only keeping their attention to the task, but also helping them to cognitively plan for it and even begin to participate as you guide them through.

Aim for at least ten reps of each of these activities and try to keep your flow as smooth as possible, engaging your baby as you go. Progressing from one set of ten to two sets and potentially more is something for you to gauge as you go with your baby. Remember, your baby's brain is like a little sponge, soaking in experiences and organizing that info, learning by the movement and the moment.

Range of motion is just one tool you can use to introduce more movement. Keep in mind that the time your baby spends on their tummy and on their side will give them additional experiences of pressure and other movement sensations, and this all works together.

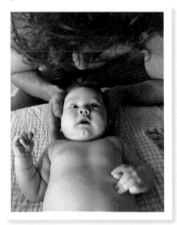

Before you begin moving your baby, take a moment to still and center them in neutral alignment. Here you see Eric's hands gently guiding Sunny (seven weeks) to position her chin in the center of her chest. His palms contour from the sides to the back of her head, with thumbs along the edges of her face and pointer fingers acting as measuring sticks to help him visually assess that her ears are spaced evenly from her shoulders and equivalently on both sides.

Guided Neck Movements

Neck Flexion with Head Lifting

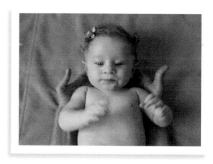

In this image, the baby is lying faceup on a flat surface that's elevated (in this case, a couch). The caregiver here is in a kneeling position on the floor at the edge of the couch so that their body is close to baby's, making both eye contact and caregiver mechanics easier (for this the Kneeling Founder exercise would be excellent prep or recovery work; see Part III).

Caregiver's fingers are supporting the ridge at the base of the baby's head, helping to maintain a neutral alignment.

Baby's posture is excellent: her chin is in the middle of her chest; there's roughly the same amount of space between the bottoms of her ears and the tops of her shoulders on her right and left sides; and her tummy is smooth and relaxed, with no visible sign of muscle contraction. In addition, she's making solid eye contact and appears mellow enough to be open to the movements.

With this setup, it's safe to begin guiding her through either of these next two neck movements.

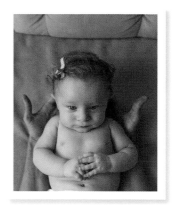

Use the flat pads of your fingers (careful not to use the pointy, pokey tips or your nails) to subtly flex your baby's head forward as you see here.

Moving her chin to her chest shortens the muscles in the front of her neck—which is the uppermost part of her anterior chain—and this ignites a wave of contraction down the front of her body (which may not happen in a younger baby until more strength is developed). This can be seen by the crease that now appears above her belly button. In other words, the baby moving her chin toward her chest engaged more than just her neck flexors; it also engaged her upper abdominal muscles to begin to lift her torso. Chin to chest is an important skill to master. For babies to sit up on their own, they must learn to lift their heads and then manage the wave of action and contraction that travels farther down the body chain. You can think of this "yes" nod as a "pre-sit-up" exercise.

Practicing this with your baby in neutral alignment helps to develop equivalent length and strength in their neck flexors, which is important for their developing ability to control their head, their overall neck alignment, and it also adds stability to their cervical spine. As their head lifts, their chin should tuck toward their chest rather than point toward the ceiling.

Baby responds beautifully here by bringing her hands together in her midline. This helps to self-stabilize and still her body so she can better control her movement.

Bonus: These and the next activities will not only help prevent the developing neck musculature from imbalances (torticollis) but will also help to prevent your baby from developing a "flat" area to their head (plagiocephaly). If either of these conditions are present, we encourage you to work directly with a pediatric physical or occupational therapist, and to also consider working with a pediatric chiropractor, as promptly as possible. Their resolution is a time-sensitive matter.

WHAT DO YOU SEE AND FEEL?
HOW CAN YOU MOTIVATE YOUR BABY?

With range-of-motion activities you are essentially doing the moving for your baby in the beginning, and you should gradually see and feel them participating more. Your hands being present will help you to feel how much muscle your little one is engaging, as well as how the weight of their head shifts in your hand. This should be expected to wax and wane with their energy throughout the day, so if their skills seem to fluctuate from practice session to practice session, don't presume something is wrong. Muscle strength and endurance take time to build, as does the movement control center within your baby's brain. Play, encourage, observe, take note . . . and curtail the support you provide as you go.

Be aware—some babies will raise their eyebrows or engage other facial muscles while trying to figure out how to lift their heads and necks. If your baby is grimacing or using a lot of facial muscles during their efforts, there's a chance you're not providing enough support for their head. Observe. Steady them with your support so they sense stability, then continue.

Encourage your baby as you go—get them to visually lock in on you if possible and try to keep their gaze through the activity. Having a smiling, happy, encouraging facial expression and using a lower volume and a soft yet positive tone to your voice can do wonders for keeping a baby engaged. As you go, you could say things to your baby like "look at me . . . 1-2-3 . . . lift [or 'turn'] your head and look at me." And if a partner is available to join in the practice, they can engage and attract the baby to visually or auditorily track to motivate the movements you are guiding.

Side-Bending aka "Lateral Flexion" of the Neck . . . and Why We Don't Encourage You to Stretch Your Baby's Neck Without a Clinician's Guidance

This movement takes the ear toward the shoulder and, while not pictured, is being mentioned as another range of motion to consider. It's commonly included in pediatric physical therapy treatment of torticollis as a stretching activity; however, since it's not a movement we often perform on its own functionally in life, rather than practicing this movement as an exercise with your baby, we are including it for you to consider utilizing as an assessment tool for their continued symmetrical mobility and developing postural alignment.

For this activity you position your baby exactly the same as you did for the neck flexion range of motion while you sit in front of them. Use one hand to gently cradle their head at the base of their skull and your other hand atop and slightly around your child's opposite shoulder to gently hold it stably in place. The hand cradling the head will be moving as you guide them to bring their ear toward their unstabilized shoulder. Take care not to lift their head upward, as flexing their spine could alter what you see and adds movement that may not be beneficial for your little one.

As you go through your child's range of motion, think of the neck and shoulder as being at right angles to each other. Within the space between them, try to visualize twenty-five-degree increments. Much like the movement of rotation, we are not aiming for 100 percent (this would be where the ear meets the shoulder); rather, somewhere between 75 and 100 percent with equivalent movement between both right and left sides of the neck is the goal.

As you go with neck range of motion in general, you are learning to feel how your child moves in this region of their body. One benefit of this is that it will help you to be better equipped to detect any tight areas should they occur. You'll want to move with mindful attention to whether their movement is smooth or if you encounter tight spots or restrictions on one side as compared to the other. Does the child move and posture differently with different levels of energy? Meaning, do they have a tighter or weaker side, or do you notice that they tend to position one ear closer to one shoulder when they are sleepy? Regular practice will help to tune your hands in for feeling where your baby is strong and where they may need more guidance. It's important to recognize that these things can shift with their energy and, much like if you slept in a wonky position, if your baby had their neck kinked to one side in your arms, their car seat, carrier, or some other container, they can certainly experience nerve irritation that could impact them until the area is moved and better positioned. And sometimes these irritations persist and dominate how your child's muscles hold their alignment. If left unaddressed, such shifts in joint alignment can negatively impact movement patterns and hinder progression toward motor milestones.

Remedying imbalances can and should have both active and passive components, but we want to be sure to mention that we do NOT encourage that you begin to just crank into stretching your child's neck. Microtears to the muscles can result, and those could lead to scar tissue and further exacerbate poor alignment and movement patterns.

Because this book is not about the treatment of imbalances or movement delays, we are not covering the subject matter of stretching tight muscles. For more specifics on this, especially if your child has discrepancies in their range of motion, we encourage you to work directly with a pediatric PT or OT, and, if possible, a chiropractor skilled in pediatric treatment. When it comes to stretching, sometimes more damage can be done than helpful correction; and we highly recommend working with professionals who can guide you with your child's specific body and needs in mind.

Neck Rotation

This image shows me guiding the baby to turn her head and neck as if shaking the head to say no.

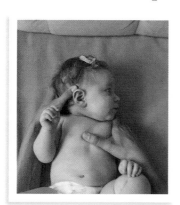

From neck flexion practice you can smoothly transition to moving your baby's head from side to side as you see me do here. This rotational activity is important as it works on the movement your child will need to use to view the environment around them. This movement is also essential for helping your baby to clear their airway while on their back, belly, seated, and anywhere in between.

To set baby up for this, I first place my left thumb above the baby's right ear so that my left hand gently grasps the base of her head. At the same time, I place my right hand over the baby's left shoulder and upper arm, and drape my thumb across her chest, to still the area she'll be turning toward.

My left hand gently lifts her head from the floor, just enough to make sure her ear doesn't drag as I then gently turn her head and neck to face her left. This movement is aided by my having placed a cute toy to the baby's left, which is what she's staring at here. The goal is her cheek resting flat upon the surface. As we go, I'm careful to not let her chin compress downward toward her body. I'm also cautious that her ear doesn't rise much closer to her chest. The goal is to keep the neck in as close as possible to a horizontal line with the rest of the spine.

When you reach the end of the child's range, pause to allow them to spend a few moments taking in the new alignment and shift in visual perspective before switching hand positions to rotate the opposite direction.

If your baby's head doesn't rotate so that their cheek is flat to the surface, keep practicing and aiming for equivalent skills to both sides. An easy way to look at rotation is in percentage increments of twenty-five (25 percent to 50 percent to 75 percent to 100 percent). Looking fully over the shoulder, or 100 percent rotated to one direction, is not a hard-fixed goal. Instead, aim for 75 to 100 percent of rotation with relative symmetry of movement capability from left to right. If you note discrepancies or limitations, discuss with your child's pediatrician right away so it can be addressed promptly. Issues with neck rotation can impact your child's rolling skills and have further down-the-line effects on development of trunk strength essential for building higher-order skills like sitting.

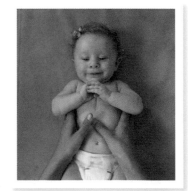

Before proceeding to guiding arm ranges of motion, I take a moment to still the baby's whole body once again. I keep my hands in contact with baby's body and slide them down her torso, pausing along her rib cage, ab-dominals, and upper pelvis.

Baby continues to respond with superb posture. Her head and neck are in neutral alignment, her eye contact remains solid, and her hands are together in the midline of her body.

Centered, still, and connected, she's ready to move on to the next set of range-of-motion exercises—which focus on her arms.

Guided Arm Movements

This activity shows you how to perform a few simple range-of-motion warm-ups for your baby's arms. These general maneuvers take the joints of the shoulders through their available movements—up and down, in and out, and rotationally. Since a baby gains control from their core outwardly, from their shoulder distally toward their hand, we begin with movement through the shoulder joint first. This joint will eventually move through multiple planes with more control, much of that coming as your baby unfurls further from physiologic flexion. For right now, in these early days of motor learning, general, gentle movements will be helpful guidance for premapping those moves. The elbow, wrist, and hand are along for the ride, so to speak; and, while they don't get direct range of motion, the arms as a whole will benefit from the movement and blood and lymphatic circulation.

As with the neck-range activities, describe for your baby what you're doing as you do it; that is, "arms go out to the sides," "reach arms up and bring your hands together," "arms go down, hands by your hips," "arms go up, hands by your head," or "one arm up and one arm down."

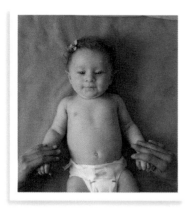

Baby starts off with excellent neutral alignment of her head, neck, and torso.

I offer the baby my thumbs to grab hold of, and at the same time I wrap my fingers over hers, so we're effectively holding each other's hands. My index fingers apply pressure to add stability along the ridge of the joints where her fingers meet her hands. My three remaining fingers stabilize the back of the baby's hands, wrists, and lower forearms, keeping the wrists from extending backward and the forearms from rotating inward. While all this is going on, I subtly bring her arms down to the surface beside her body. I'm careful that her elbows are as straight as she can comfortably allow without applying any force or stretch. I am equally mindful to pause and proceed slowly when I sense any resistance or attempt to recoil and elevate or roll her shoulders inward.

In this position she is neutral and relaxed out of physiologic flexion. This is teaching her body while also providing a great centered position from which to move forward with more arm maneuvering.

Meanwhile, the baby's head tilts down to look at me (as indicated by her beautiful little double chin and downward gaze). As she makes excellent eye contact, she also lengthens the muscles in the back of her neck, and subtly provides some practice of the previously focal neck range-of-motion work (flexion). She is engaged and happily participating. I'm smiling at the baby and encouraging her with a positive and gentle tone.

Note: I'm not using a bumper roll to support the baby's neck and head in this series, but it's perfectly okay for you to use one if your baby shows improved alignment with the extra support. When you move the arms via directing the shoulder joints, keep an eye on what happens to the alignment of your baby's head, neck, and upper torso. This can give you subtle clues about where your baby is strong and stable or possibly tight, weak, or imbalanced. If a neck roll and more practice of neck and arm range of motion don't improve this, there is a chance they might need a little more developmental guidance. Habitual malpositioning is something to watch for and discuss with your pediatrician sooner than later.

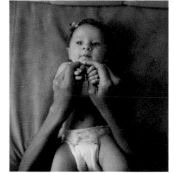

Next I bring the baby's arms from down by her sides to straight up in front of and over her. Her hands are close together, almost touching; and her alignment remains strong. This position lengthens muscles throughout the arms and shoulders. It also puts the baby in a hands-together-in-midline position, which is great for communication between the two hemispheres of the brain and helpful for her developing the visual skill of midline orientation.

From here you can repeat those same two moves or flow forward as you see next before returning the arms down and then alternating one up and one down as you will see ahead. This is not a rigid routine, rather a flow that can dynamically shift with your baby's mood from one session to the next.

In this particular session with this girl, I chose to guide her arms back down toward the surface and out to the sides of her torso. Her shoulders roll outward to make a T of her arms with her torso, with her forearms and hands facing up.

My grip remains the same and I proceed slowly, bringing her arms as close to the surface as is comfortable for her.

This movement allows the baby's shoulder joints to rotate outward and subtly open up along with lengthening her chest muscles. This is also helpful for introducing a baby to posturing out of physiologic flexion.

You can see here that she has rotated her head and neck to her right, as indicated by her chin and face direction. She was visually tracking her mother, who was shaking a rattle from where she stood behind me as I knelt in front of the baby (who was on a couch for this). This exemplifies how this activity can easily be combined with visual tracking to elicit neck-rotation practice, if another caregiver is present and participating.

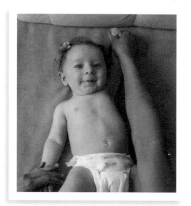

From here you may choose to flow back to the previous position with arms and hands together above the torso, or you may return to both arms down by the sides before then proceeding to what you see me do next with this sweet girl.

After having brought her arms back down by her hips, I then move the baby's left arm up near her ear, with her palm facing up, as I simultaneously bring her right arm down by her side, with her palm facing down.

I then repeat the movement, alternating arms to switch their positions. This lengthens various muscles in the arms and introduces reciprocal action, which will later be a familiar thing when your baby begins crawling.

After guiding the baby through a few reps of each of these arm ranges, I shift my focus from her arms farther down her body to her torso.

Guided Trunk Movements

APPROXIMATE AGE RANGE: 4–6 MONTHS

Our next focus is a form of baby sit-ups that engage and guide toward strengthening the muscles that support the baby's torso. Strength gains in this region enhance overall core stability. These next activities will be performed by the baby's mom. The baby seen here is four months old.

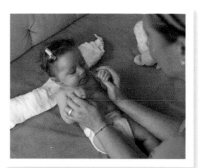

Baby will begin on her back, then sit up as her mom holds her hands and guides her. In this session, because the baby had become tired, we placed a bumper roll under her neck to encourage neutral alignment in her setup.

Mom's grip is the same as used with the arm maneuvers, where we elicit the baby's Grasp Reflex to encourage holding on and participating. At the same time, Mom's forearms rest gently atop baby's thighs, keeping them from rocking up as baby shifts upright. This encourages the baby to use her abdominal muscles to flex her trunk over her hips more than allowing her to use her hip flexor muscles to assist (as is the natural tendency and okay for some practice reps, but we encourage doing this both ways).

Mom brings her baby's arms out in front of her shoulder joints, and you see here that baby keeps her elbows flexed near her body. This is to be expected because of physiologic flexion; but as you give a slow and gentle upward pull to lift your baby from the surface in the direction of sitting, make sure they are not relying on their arm muscles (which you would note by them pulling their fists closer to their shoulders and their tummy not engaging).

Here we see this baby shift her chin down to her chest, which engages the upper parts of her abdominal muscles. Because she's so young, her abdominals aren't yet developed enough to fully engage, though, and she naturally compensates for this by bending her elbows, making performing the sit-ups a bit easier since it gets other muscles to assist her abs. This compensation is something we want to see going away with time and practice as the abdominal muscles grow stronger.

As you proceed with this activity, watch your baby's reaction from the top of their head downward. During the first three months, your goal for your baby is for them to begin to keep their chin tucked toward their chest through the transition, an equivalent grip strength from both hands, and maybe even beginning to feel some upper abdominal muscle activation. Over the days, weeks, months to come, your baby will grow stronger with this activity and begin to not only pull their chin toward their chest, but then further activate the muscles that pull their chest toward their pelvis. This will increase their ability to come out of the horizontal plane of lying on the floor into an upright position.

It's important to note that this activity would not be done with a newborn. Wait until the baby is able to lift their head in neutral midline alignment while on their back. This is because your hands will be holding theirs and, because they lack neck control, their head could flop backward with the challenge of gravity and injure their delicate spinal nerves. That said, if you have a partner to go through this activity helping you to help the baby, you can approach this as a team once your baby shows some participation in the chin-to-chest head nod from the neck range-of-motion work. For this you would keep your hands guiding the same way and your partner would position behind the baby's head, using their hands to help the baby maintain a neutral head and neck and tuck their chin toward their chest as you guide them to lift their torso.

Baby sits all the way up, eye to eye with her mom. She exhibits strong posture for a four-month-old. This is indicated by her relaxed shoulders, chin centered in relation to her chest, and an even amount of space between her ears and shoulders. Said differently, her spine is neutrally aligned with her neck tall atop her torso.

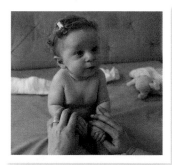

Mom helps the baby perform several reps of sit-ups and then gives her a break by switching things up.

Because baby was trying to pull and thrust herself upward toward standing, Mom lifts her and places her on her feet, with her hands and palms around her baby's hips, and her thumbs adding additional torso support at baby's abdominals.

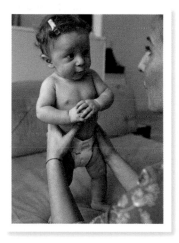

Because the baby is still learning to fully engage her abdominal muscles and is not truly ready for standing practice to be focal yet, this was just a brief moment of eye contact and connection spent here. In this final image we see her use an adorable self-stabilizing strategy as she brings her hands together in her midline.

This is an activity you can continue to use throughout the whole first year and beyond. If done with attention to neutral alignment, and avoiding completion of the sit-up if there is a side-bend occurring in the neck, this can make a positive difference in the development of postural control muscles, trunk alignment, and benefit your baby's sitting skills.

Guided Hip and Leg Movements

Mom is now ready to help her baby perform activities that address joints farther down her body, including her lower trunk, hips, legs, and feet. She begins by placing the baby on her back with her legs straight down to the surface below her and her body in a neutral alignment. She then places her hands around the ends of the baby's limbs, with her thumbs on the baby's heels, her fingers on the baby's lower legs, and avoiding putting pressure on the actual ankle joints themselves.

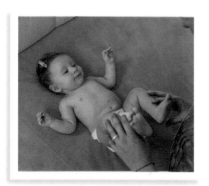

From the baby's feet, Mom gently exerts pressure as she guides the baby's legs to flex at both hips and knees, and brings the baby's legs up to about a ninety-degree angle of hips to torso and ninety degrees at the knees. Mom is mindful that knees point upward versus out to the infant's sides or in toward each other.

Mom can flex the legs farther if the baby is happily engaged and tolerating the range of motion. Going so far as to apply pressure from the legs to the abdomen can have positive impacts on digestion. A watchful eye should be kept on the top edge and inner thigh portions of the baby's diaper to ensure they are not rubbing and irritating the skin.

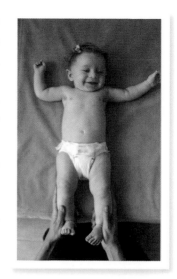

From this upper flexed position, the mom maintains her hand contact and guides the baby to extend her joints and bring her legs back down to the surface.

This alternation of motion (extension to flexion and back and forth) is great for educating the joints about what they can do, lubricating their surfaces; and, if the baby begins to actively participate and reach for her feet in the process, this can serve to further engage and strengthen her abdominal muscles as well.

Here we see a way to guide hands-to-feet play. Mom places a few fingers gently atop baby's hands and encourages baby to bring her hands to grasp her toes. Such movement skills don't tend to occur independently until a baby is six or seven months old, and this four-month-old shows her struggles by falling out of neck and hip alignment (as noted by her right ear leaning closer to her right shoulder, her chin subtly pointing to the left of the midline of her chest, and her right hip hiking subtly closer to the base of her rib cage on her right side).

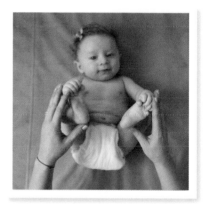

It's certainly not too early to introduce her to this sort of play, though. It will teach her muscles and body to coordinate this move and therefore spur development of the skills that eventually allow the baby to excel at this on her own.

If you feel your baby resisting your movement, pause, check in on their facial expression, and listen to their noises. Are they grimacing or grunting? Discomfort in the abdomen due to digestion is possible, so, like all activities done horizontally, it's important to consider the timing of this activity in relation to feeding. Resistance can also occur if the baby is tired or simply not interested in this activity.

This is where it becomes important to really tune in to your baby. Before letting go of the limbs, pause and reapproach the activity. If both legs moving together in up-and-down repetitions is upsetting, don't force it and risk further upsetting your baby. Simply flow into another activity. You may even find that you can easily return to this again later in your practice session.

From here you might consider alternating the legs in a reciprocal bicycling pattern or performing lower trunk rotations, two moves that can later translate benefits to your child's rolling and crawling skills. You saw these activities earlier with a newborn, but in these next few shots you'll see me step in to coach the mom through how to do this with her four-month-old.

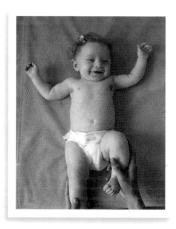

There are notable changes in how this looks in an older baby who is coming further out of physiologic flexion, making and maintaining more eye contact, and moving their spine more segmentally (versus logrolling).

With my index finger along the side of baby's left knee, my thumb across the top of her foot and shin, and my palm cupping the side of her heel, I guide baby's left hip and knee upward while also making sure her leg tracks in a neutral alignment (knee up versus pointing out to the side of her body). At the same time, I'm holding the baby's right leg straight with a similar grasp around the lower aspect of her limb.

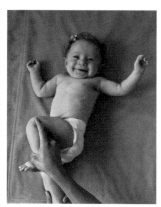

From there I flow into shifting the baby's left leg to the opposite side of her body, bringing the knee across her midline, and thereby initiating a roll from her back toward her right side.

Moving the lower body slowly and steadily naturally guides the baby to rotate her upper body in the same direction. Where you saw a younger baby immediately logroll their body as a unit, from the photo at left to the one on the next page you can see this baby moving her body more segmentally. Her lower body rotation is led by her guided upper leg, her hips, and her stomach; and then her upper body and arm follow to complete her full body rotation. Here we can see that her left arm, which was previously on the floor, is now in the air.

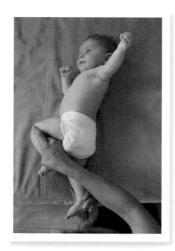

Keep directives to your baby simple and step-by-step. For example, you can say "leg goes up" slowly and with emphasis as baby's leg is bent upward; and "leg goes over" as you guide your baby to rotate. Saying the words slowly drawn out and paired with the particular action or direction allows the baby's brain a moment to register and commit to the action along with you. They may not understand on the first few attempts at movement, but repetition is a great way to teach and train. You may find it helpful in terms of both educating their body on the movements as well as keeping your baby engaged if you turn your directions into a song and make the movements almost like a rhythmic rocking action. As you do so, watch and feel for your baby's increasing muscular engagement and participation. This should feel like them pulling their leg up toward their body, flexing their hip and knee, and maybe even engaging their tummy to initiate some of the rotational action along with you.

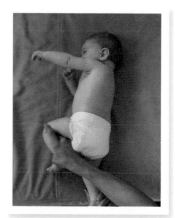

Baby rotates farther toward the floor. Her left knee is now in contact with the surface below her. My hands remain still while she figures out how to bring the rest of her body over to the opposite side. The raised arm that was trailing her body is now reaching forward toward the floor.

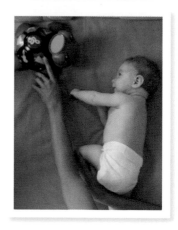

Placing a desirable toy on the side of the baby that you want them to rotate toward can be very helpful in providing them the visual stimulus and motivation to turn their head in the first place. It can also persuade a child to reach out for the toy and remain in the rotated position for a few minutes to soak in the new perspectives it provides. This provides benefits to eye-hand coordination and visual perception, fine motor skills of reaching and potentially attempting to grasp, and it also gives a different degree of pressure to the side of her body and stomach upon which her body's weight is now distributed. (So if you're wondering if this can be beneficial for your baby's digestion, too, yes, you're right!)

With an older baby (four-plus months), all these activities can easily flow into doing more movements that focus on trunk strengthening (such as those in the previous pages), whereas the younger baby who still lacks neck strength and stability won't be physically ready for the trunk work. To introduce it too early could result in an unsupported, weak neck flopping about, which can potentially put too much stress and strain on delicate structures and lend to irritation or injury, or just totally frustrate the baby (remember, you want positive experiences). You'll know your baby is ready when they begin to tuck their own chin and lift their head subtly from the surface.

Hands-to-Feet Play

This is another great activity to do with your baby while they are on their back, starting around four months of age. It's a dynamic mode of play that incorporates eye-hand coordination, arm reaching and fine motor grasping control, hip mobility, and core-strengthening work. Fun engagement like this for your baby means the work is hidden in the play. This is a great option to flow toward from your range-of-motion warm-up activities as it takes baby's attention from being jointly shared with the involved caregiver to placing it on a toy and their own body in a way that continues to engage many core muscles while they are on their back.

Notice the strategically placed teething rattle ring around Sunny's right lower leg. I had placed her on her back with her legs down to the floor and shook this rattle above her to get her eyes locked on it. She responded by first reaching her arms, so then I flexed one leg up and put the ring around her ankle, where she could see it. She responded by bringing both legs up, just

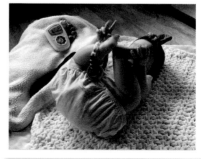

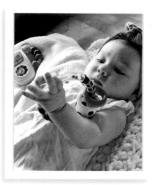

like she had done in our hip range-of-motion practice that preceded this activity, and rocking side to side in efforts to grab her feet to figure out how to get the toy into her hands.

Success! Baby has managed to get the ring off her leg and she is seen here holding it in the midline of her body as she examines it with both hands. Her spinal alignment is neutral and strong. Note: This is a great strategy that allows the caregiver to engage the baby to initiate movement and then step back to allow them to problem solve during some solo playtime (which can free their hands up to either join baby in some exercise or tackle some other nearby task). If baby is showing signs of frustration, the caregiver could step back in and provide more guidance in a hand-over-hand fashion to help baby achieve success with bringing hands to feet or to their toy. They could even bring feet to mouth.

It should go without saying that caregivers should be judicious about the toys they choose as well as observing the little one for safety.

Rolling Back to Side

APPROXIMATE AGE RANGE: 4–6 MONTHS

H ere we see a nearly four-month-old baby beginning to integrate all the things discussed in the
supine skills chapters.

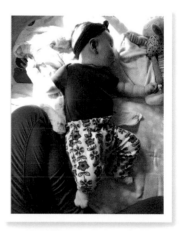

She starts on her back with the item of interest
placed to her left. We see she has fully rotated her
neck, and her left cheek is flat on the surface. We
even see that she is exhibiting an ATNR here as she
reaches her left hand toward the toy. As she goes, we
see her arms move through the ATNR (meaning she
is able to move out of the "fencer's position"), effectively showing that this reflex is integrating (disap-
pearing).

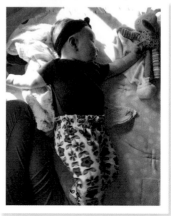

In the second image we see her right hip starting
to flex up, rotate across her body's midline while her
left leg extends and she rolls onto her left side. Her
right arm still remains on the surface.

This third image shows baby's right hip and knee
flexing and rotating further as her torso and upper

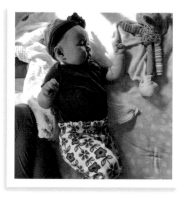

body follow, logrolling with her. Her right arm is now off the floor and approaching her midline as she reaches toward the toy. She hangs out in side-lying on her left side. This position offers her new visual perspectives and muscle use patterns, and it's great midline orientation practice.

This is a great place to conclude this discussion of supine-based activities. As previously stated, once your baby has built substantial-enough core strength, hip and spinal mobility to roll out of supine to their side and beyond, you are less likely to keep them there for play.

The next chapter will show you ways you can support your newborn in the side-lying position and work on skill building from there.

Positioning Baby in Side-Lying

Although newborn babies are not likely to find and stay in this position on their own, it's wonderfully beneficial for them to spend
time here. Being in side-lying is an excellent opportunity for your
baby to learn more about where their body is in space. It encourages their hands coming together in the midline of their body, a task
that is beneficial for the communication between the right and left
sides of their brain; and it also encourages visual convergence (eyes
coming together to focus). These things combined are powerful for
your child's developing eye-hand coordination. As they begin reaching, they will experience shifts in their body weight, which is beneficial as an early rolling practice. This also provides varied degrees
of pressure to their joints and abdomen, which can have impacts on
developing muscle tone and digestion.

To safely position your baby in side-lying, you'll want to consider
their spinal alignment and utilize rolled blankets as bumpers, similar to how you have in other positions.

A few tips to set your baby up for success here:

1. Prevent side-bending of their neck with a rolled blanket supporting the space between the downward shoulder and the ear. Be sure your baby's ear isn't folded and smooshed.

2. Prevent excessive extension of their head and neck. Looking down at your baby from their head toward their toes, their ears should be lined up over their shoulders. If their mouth is wide open, there's a fair chance they are overextended. That position does their developing "oral motor" muscles and feeding skills no favors, meaning it won't help their ability to strongly latch, suck, or swallow. It can also compromise their airway. Use a hand to realign their spine.

3. Prevent bending or rotation of their spine through their trunk with bumper rolls behind their back and in front of their chest and abdomen.

4. Support their hips in a neutral position with a bumper roll or folded blanket between their legs. You can use one roll in front of their body starting at their chest and going down through their legs. Encouraging their arms to hug this blanket will also help to keep their shoulder joints more neutrally aligned versus allowing the top arm to roll excessively inward with gravity.

Of course, as your baby begins moving and exploring, all these rolls are likely to shift. Keep a watchful eye, and be sure to spend equivalent time positioned on both sides. Remember, aligning them well educates their body well, and the input their brain receives from each session's experiences all adds up in the bigger picture of their motor learning.

The focal activities for your baby to practice in the side-lying position are centered first around neck movement and visual or auditory tracking as you've learned already in other positions. Once your baby begins exploring their environment with their hands touching and arms reaching, this opens up more play. These are precursors for reaching and grasping skills and will contribute to your baby's efforts with rolling.

Seen here is a newborn, ten days old, exemplary in position with the bumper rolls in place as described. While it is not visible here, note the baby's bottom arm; your baby's arm should have its upper portion on the surface, slightly in front of their chest as opposed to directly under their side, and not elevated with a blanket. Ensure 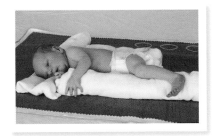 that their shoulder joint is not rolling inward underneath them into a poor position that could compromise their blood flow, nerves, or muscles.

Here is a three-week-old baby being positioned by her mother with the same principles in mind. Rolled blankets under the neck for support and behind/in front of the torso will help to prevent rolling over. This image beautifully captures the mom using a broad touch with both hands to keep her pressure gentle and diffuse as she positions her baby. It also captures the closeness with which 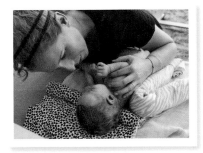 she positions herself to her baby, coming face-to-face for eye contact at a range that her daughter's visual skills can handle. Mom is in a kneeling position in front of a couch, where baby is positioned atop its seat. Because this might lend to bringing her neck out of alignment, Mom would be well advised to prep her own body for this with a few Foundation Training Kneeling Founders (see Part III for details). She can also set her baby up in side-lying and then layer in her own work to decompress and lengthen her spine as she goes.

With no roll placed in front of her, here we see the baby exploring the neck roll with her own hand. Her top shoulder and arm are extended outward and her hand is engaged in touch exploration. Her bottom hand is to her mouth, which gives her sensory system great feedback. Her top leg is active, exploring her bottom leg with her foot. This whole scenario provides a ton of sensory feedback for the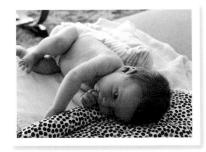

baby about where her body is in space, helping to build her spatial awareness as she gets active practice with eye-hand coordination and reaching. Note the action of her upper arm from this photo to the next as she explores her environment and what her body can do.

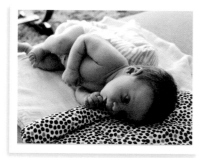

Baby has gone from reaching to retracting her top arm, which is now relaxed against her body. While a better resting position for babies would be with a roll in front of them, the reality of awake and alert babies is they may not stay still enough to keep it in place. Selectively placing toys on the surface ahead of them or attracting their attention with visual or auditory tracking games can provide stimulus and engagement for babies in this position.

This is an image of our daughter at two months, taking a nap in side-lying. At this stage Sunny had shown us that she could turn her neck both directions while on her tummy, while on her back, and while on either side, so we felt confident in her strength and ability to clear her own airway. Regardless, she was never left unsupervised in this position. (Babies can move in their sleep and easily become entangled in their blankets, so we want to be clear that we never advise leaving your baby unattended in *any* position.)

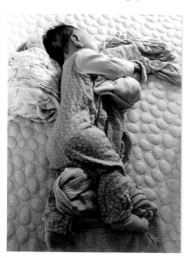

Here we see her supported by three blankets and one folded "lovey" toy. She has one blanket loosely rolled and tucked under her neck, one blanket in a loose fold behind her back, the darker pink blanket taking up space between her legs and preventing her upper knee from resting on the ground, and the light pink lovey folded under her upper arm.

This is less polished than the previous images but effective in getting the job done.

Before we progress to what your baby should be able to do in terms of sitting upright, let's take a moment to tie together these first three fundamental positions (prone, supine, and side-lying). Because your guidance can make all the difference in the quality and symmetry of how these acts are practiced, we're going to show you rolling in shorter activity segments first—that is, from the side to the tummy and the side to the back—before then tying the whole flow together.

Visual Tracking and Reaching to Roll Side-Lying to Tummy

This activity is a great example of how positioning time is now becoming more dynamic playtime for your baby. Not only does this activity help your baby practice visually following an object, working their neck mobility, eye-hand coordination, reaching skills, and hip

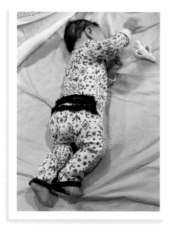

mobility; but it also helps your baby to strengthen their arms, core, and controlled mobility with transitioning from being on their side to being on their belly. You'll know your baby is ready for this when they show control of their neck to visually track while on their back and interest in looking at and batting at toys.

Here is our daughter at three months without any bumper rolls, placed on her side and initiating her own rolling practice via her upper arm reaching for her (strategically placed) teething toy as her upper leg is simultaneously flexing forward.

To replicate a similar situation, caregivers can consider tucking a bumper roll along the backside and slightly under their baby's body to position them subtly biased between side-lying and tummy time. This roll placement will prevent your baby rolling backward to their back and support their spending time in this "in-between position," which will encourage your baby shifting their body weight to roll to their tummy. This offers yet another play option for during awake time. As with everything else being encouraged, be sure to do this on both sides.

Next you see what is essentially the same activity with an older six-month-old baby. The previous version with the younger baby is a setup that allows the baby to have independent playtime and ex-plore their movement within their strategically staged environment, whereas this next version entails a caregiver motivating the baby to move by enticing their visual tracking and reaching with a small toy.

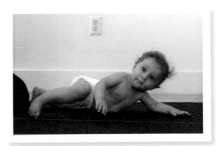

Baby starts placed in side-lying and she im-mediately begins propping herself up on her left arm as she flexes her right hip to bring her right foot to the ground ahead of her. She's looking straight ahead because a toy is being presented in front of her.

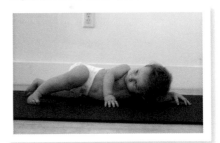

Mom raises the toy above her baby's head and to her right. Baby responds by rotating her neck to follow the toy—which is our goal.

Baby's released her propping arm and dropped lower to the ground, using her right hand and foot to help maintain her position on her side.

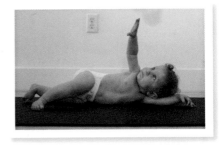

Mom moves the toy almost directly above the baby. Baby responds by rotating her head far-ther up, and reaching straight up with her right arm. Baby's right toes claw at the floor, showing she's trying to create more stability for herself as she stretches and reaches. This is a totally normal reaction, so if your baby also claws their toes, no need for concern.

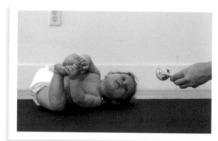

Mom brings the toy down in an arc, encouraging the baby to continue rotating her head and neck. The toy is now lower to the ground, but slightly above her head if you look from a head-to-toes perspective. In response, the baby lifts her chin and dips the base of her head back to get a better look.

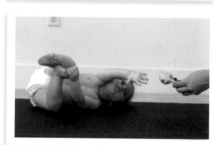

At the same time she engages her tummy muscles and hip flexors, bending her legs at the hip and knee joints, and then grasping her feet with her hands. This position helps her to roll as she follows the toy, and also provides stability, which she may have been craving if the extra neck extension to view the toy made her feel a little less stable. (Note: Just like being prone on the floor, to lift the head to view levels above the surface and horizon level is more work for the baby, and more work can often lead to subtle instability if the muscles are not yet strong and steady within the action.)

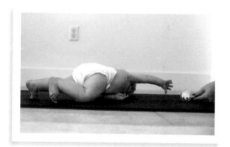

Overall, the baby is in a relatively neutral position, with her chin and spine fairly well in line with the center of her chest. So far, she's doing great.

With her vision locked on the toy, and quite possibly now feeling more balanced, the baby releases her right foot, and she reaches for the toy with her right hand.

Mom lowers the toy to the floor.

Baby reaches farther still with her right arm, brings her right knee and foot to the surface as she extends her left leg, and rolls over her left side.

Take notice of her torso still midroll with her left arm essentially stuck underneath it. This is not necessarily problematic. In fact, what she is executing here is basically the definition of segmental rolling, where her hips and lower trunk roll first, followed by her abdomen, and then, last, her chest, shoulders, arms, head, and neck will follow.

The side-lying discussion as a whole will conclude in the next chapter with an activity that will show you how you can take your baby from a position like this into tummy-time practice. But first, the next photo series shows the same six-month-old practicing going from her side to her back.

Visual Tracking and Reaching to Roll Side-Lying to Back

APPROXIMATE AGE RANGE: 3–4+ MONTHS

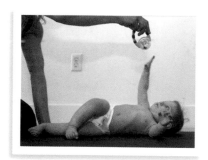

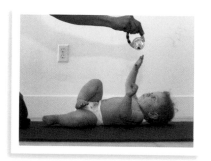

Baby lies on her left side. I hold a toy over her head and, once it catches her attention, slowly move it to her right.

Baby first rotates her neck as she visually tracks the toy. At the same time, her rib cage opens up as she rotates her upper torso to her right. Her right foot is resting across the midline of her body, pressing down flat on the floor with her toes clawing the surface. This gives the baby feedback about where her body is positioned and also helps to both keep the lower portion of her body stable and provide a push-off position to help her roll.

Baby pushes to lift her right foot off the ground as her hip flexes and pulls the leg across her midline. This rotation of her lower body causes a wave of motion to complete her roll toward her back.

Baby has rolled entirely off her side and onto her back. Her spine is in alignment, with her head and neck in neutral rotation looking directly above. And now that she's in a stable position, she's reaching for the toy over her head.

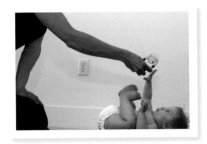

From here the baby's caregiver could choose to let the baby experience success for her efforts by giving her the toy she worked so hard to move toward. Or, to make this one step more engaging and challenging, the toy could be placed over one of the baby's feet to entice hands-to-feet reaching play.

These next few images of a five-month-old will show you how you can incorporate visually tracking and reaching for a toy into guiding the full dynamic flow of rolling from on the back to the side to the tummy, and then setting up for practicing propping skills from there.

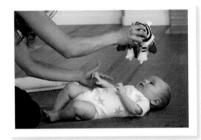

In this particular play session, this baby boy was tired and not very interested in reaching for the toy with his right arm (though you can see his left is starting to reach up from the surface toward the toy). So here you see me using one hand to get his eyes locked on the toy while my other hand gives his right arm encouragement by giving him something to grab. See in the next photo how I then guide him toward reaching.

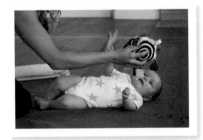

Baby has started to transition from being on his back toward his left side. We see his right arm is being led, palm to palm, by my hand; and his right heel is pressing into the floor. His whole body starts to logroll along with his neck rotating toward his left as he visually tracks the toy I am bringing farther toward his left periphery, toward the floor.

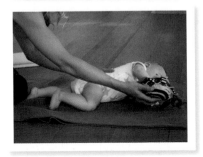

The toy is now down to the surface and baby boy has logrolled to bring his right knee in contact with the floor and his right hand in contact with the toy. Along the way, once his arm crossed the side of his own body toward his midline, my left hand shifted from his palm to provide subtle stability at his low back, behind his pelvis on his right side.

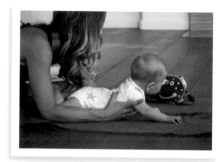

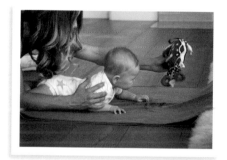

Now we switch it up a bit to keep baby boy's attention on task and allow me to get into a position to better support and engage him. My forearms are now sandwiching in his torso and legs. My left hand holds the toy to his left periphery because on the way here to his tummy he had tracked from his right to his left; I'm now switching it to encourage tracking from his left to his right so his neck muscles get a chance to work both directions. My right hand provides stability with my thumb to his mid-back, just below his shoulder blade; my middle, ring, and pinky fingers are along the side of his rib cage and providing support under his upper arm, while my pointer finger is atop his upper arm, acting to subtly direct it into the position you see in the next photo.

This final image shows the toy being moved to the front and center of the baby's visual path. It is elevated from the floor to encourage baby lifting his head, neck, and upper back. Here you see my (right) hand has shifted almost entirely to his arm. My forearm provides a bumper along his whole right side from his knee to his midtrunk, offering a subtle sense of stability. My thumb rests on his upper back, behind his shoulder, giving stability to his shoulder blade and posterior aspect of his shoulder girdle. My pointer, middle, and ring fingers are widely spreading their support from the front of his shoulder joint down around the front and side aspects of his upper arm. My pinky finger gives subtle downward pressure to his forearm as the whole of my hand is subtly encouraging his arm to press down into the surface. This manual assistance will help babies to feel stable as they are challenged to look up, giving them encouragement to press down and prop higher, stronger, taller.

Note: To execute this, I was between a kneeling position and being on elbows and knees behind the baby. A great warm-up for the caregiver prior to this activity, or reset exercise following this, would be an 8-Point Plank and a Kneeling Founder (see Part III).

In the chapters ahead you will find more guidance for helping your baby to come from propping on elbows as seen here to pressing up on their palms with their elbows extended, among other advanced tasks for building trunk, hip, and leg strength to prepare for upright skills. But first, a few words on sitting and standing with a baby under four months are in order.

Positioning Baby in Sitting

Your newborn's body is simply not ready to sit fully upright on its own. Physiologic flexion will dominate and the lack of strength in the baby's body make doing so too early a recipe for microinjuries to various soft tissue structures by the sheer force of gravity impacting their weak body, and their inability to effectively resist it. This can lend to muscle imbalances and asymmetrical posturing. It is for this reason that we don't advise attempting to place your baby sitting reclined on a couch cushion or propped on your bed. To sustain safely sitting this way, a baby first needs several weeks to months of building neck and trunk strength.

You've already been shown earlier in this book how to safely position your baby in sitting on your lap while facing you. And in pages ahead you will encounter activities that will help you challenge your baby while they sit facing away from you, with tasks like reaching for a toy and recovering their balance to sit upright, as well as transitioning from sitting to all fours and sitting to standing. But first you will want to ensure that your baby starts to develop the skills to sit safely on their own.

As your baby builds more postural strength, which your early supine, prone, and side-lying work will help with, you will be able to
guide your baby's path toward independent sitting by introducing
prop sitting as seen here with a four-month-old little girl.

By the end of your baby's first three months of life,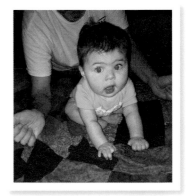
they should have increased their neck control enough
for their head to not flop around. In fact, they should
be able to hold their head and neck in the midline of
their body when you support them upright.

Their arms will gradually be involved in propping
their torso upright (subtly hinged forward over their
bottom and legs) while sitting. Arms in front of their
body with palms in fists will typically precede the
palms opening for flat hands propping, which precedes the arms coming farther out toward the sides of the baby's
body, which precedes the arms coming to the ground behind the
baby.

Before you can begin to introduce layering challenges to exercise
your baby in sitting, you should consider that the very first challenge
is the act of sitting in and of itself. Gravity is a challenge to keep their
head centered over the top of their trunk over the top of their hips.

Learning propping skills and practicing tracking from there are
the next orders of business. At first it will be a challenge just to look
up without losing balance and toppling over, so your practice should
begin there. In the previous image you see the caregiver behind the
baby, which is great for providing protection with hands ready to
catch the baby. You can consider doing this in front of a mirror or
with another caregiver sitting in front of the baby to engage them
with positive encouragement and motivation to look upward.

Eventually, as in all other positions, neck rotations while visually
tracking are among your baby's first seated challenges. This can begin with the toy at the level of the ground and gradually coming
higher, to the eye/horizon level, and then above horizon level so that
the baby is looking up.

As posterior chain strength develops, looking upward should encourage their head, neck, and back to extend farther. With this sort of practice you will eventually see your child start to remove their propping arms from the floor and reach for items you present for tracking.

As you go, keep in mind that any seat or container used is likely to position your baby's body against gravity in a way that could be potentially harmful (i.e., slumping pelvis/sacrum, twisting, side-bending or rotating the spine or large joints of the body, neck hyperextending or leaning to a side) because baby has yet to build the trunk strength and control to hold themself upright against gravity's force.

You can most efficiently and effectively build upon your child's seated skills by practicing them in neutral alignment, out of a container, and with your support first.

We encourage parents and caregivers to learn to look at where the force (of gravity and body weight) gets distributed through their baby's body. Consider the safe use of strategically placed bumper rolls to help keep your baby's posture healthfully, neutrally aligned. This mindful attention steadily in practice in all positions, sitting included, can help prevent any deleterious effects.

For our daughter, by the end of her first three months, we found that, if her trunk was given full support of our hands broadly placed to either side of it, she was able to prop sit using either hand to the side of her body or both hands in front of her. While she was unable to do this without support, with it her arms would reflexively come to the surface in an attempt to hold her weight.

At this early stage a baby cannot yet transition from the floor to sitting on their own, but we found with our daughter that when we placed her into a side-lying position and guided her body through the process of sitting up through a side-sitting position, she would attempt to help by pushing off her elbow. In the pages ahead you will find an activity that shows you specifically how to do this, as well as other activities that can help build trunk strength for developing sitting skills.

A QUICK WORD ON "W-SITTING" AND OTHER SEATED POSTURES

W-sitting is when your child is seated with their bottom to the floor, legs bent in front of them, and feet to the outsides of their body. While this is not a posture you are likely to begin to see until your child is independently transitioning into sitting (sometime after about six months), we want to mention it now so it's in your head later.

When a child assumes a w-sit, their pelvis is rocked out of neutral alignment, either forward into an anterior tilt with their tummy elongating and back shortening in hyperextension OR backward into a posterior tilt with their low spine excessively flexing and abdominal muscles shortening—all while their hips are excessively inwardly rotated, which places an inordinate force on their inner knees and hips.

While this is not an ideal resting position for your child to play in, it is fairly common as it gives a wide base of seated support; and it is probably okay in brief amounts of time if it's not habitual and simply a position your baby moves through from time to time as they shift between other seated positions.

Other common sitting positions during the first year are ring sitting (legs bent in front of them with feet together), side sitting (knees both bent and feet going to the same side of the body, weight held through the outer hip and leg on the side the knees point toward), and long sitting (legs straight out in front of the body).

Sitting cross-legged, aka tailor sitting (a term many are not familiar with, but actually originated centuries ago because it was how tailors sat while sewing; formerly known as "Indian-style"; now commonly called by school-aged kids "crisscross applesauce") is not covered in this book because it develops beyond the first year.

Around the time your baby begins to prop sit, another option to help them learn to engage their trunk for upright sitting involves the caregiver using their body to effectively sandwich in the baby's body as you see me doing in these next photos with our daughter.

Here Sunny is long sitting (with her legs out in front of her) as I am also doing with my legs, effectively creating stability bumpers along both sides of her torso. She is able to rest her hands and forearms atop my legs, and you can see that I've placed one

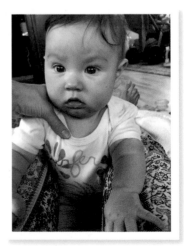

hand around her shoulder to provide an additional source of stability to help her align her torso, neck, and head atop her seated base.

From here, visually tracking up, down, and to the sides—to view the environment, another caregiver, sibling, or pet, or to track a toy—are all ways to help your baby strengthen their postural control muscles.

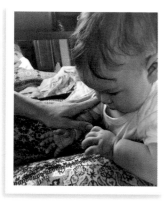

You can see here that my support hand has shifted farther down Sunny's arm to stabilize her hand and arm against my leg as she looks down and explores the interesting pattern of my pants. Simple work and simple support hidden within a position that allows for closeness and bonding.

More on how to help your baby build trunk strength for healthy posture in sitting as well as build independence with transitioning in and out of sitting will be found within the activities ahead.

Before we proceed, first a few words on placing a newborn baby into standing positions.

Positioning Baby in Standing

For the newborn especially, it's truly too soon to do this. Without muscular strength providing stability to the baby's skeletal system, you will see your baby's spine round weakly, their head and neck unable to be held upward. That said, at their early checkups, you will likely see their pediatrician doing this anyway as they check your baby's reflexes. It's actually pretty neat to observe, fascinating really. With the baby's trunk well supported, when their feet brush the floor, you may observe a newborn reflex that looks as though the baby is walking. This reflex should disappear around the end of month two. Interestingly, researchers have speculated that this particular reflex could be intimately interwoven into the brain's development of walking patterns to come.

Into the third month of your baby's life, once a little head control and neck strength have developed, you can play with introducing a few moments here and there of holding them in a supported standing position. To be clear though, their hip joints are not truly ready to support their own body weight yet, so this should be done with you supporting most of their weight. You will want to use both your hands to provide ample stabilization around your child's torso, under the level of their armpits. Try to make your grip all-encompassing with fingers spread widely and thumbs encircling your baby's back. Watch that you use the flat pads of your fingers for gentler pressure. And especially watch that your touch isn't elevating their tiny shoulders or compressing their fragile underarm or neck area. There are lots of important nerves and blood vessels running through this region.

These next three images capture early standing practice in our own home and experience with our daughter, who was two and a half months old here. Knowing she had strength and control of neck motion to look over either shoulder while on her tummy, back, and in our arms, we felt comfortable seeing how her skills with this looked while supported upright on her feet, when given solid stabilization to her midsection. There are a few details about her posturing that offer some valid teaching points as you approach trying this with your baby.

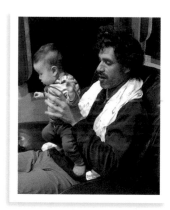

Here we see Dad in a long-sitting posture that provides a stable lap for baby girl's feet to press into. As he brought her upright from sitting, her feet and legs naturally spread widely and her arms flexed at their elbows and pulled up toward her core. These are both natural strategies that give the body more stability. What's most notable about this is with regard to what is going on with Dad's hands. As he brought her from sitting forward-facing on his lap (where he first had her to allow her to fix her eyes on a toy positioned in front of them) to standing, his grip was more with his palms to her low sides and his thumbs to her midback. His pointer fingers encircled her upper chest but his middle, ring, and pinky fingers were loose.

This was a learning curve for both of them, and by no means the goal practice posture as her arms are flexed and we see her retracting her left arm back. The goal with standing practice is to acclimate the leg muscles with experience of holding (a portion of) the body's weight without compensatory balance strategies or asymmetrical neck posturing occurring. If they do occur, this is either a sign that you're not providing enough stabilization with your support OR your baby simply may not be ready for this yet.

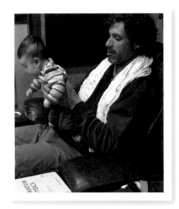

From this image to the next we see remarkable shifts in baby girl's posturing once Dad brings his remaining fingers in contact with her abdominal muscles (part of the key to stabilizing the trunk). Her arms have started to come down and are no longer retracting. Her legs have narrowed their position. Note that Dad's fingers are held closely together here.

Dad keeps his eyes to her midback, watching how she holds her head and neck in relation to this part of her spine. Her gaze has dropped, but her head and neck have not. If this position causes your baby's head and neck to flop forward, they may not be ready for this yet; and they would likely benefit from more neck-strengthening practice, especially on their tummy as it would require their posterior chain of muscles—the muscles that lift the head and upper spine in particular—to engage.

Dad changes his support by spreading his fingers widely to cover more surface area, thereby providing more stabilization to the baby's midback as well as more stimulus for the abdominals to engage.

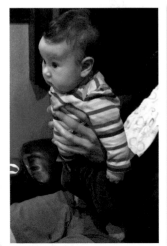

Baby responds to this by shifting not only her gaze, but her entire head and neck upward. Her elbows extend further, bringing her arms down symmetrically by her sides with her hands near her hips. Her stance remains narrow and she extends her hips and knees effectively pushing her feet down into her dad's lap.

Note that Dad is holding her in such a way that her body's weight is subtly biased forward. Her feet remain flat and she is leaning in a way that encourages her to engage her posterior chain to lift her head, neck, and trunk posteriorly so they come upright over her pelvis.

This is a job well done and a great way to practice early standing.

In the pages ahead you will encounter activities that will help your child to gain more strength and mobility in their trunk, hip girdle, and legs—all of which will benefit their ability to stand with healthy, well-aligned posture. And that posture is an important foundation for healthy, symmetrical movement skill development.

But first a quick recap on the biggest anticipated growth gains of your baby's first three months:

- Baby will develop strength to control lifting their head and turning it while on their back, belly, and side. Visually tracking with their eyes and turning their head in response to sounds will be their most important early exercises.
- Baby will begin trying to lift their head while being held in an upright position—this should include using their arms and hands to push their weight into the chest of the person who is holding them. By extending their elbows, baby begins to prop (push up) through their hands. This will happen on the floor too.
- Baby will begin shifting their gaze, their body weight, and logrolling may occur.

To help you keep it simple, narrow your daily focus to:

- Posture support in all positions—whether your baby is held in your arms or is on some sort of surface, whether awake and active or passively sleeping
- Building active muscle endurance by capturing your baby's wakeful windows for play
- Listening to your baby, meeting them where they are, and gently guiding them with safe handling and a mindful eye to how gravity impacts them

And remember, "work" or "exercise" for baby is play based and should be fun . . . if your baby is upset, do NOT waste your time pushing and upsetting them further. Reapproach again at another time.

Activities can and should be practiced throughout the day, several times, and of course at times when your baby is at their best for it.

The positioning and early activities you've been introduced to thus far will help your baby to build a fundamental baseline of strength, endurance, and mobility that make for a solid foundation moving on to months four to six and beyond.

Without this focused attention to the first weeks and months of life, what I often saw clinically was weakness in the uppermost portions of the spine, which babies are essentially meant to strengthen first. This presented most frequently with some form of muscle imbalance that caused asymmetrical head and neck alignment, and often had accompanying changes to head shape (flat spots aka plagiocephaly). Unfortunately this also frequently presented with delays in pushing up from the floor, delays in rolling, which delayed building core strength and led to delayed sitting skills, and sometimes other progressively built skills like crawling, standing, or walking.

As you move forward with the activities ahead, it's important to keep in mind that the focus is more on quality movement and strength building than on the chronology or your child hitting each milestone at a particular time. Build the fundamental baseline first.

While an age range for each activity will be provided and this can help you gauge if a "delay" is occurring and intervention would be beneficial, the reality is that no two kids are on exactly the same trajectory of growth and skill development, thanks to a multitude of factors from genetics to nutrition to practice exposure and quality. So it's important to note that not all kids are going to be ready for each activity at the same time. Also keep in mind that the activities are going to overlap in terms of what you might be practicing at any given time, and it will be up to your judgment and familiarity with your child's strength, skills, energy, and comfort as you choose your exercise-play.

Some babies will do better with a directed activity almost immediately upon waking when their energy is fresh, while others will not be keen to work until after they've eaten or been cuddled with sufficient skin-to-skin and face-to-face connection time. Most will protest activities if their diaper is soiled and feeling wet or heavy. (Note: This may not necessarily be a cry or apparent verbal protest; they may simply seem to refuse to move, focus, or participate.) You may do better at times to allow your child to experience floor exploration time with toys in their environment before you begin introducing touch and task direction. Remember, go with the flow and keep a rotation of activities and environments throughout the day. You may also consider doing some activities diaper-free to see if the freedom of moving without it changes how your child participates.

Building Upright
Sitting Skills

Once your baby has solid head and neck control to initiate lifting their own head from the surface while on their back and they can prop their head, neck, and upper back up from the surface while in tummy time atop their forearms, the progression of focus shifts to building muscles necessary for upright sitting skills.

From the head-down approach, the focus is now on the trunk—front, back, sides, and not just the muscles above the seated base but also the muscles just below the pelvis that help to keep the baby stable atop their bottom while they sit.

So as you approach this, think: the baby's seated base is their bottom, their bottommost body portion currently in contact with the surface and upon which everything else is stacked. As bones go, you're looking at the baby's pelvis and where it joins the top of their leg bones. You're also looking at how their spine stacks, or aligns, atop this base, and leading up to your baby's head. For their head to sit nicely aligned atop their spine, it is essential that the spine sit well aligned atop the seated base. And to have a stable seated base upon which to balance, it's also important to note how your child positions their legs. It sounds like a lot, and it is, but the activities to help guide this can all be made playful and fun.

The activities ahead will help you to build your baby's strength and confidence with the important skills of sitting, reaching out and recovering back to upright balance while sitting, and transitioning from sitting to other positions. This is, in itself, fundamental baseline work in terms of creating a solid core that will provide stability for your baby as they begin moving their lower limbs more (both with their arms to crawl and solo for stance and beyond) to control their advancing movement skills.

Some of the activities to come will have your child sitting; other activities will have your child low to the ground practicing precrawling maneuvers. All of them will be challenging muscles attached in some way to the pelvis and will help to build a strong and stable core from which your child's limbs can be more strongly controlled and freely move toward crawling, cruising, and walking.

The Baby Sit-Up

The baby sit-up is an activity that does a great deal for building abdominal muscle strength and stability of the torso (which, as previously mentioned, is essential for a strong base from which the limbs extend and move).

Sit-up practice can be easily layered into everyday tasks you're already doing with your baby throughout the day, such as diaper and clothing changes. It can also be combined with bathtime if you are using a semireclined bath seat (just recognize that this actually assists the baby since they aren't starting out fully on their back).

When a baby is first learning to sit up like this with you, they are going to recruit all the muscles they can to help them bring their upper body up from the floor. This means it's more than just their abdominals doing the work of bringing their chest toward their pelvis.

You're likely to see and feel their arm muscles doing a lot of pulling, flexing their elbows to literally use the arms to muscle up. You are also likely to see their legs come up off the floor, their hip flexors aiding their tummy muscles to rock their body upward. This is totally normal, to be expected, and will make first attempts much easier on your baby (read: less challenging and therefore less potentially upsetting). However, the unfortunate reality of this compensatory muscle assistance is that it doesn't optimize the development of the muscles that should be leading the way; and, if it becomes habitual, it can hinder your child's sitting skill development and structural alignment.

So let's take a look at this with this adorable little five-month-old girl.

Baby starts out with her back on the floor. Her hands are held with the caregiver providing a finger to her palm for her to grasp and the caregiver's thumbs securing her grasp across the top of her tiny fingers. From here the caregiver gently pulls upward in the direction of sitting. Baby attempts to lift her head, but you see here that her hips both started from a flexed position. This means her hip

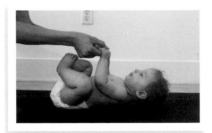 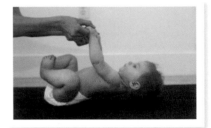

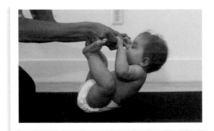 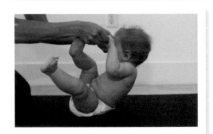

flexor muscles are starting in a shortened position and her tummy muscles must figure out what to do. Because her abdominal muscles aren't yet strong enough to accomplish the sit-up, she arches her back, lifts her legs, and bends her elbows. It's natural for a baby to do this; bending legs and arms is basically the default choice at this age (essentially using physiologic flexion to compensate for core muscles that have yet to develop strength to control the transition). And it'll get the job done—she will be sitting upright in another moment, as her caregiver gently pulls her forward and her legs come down again. For the sake of baby's optimal development, though, we instead want the baby to activate her core by more focused use of her abs. The next set of photos represents this idea, and it will be challenging for your baby, so practicing both ways is encouraged as you start out.

The key mistake in the first example was starting from a position where the caregiver was not exerting enough control over the baby's legs to keep them straight and down to the ground. Fortunately, this can be easily improved upon by either lowering yourself closer to your baby on the floor, or, more ideally for your body, placing your baby on an elevated surface, such as a bed or couch, to bring the baby closer to you. This will make it easier to position the baby's legs. This is demonstrated next with the girl's mother leveling up the situation.

Note: Mom is seen partially in frame, where she was in a strong kneeling position in front of the couch. A great caregiver warm-up for this activity would be a Founder and a Kneeling Founder. The same would make great reset activities for the caregiver following this practice, with the addition of Standing Decompression if time allows. (See Part III for these exercises.)

Baby starts out lying on a couch. Being a couple feet up from the floor brings her closer to her mom, which will make it easier for the mom to position more optimally as she helps the baby work her abdominal muscles.

First Mom lovingly engages and motivates her baby before getting down to "work." She hides gentle pressure in kisses and raspberries to the baby's belly, which results in the baby laughing and using her tummy muscles, the very muscles she is about to exercise (think: hidden muscle-engaging warm-up). In the next image you can see how Mom, engaging her baby first and then pulling back to start the activity, motivated baby to look and lift up.

Mom begins by saying to the baby, "Hands to me, it's time to sit up!"

Baby's legs should be as close as possible to flat on the surface, as this will force her abdominal muscles to do the work of bringing her torso upright. Instead, we see her elbow, hip, and knee joints are all currently bent. Mom addresses this in the next photo.

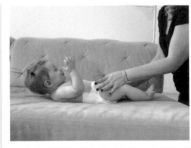

Mom comes closer to the baby, offering her thumbs for the baby to grasp as she wraps her fingers around the baby's hands, wrists, and forearms. She uses her forearms to gently weight her baby's legs down to the surface as she begins to pull her up. (Note: Aim for the knees and toes pointing upward to slightly outward, where they naturally and comfortably fall without forcefully pushing the joints to be perfectly straight.)

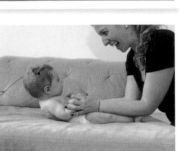

Baby responds by lifting her head, neck, and starting to lift her upper back.

She is also strongly flexing both arms to assist her transition upward, which you can see in her elbows. From this image to the next you will notice that the amount of flexion doesn't change. Her mom does a great job of resisting this pull and not allowing the baby's hands to get any closer to her shoulders.

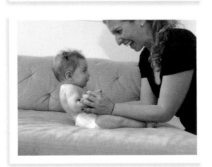

Baby is roughly halfway through sitting upright. She's looking strong, with her eyes now locked on Mom's necklace.

Mom is steadily cheering along the baby to keep her playfully engaged.

Mom stops pressing with her forearms, allowing the baby to bend her hips and knees to start to create a ring-sitting position as she shifts farther upright.

At the same time Mom notices the baby's eyes have shifted down from her face to her necklace; and she verbally encourages her baby to reach out for it (which is great adapting on this mom's part as it keeps the baby motivated during the task).

Baby sits fully upright and brings her heels together to form a ring-sitting position. The urge to reach has created the final impetus to shift her weight; and, from this image to the next, we see her trunk hinging forward over her seated base.

Mom still holds the baby's hands, which we see starting to open.

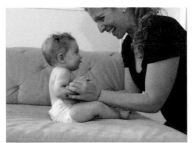

Baby's urge to reach creates the final impetus to shift her weight to be centered well over her seated base, and her thighs are now resting down on the ground.

Baby's eyes continue to be glued to her mom's necklace. Mom leans in farther to encourage the baby's interest.

As soon as Mom lets go of her hands, the baby reaches forward for the necklace.

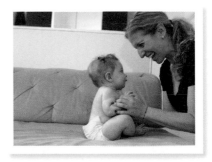

Mom responds by placing her hands loosely on both sides of her baby's torso with just her thumbs and distal finger pads in contact. She is ready to provide the baby additional stability if she continues to lean farther forward over her seated base. From here Mom can even guide the baby to shift to kneeling in front of her if their session were to continue. More on that sort of activity to come ahead.

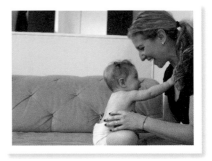

First let's go back to the concept of prop sitting and go over a few ways to support your child and help build their trunk strength in that position. This is important because it is your baby's first independent seated posture and therefore a very important stepping-stone to independent sitting without hands.

Prop Sitting with Caregiver Support

As mentioned earlier in "Baby Fundamentals," reflexive arm prop-ping to the front of the body should naturally begin around three or four months of age. The photos in this series are with a baby boy who was between five and six months of age at the time.

The stronger your baby becomes with this skill in terms of trunk strength and arm strength, as well as balance over their seated base, the more you should see their fists opening.

Their ability to visually track a toy or something moving about their environment is how you challenge them in this position, regard-less of how the arms are planted.

Looking at the level of the floor first is easiest; and your baby is challenged further the higher the tracked items are elevated. This might first mean just a couple inches above the floor with a toy, something that doesn't require them to extend their head, neck, and upper trunk too far as they track side to side, as that would make balance more challenging on their muscles.

As their posterior chain grows stronger and extension of the back to bring the trunk more upright becomes stronger, you'll be able to bring toys to their eye level, or the horizon, and gradually higher.

As trunk strength increases, their stability and balance increase, and eventually you will see them lifting one arm at a time and then both.

Lifting arms to reach brings a whole new layer of trunk challenges because you then challenge the balance of the core to remain upright. In activities to come you will see more ways to challenge your child's sitting balance with reaching outward from their centered base of support, grasping a toy, and returning to upright sitting. But, first, simple prop sitting with stability is our focus.

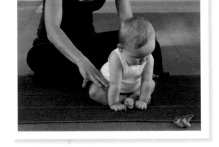

Stabilization to the low trunk and the hip is provided with the hands' web space (between the thumb and pointer finger) placed behind the upper aspect of the back of the pelvis, and three fingers to the lap with gentle downward pressure.

The baby is in a ring-sitting position with his heels together and his arms propping into the floor ahead of him on closed fists.

The toy is centered ahead of his body for him to track on the surface of the floor, which he can do while still maintaining a neutral midline alignment (chin in center of his chest). *However*, his arms are slightly skewed to his right as opposed to central (this is more obvious in his left arm than his right).

The caregiver is tailor sitting on the floor behind the baby. An alternative for this would be to have a second caregiver in front of the baby moving the toy of interest to motivate the baby to look up.

The toy is brought closer to the baby's body and he continues to maintain neutral head alignment fairly well, but he loses his extension and begins to round his head and neck down.

Because his trunk began to follow his upper spine, stabilization being provided was shifted to his upper trunk via three fingers to the front of his shoulders, upper arms, and chest.

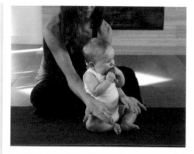

In the next few images you will see how the activity was shifted to visual tracking, and assistance was provided to help the child sit with improved trunk alignment.

Note: The baby's body is naturally much lower than the caregiver's body will be, so the caregiver should be mindful to also keep a tall torso and expanded, elevated spine atop their own seated base.

A few shifts have been made to help improve the baby's alignment and keep flowing into another activity that can help to strengthen the same skills.

I've given the item of interest to the baby and returned my arms and hands back to where his trunk alignment was at its strongest—the backs of my hands now to his lap and my wrists and forearms to his low side trunk.

His alignment is more or less neutral, though if you look closely you can see he is subtly leaning everything from his head down his trunk and into his right leg closer to the floor as compared to his left side. While we will be moving on with the visual tracking activity and skipping over how to treat an imbalance like this, subtleties of this nature are things you'll want to be keenly aware of with your

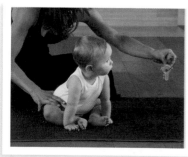

own child to ensure they don't become habitual.

Note: As far as caregiver posture goes, you can see I've had to lean forward farther and my own neck is flexing forward. A good follow-up to this position would be a Founder and a Standing Decompression. Any prone work such as a Prone Decompression or an 8-Point Plank exercise would also be beneficial.

Here we go with visual tracking. I've taken the toy from the baby and helped him plant his hands to the floor again, one on either side of his feet to create a prop that allows his arms to be tall and straight over his palms (which I opened and he has again closed).

I kept one hand to the baby's low trunk and upper thigh and the other hand brought the toy to eye level in front of him, biased to the side opposite of where I'm providing stabilization. If we are being precise about what he is exhibiting, as the baby turns his head to his left periphery, we can subtly see that his right ear is dropping toward his right shoulder as a result of his neck side-bending to his right. Again, we will not be discussing how to treat such asymmetries, but these are pointed out so that you, as a caregiver, become alert to looking at your own baby's movement in such detail. If such maneuvering becomes habitual, be encouraged to discuss it with your child's pediatrician and seek the assistance of a pediatric PT or OT as well as a chiropractor skilled in work with infants.

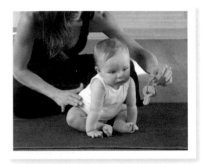

The toy is now directly in front of the baby and it is more apparent that his neck is side-bending to his right. If you look at the alignment of his chin, you can see that it is subtly pointing to his left shoulder.

My hand provides the same stabilization.

I switch my hands so that my right is now holding the toy up to his right periphery for the baby boy to continue to track. My left hand is now at

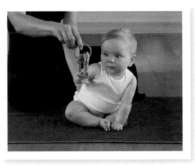

his left low trunk, positioned more toward his backside to provide additional stability as he reaches with his right arm. Going beyond just visually tracking and adding in reaching is a big move for this guy and a wonderful effort, but he is notably leaning his whole body to his left with this effort. This is another shift a parent or caregiver would want to keep a keen eye on during practice.

Ideally, with practice and stabilization provided, your baby will develop the ability to prop on their palms and track in a full arc of about 180 degrees from their left to their right and back again. This should progress to their ability to unweight their arms and sit taller, reaching with either hand without losing their alignment over their seated base.

Practicing visual tracking in prop sitting is a great challenge to your baby's seated alignment and muscular stability. These photos have shown ways you can assist your baby with your hands providing additional stabilization as their muscles grow in strength and endurance, and their trunk range of motion becomes more controlled.

Once your baby has built substantial trunk strength in prop sitting (which is a combination of all earlier mobility skills, especially rolling, propping in prone, and visual tracking while prop sitting), they will naturally begin to remove their hands from the floor to reach for items of interest in their environment. This opens the door for the next set of activities that will further challenge their seated balance and help to build more trunk strength and hip mobility—specifically, work with reaching out and recovering upright balance.

Sitting and Reaching

APPROXIMATE AGE RANGE: 4–8 MONTHS

This activity guides your baby to sit and reach for toys. It helps your baby practice their sitting balance, visual tracking of objects, eye-hand coordination, reaching, and grasping. This movement over the top of their seated base enhances the strength, mobility, and stability of their core, pelvic girdle, hips, and upper legs, all of which further prepare your baby for shifting from their seated base into other positions.

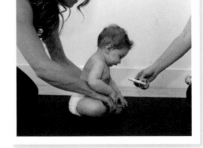

Seen here is a seven-month-old baby girl.

We begin with the baby girl sitting on the floor. I guide her to bring her feet together to form a ring as I use my forearms along the sides of her torso and my palms to the top of her lap to provide stability. She puts her hands on mine, creating additional stability for herself as she finds her balance.

Note: Her body weight is subtly shifted forward, making her center of gravity (the bulk of her weight) fall in the center of the ring.

While she is looking down toward her feet balancing herself, her mom presents a toy near her visual path and the baby's eyes quickly lock on it. Throughout this, her spine is nicely aligned.

Mom moves the toy up.

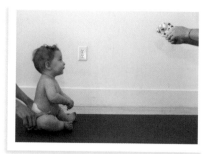

Baby's head moves upward to keep it in sight, maintaining a strong and neutral spinal alignment with her chin in the center of her chest and her ears remaining over her shoulders without any side-bend of her neck. As she does so, she widens the space between her feet to increase the base of support keeping her balanced. She also moves her hands up and together, which gives her body additional stability.

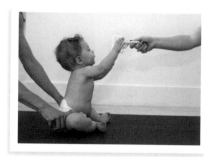

As she goes, I move with her to challenge her skills and see how much stability she actually needs me to provide. I remove my forearms from her torso, and place just one finger on top of each of her thighs, gently pressing downward with the whole length of my flat (be sure not to poke!) index fingers. This proves to be sufficient as we see her reach up for the toy in the next image.

Mom raises the toy above baby's shoulder level.

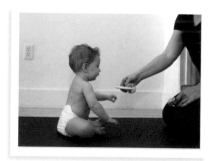

Baby raises her head more to keep an eye on it, and goes a step further by reaching for it with both hands! This is more extension of her head and neck, which shifts her body's weight toward her back, which challenges her balance and stability further.

Note: Baby's legs elevate slightly from the surface (as noted by her knees) and I respond by gently flexing my fingers and applying more firm downward pressure to help her find her stability. Baby doesn't grab the toy yet, which is possibly because she doesn't feel sufficiently stable to do so.

Mom lowers the toy to right in front of her baby at eye level. From here the baby no longer has to extend her neck and she can more easily maintain her balance.

Baby lowers her hands and her legs, and she shifts her body weight forward as she once again reaches toward the toy. From the last image to this one you can see a subtle shift in the engagement of her abdominal muscles (the lower portion of her tummy is flat here as compared to more rounded in the previous image) as she contracts them further and improves her self-stabilization.

This is happening in real time, a flow of mere seconds; and since the baby is doing great on her own, I remove my hands.

Baby has successfully grabbed the toy and she now exhibits a great show of her advancing fine motor skills by bringing it together between both hands and raises it in what looks like celebratory triumph!

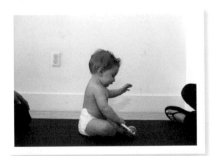

At the same time she moves her feet closer together, her legs still forming a ring. Her spine is in a nice, tall stack over the top of her pelvis such that her ears are over her shoulders and her shoulders are over her hips.

Baby lowers the toy to the ground with her right arm, while keeping her left arm up for balance.

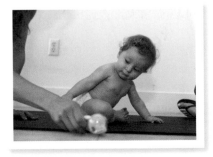

I move the toy to baby's right, challenging her to visually track it outside her base of support. Baby responds by bearing her body weight on her left arm while rotating her torso to her right. This is fantastic single arm propping to maintain her balance as she works her neck and trunk mobility.

Her spine is still in great alignment from head to tail (pelvis); and her feet are brought even closer as she presses her soles and toes together, further enhancing her stability.

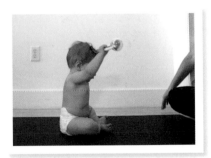

This activity can be made more challenging by raising the toy to a height that requires your baby to extend their head, neck, and trunk farther as they go; or by moving the toy at angles that make your baby rotate their head and body to track it. Moving the toy far enough away may serve to motivate your baby to stretch out their arms to reach for it. The farther they reach, the more work they'll have to do to recover their balance and return to an upright sitting position. Reaching and recovering ensures that they work their core in the front, back, and sides. This challenge to their muscles enhances strength and overall stability as they learn to control their maneuvers.

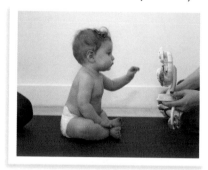

Here we see Mom keep baby engaged by presenting a new toy at her eye level, just outside her reach. Baby reaches cautiously at first with just one hand, keeping the other hand to her lap to maintain her stability as she decides if she's interested in this new object.

Baby is sold on the toy and she reaches forward with both hands as she shifts her center of gravity forward to grab on and turn the wheel before her. She is sitting tall and strong, her ears over her shoulders, over her hips; and her seated base is a solid little ring.

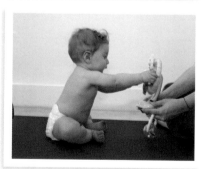

This activity is more or less the same as the last one, except that the toy is held higher, which forces the baby to keep her trunk in a more upright position and is therefore a different level of challenge to her seated balance.

Incremental challenges and subtle gains like this one give your baby more variety of playful challenging work and ultimately more independence when sitting and shifting their body's center of mass to reach for objects. This, in turn, helps prepare them for the control they will need when shifting their weight even farther over their seated base to transition into other positions like hands and knees, kneeling, and for more advanced motor skills like crawling.

So far, we've staged this sitting activity on the floor. However, you can also perform it with your baby sitting on your lap, which can offer more stabilizing support, closeness, and comfort depending on the degree of energy and behavior your baby exhibits at any given time. Lap sitting can either be with the baby's bottom directly atop your legs and their feet flat on the floor as shown in the final three photos from this session, or, as shown in one of the next activities ("Placing and Retrieving Rings to Practice Reach and Recover"), it can be done with the baby straddle sitting your leg and their feet atop a surface or dangling in the air (which could be more challenging).

I kneel and then guide the baby to sit on my lap.

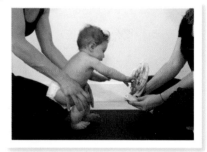

I place my hands on the baby's thighs, with my fingers lightly cupping her knee joints, as I guide her to align her upper leg to point ahead of her (instead of rolling outwardly with gravity). At the same time I subtly bias her weight forward over her bottom and heels. My wrists and fore-arms provide gentle stabilizing pressure to her lower torso.

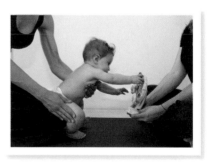

Mom presents a toy at slightly below baby's eye level. To encourage the baby, I exert subtle pressure to shift her body weight forward over her feet. Baby responds by immediately diving forward for the toy, and my hands shift with her in response.

As her trunk hinges farther forward, I want to encourage the baby to take weight into her flat feet to help her find balance as she, at the same time, figures out how to find balance between the front- and backside of her body (of course, none of this is exactly conscious on the baby's behalf, she simply knows she wants that toy).

So I place one hand in front of her torso as a platform to prevent her from diving too far forward. I'm at her upper chest more than her abdominals and my hope is that she will engage her backside and gluteals (if the toy were higher and she did engage those muscles, I'd anticipate seeing her rise to stand—which would be a great age-appropriate activity to flow into if it occurred).

My other hand is along the outer edge of her hip, bottom, and leg to give stability and prevent an outward roll.

If you look closely, you can see that her right foot has come down and her knee has rolled slightly outward. Her left foot remains planted on its heel with toes upward.

Baby girl really wants this toy and continues to reach and pull forward, trying to get both hands on it as her body shifts down into a squat.

A squat is a great position to introduce more variety for play. It's not something babies this age can do on their own, though, so I continue to shift with her to provide stability and encourage her body to engage appropriate muscles to self-support as much as possible.

Remember, the young brain may not be able to execute this maneuver or position on its own, but it can certainly learn valuable information for how to do so by a baby's practicing it with your guidance.

I centralize both my hands around the sides of the baby's torso, 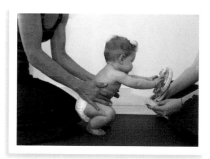 bringing my stabilization force more focused to her core, to see if this more proximal (closer to her core) versus distal (farther from her core) placement gives her the stabilization she needs to successfully find balance and plant her feet.

My fingers wrap around her abdominal muscles to encourage her core to continue to engage. My pinky remains on the outer edge of her thigh to encourage its forward tracking (knees ahead) versus outward rolling, and my ring finger is atop her thigh with a gentle downward pressure to encourage her keeping her weight down through flat feet.

Feeling stable, the baby places both her hands on the toy.

This looks great, so we continue to let baby girl play with the toy as is. The work remains nicely hidden as long as she is having fun!

Her head-to-tail spinal alignment is neutral and strong, her legs are well aligned without excessive outward rolling, her feet are flat, and she makes contact with both hands as her arms strongly and symmetrically reach forward.

If we'd kept going, my next move would've been to exert gentle lifting pressure on the baby's lower torso, while her mom simultaneously raised the toy. This would serve to encourage the baby to shift to standing upright while visually tracking the toy.

Another option from here, given the baby's position, could have been to guide her to kneeling; however, in this particular session she had grown very tired and lost interest in the toy, so we ended the play here—which was more than fine as we got a great deal of excellent work done.

The next activity is very similar, with a few subtle advancements. You'll see the same baby model, but she is two months older in the next session. If you found that your baby did well with this activity, they may be ready for the next.

Placing and Retrieving Rings to Practice Reach and Recover

APPROXIMATE AGE RANGE: 6-9 MONTHS

This activity is similar to the last in that our focus is working the trunk muscles as the baby is reaching outward for a toy and then working to muscularly recover their balance back to a tall, seated upright position. In this session we used a ring-stacking toy, which nicely challenges the age-appropriate fine motor skills of grasping and releasing. What you cannot clearly see in these images is that the baby's feet are not in a closed-chain position bearing her weight into a surface; instead, they are dangling free in an open-chain position. This puts more challenge on her core muscles above her pelvis to provide stability and balance.

Hiding work in this form of activity helps your baby to build control with shifting their body weight over their seated base. It strengthens the surrounding muscles of the arms, core, pelvis, and upper legs. It builds mobility in the joints as the baby also gets practice beyond just remaining balanced while sitting, as they work on visually tracking objects, enhancing their eye-hand coordination, and their grasp and release as they work to reach forward to place and remove objects.

Pictured here is a nine-month-old baby girl.

Mom sits on the edge of a couch. Baby sits astride her mom's leg, facing outward. Mom keeps a careful eye on ensuring that baby's hips are level as opposed to one side hiking higher than the other as that would put asymmetric forces across the baby's hips, tummy, and back—the kind that could lead to imbalances developing if she remained there and did muscle-building work.

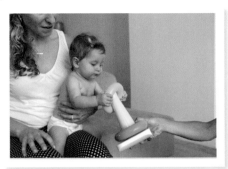

Mom's left hand wraps around the baby's tummy to provide stability and encouragement for her abdominal muscles to engage. Being positioned so closely also provides the baby a sense of comfort and security, making her more willing to reach out from her seated base and perform challenging tasks.

As they got set up, I gave the baby a bright green ring to hold. I now present a stacking tower with another ring already on it in front of the baby, just a small reach away, and encourage her by simply saying "put yours on too!"

Baby accepts the challenge, hinges forward slightly, and places her ring onto the stack.

While this activity might at first seem straightforward, it has a wealth of variations because I can move the toy anywhere. For example, I can place the stack directly in front of the baby, or at any angle from her left or right; at the baby's hand level, or below it or above it; and close to the baby or farther away from the baby.

Starting with a position that's easy for your baby and then moving the stack to slowly but steadily increase the level of difficulty is how you hide the muscular "work" for their muscle chains and also help to keep them interested.

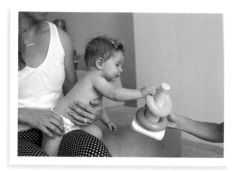

I move the stack farther away from the baby, and slightly to her left. Baby rotates her torso and extends her arm to reach for the ring. This is great visual tracking and trunk mobility work, *and* she has executed her reach by bringing her right hand across the midline of her body—which is an advanced maneuver that speaks to the healthy communication between the two hemispheres of her brain (a small detail to note that can offer you a legitimate cause for minicelebration within your days!)—to successfully grasp the ring once again.

While continuing to hold her baby's trunk securely with her left hand, Mom places her right hand on top of the baby's thigh and applies a small amount of weight to keep baby's leg still and stable. This provides her daughter assistance with anchoring her pelvis to the surface below her as she reaches farther out and then continues on to utilize other muscles (also attached to the pelvis) to return back to upright sitting.

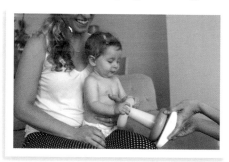

As the baby bends her elbow to pull the ring, I shift with her, bringing the toy back closer to her and at an angle that makes removing the ring a bit easier for her. This dynamic flow leads her to sit upright as she takes the ring back off the stack.

This action is just as important as her reaching for the ring as it works other important muscles around the baby's trunk—all of which build upon her strength, stability, and balance to help prepare her for shifting out of sitting to other more advanced positions.

This middle part of your baby's first year of life is very dynamic. It may seem they are limited in what they can do since they are still not "mobile" in terms of crawling, standing, or walking; but the important thing to keep in mind is that they are building up essential trunk and hip mobility skills to prepare them for the next advances in their milestone acquisition.

Upright sitting skills are about more than just balance with sitting. During this time you can and should also work on helping your baby to feel what it's like to be out of balance—to shift their upper body weight up and over their lap or "seated base" to find other positions, such as moving back down to the floor (and how they can move in more advanced ways once there; i.e., crawling) or up to standing, to all fours, and to kneeling.

These next activities will offer you guidance with these skills, and you may note that the age of the models involved fluctuates a little (because, again, not every child is on the same developmental trajectory). You'll know your baby is ready to begin this play when they start to show decent control of their balance with the sitting and reaching work—meaning they can maintain a neutral head-neck-trunk alignment while shifting their trunk over their seated base to grab or activate a toy and return to sitting without toppling over. Protective extension of the arms need not be fully developed to begin practicing these types of activities as you, as caregiver, will provide stability and protection. Some of the work ahead will also serve to help you to guide your child in building those skills.

From Sitting Up to Lying on Stomach (Moving Toward Front)

APPROXIMATE AGE RANGE: 6–9 MONTHS

This activity helps your baby transition from sitting upright back down to the floor, to being prone atop their belly, using a forward motion. Practicing this maneuver helps to build your baby's strength, mobility, and balance while seated while also helping them to build comfort and independence with their transitioning skills. This activity gives babies the option to switch to being on their tummies, a position requiring less effort to sustain than upright sitting and for

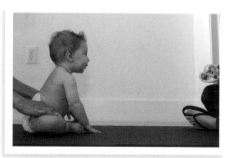

which, by this age, they've already developed months of independent movement skills.

Pictured here is a seven-month-old baby girl.

Baby starts off in a ring-sitting position with her right hand on the ground to help steady herself; and my hands are atop her thighs and the sides of her hips for additional stability as her weight hinged forward. Her left hand was beginning to raise for the toy her mom is holding in front of her; but I'm about to shift my hands farther up her torso and shake things up a bit.

Note: I waited until her eyes were locked on the toy ahead of her before bringing the challenge of more imposed movements.

I slide my hands about midway up the baby's trunk with my fingers stabilizing her abdomen, my palms supporting the sides of her torso, and my thumbs supporting her back.

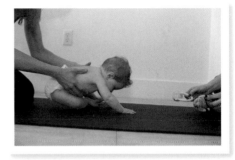

As I do so, I simultaneously start to shift the baby's body weight forward as I also lift the baby so that her bottom rises to provide just enough space for her legs to extend back and slide underneath.

The baby responds exactly as I'd hoped, by bringing both of her hands to the floor ahead of her, shifting her gaze momentarily to the floor and keeping her spine in a neutral alignment from head to tail. She has also begun to lift and shift her legs, which becomes more apparent in the next image.

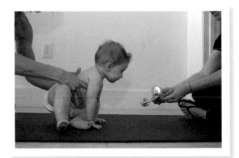

Mom shakes and taps two rattles together to regain the baby's attention and motivate her to lift her head and continue to move forward.

My hands remain in the same places, and I've broadened the space between my fingers to provide more all-encompassing trunk stabilization and pressure to the baby's abdominals. My goal with this is to encourage her to engage these core muscles throughout the maneuvering.

Baby looks up and slides her arms toward her core into a tall prop with her shoulders strongly stacked over elbows over wrists over palms. She then moves her legs to her right, rotating her lower torso to begin shifting her legs underneath her.

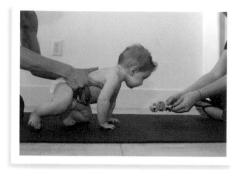

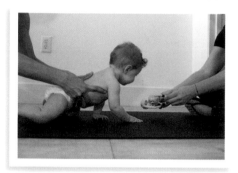

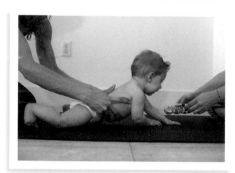

Mom lowers the toys to encourage the baby to lower her body farther down.

My hands remain steady, in the same position.

Baby continues to shift her legs under and behind her.

Mom and I remain steady, allowing the baby to continue to shift.

Baby's legs extend farther back, and she now begins to support some of her weight with her knees and toes. She also begins to bend her elbows to lower herself farther toward the floor.

She has achieved a precrawling position and begins to slide her left hand along the floor to reach for the toy.

Once I gently let her go, the baby will be on her tummy . . . and free to move closer toward the toy.

If Mom were to move the toy along the floor, just outside the baby's reach, this could provide an opportune setup from which to introduce precrawling movements and take the play session in a new direction.

More on how to introduce those crawling movements to come; but first, let's look at another way to guide your baby to transition from sitting upright back down to the floor.

From Sitting Up to Lying on Stomach (Moving Toward Side)

APPROXIMATE AGE RANGE: 6–9 MONTHS

This activity is another way to help babies practice transitioning from sitting upright to lying on their tummies. While the previous activity showed how your baby can do this by leaning progressively forward, in this exercise your baby instead leans progressively to their side (either right or left; be sure to alternate to strengthen your baby's muscles equally on both sides).

Seen here is a seven-month-old baby girl.

Baby again begins in a ring-sitting position. She has her right hand to the side of her lap and left arm elevated in the air to help give her trunk extra stability.

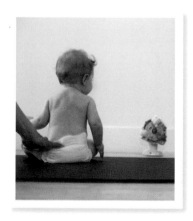

To help keep her stable as I prepare to introduce more challenging movements, I place my left hand atop her left thigh with my thumb behind her pelvis, the web space between my thumb and index finger to the side of her hip, and my index finger to the front of her hip bone.

Baby's attention is on a strategically placed toy set off to her right. Her mom is sitting to the right of the toy and will be using it shortly to help entice the baby to move.

My left hand shifts up and my fingers gently apply pressure to

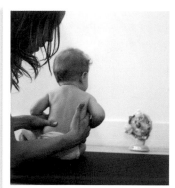

the baby's abdominals to both provide stability and encourage her to activate her core.

At the same time, I press my right palm and fingers to the right side of the baby's torso and use both hands to start gently guiding the baby toward her right.

Baby responds by bending both elbows and bringing her arms closer to her core for stability, while at the same time starting to lift her left leg and putting more weight on the right side of her buttocks.

As we lean farther toward the baby's right, my left

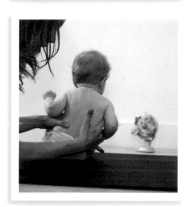

hand position doesn't change and baby's left arm begins to raise and retract (as she seeks more stability).

I keep my right palm to the baby's right side, between her arm and upper torso. If you look closely you can see that my middle and ring fingers are pressing into the baby's forearm and my pinky finger is starting to lift away from her side to initiate shifting her right arm away from her torso, toward the ground (this will become more apparent in the next image).

As her center of gravity shifts, the baby puts even

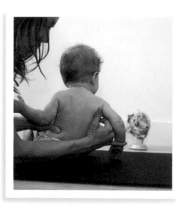

more weight on her right buttock.

Her head and neck remain rotated to her right with her eyes still locked on the toy.

My left hand provides the same gentle pressure to continue to shift the baby's center of gravity toward her right. With my right hand, I use less of the palm and more of the area by my thumb as my hand shifts to create more space between the baby's arm and her trunk. I use the knuckles of my pointer, middle, and ring fingers to create outward pressure on baby's arm, while my pinky finger wraps around baby's lower forearm to guide it farther outward.

Baby's right bottom cheek, upper thigh, and right-side lower trunk are in contact with the floor now as her right fingertips start to graze the surface.

If you look closely between my arms, you can see that her left leg is now starting to lift from the surface, showing her increasingly shifting toward her right and a subtle beginning of rotation of her upper body in the same direction.

As we subtly shift farther toward the baby's right, she plants her right palm to the ground and my right palm returns to cupping her right low trunk.

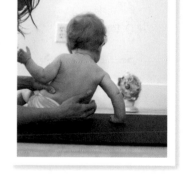

With my left hand I gently exert pressure guiding the baby's left side to rotate toward the floor. My fingers don't touch her thigh, but instead point toward the floor as a visual cue.

My right hand has shifted back to baby's right low trunk with my palm behind her pelvis, my thumb spanning the lower half of her back, and, if you look very closely, you'll see my fingers close by her right hip, but not in contact. I'm here for stability if she needs me but the guidance/pressure/support that I provide is coming from my left hand at this point.

Looking between my arms you can see that the baby's left leg has lifted more and begun to inwardly rotate—this is necessary to help her body rotate toward her right.

Baby makes a big shift to her right, rolling onto the outer side of her right hip and bottom as she bends her right elbow and comes down to prop on her right elbow and forearm.

Her left arm remains bent at the elbow and pulled close to her side, though it is lifted in the air to provide a degree of counterbalance. Her left leg can be seen between my arms, and it is no longer in contact with the ground.

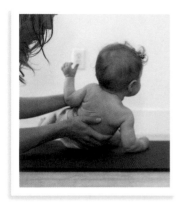

My left hand remains in the same position, providing the same subtle guidance to rotate toward her right.

My right hand continues to stay in the same relative position, ready to provide stability if the baby needs it as she presses her right low trunk and hip backward as she rotates farther over her right side toward her stomach.

While it can't be seen in this photo, her mom has picked up the toy with flashing lights and started to move ahead of the baby, toward her right, further encouraging her to rotate her body.

Mom has placed the toy on her lap at her baby's eyeline, allowing the baby to keep her neck in a neutral alignment instead of having to look up or down. Baby spots this and starts to make a big maneuver.

My hands remain in the same positions and simply move with the baby, no longer providing guidance so much as just being there for stability as she goes.

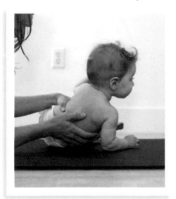

Baby rotates over her right hip, bringing her left side closer to the ground. Note: There is a big shift in her left arm; if you look closely, you'll see that her elbow is no longer at the side to slightly behind her torso. Baby has brought her arm in front of her and is beginning to reach it ahead of her toward the toy. (Some little ones might not feel secure and balanced enough to reach out, and they might even hinder their rolling by pulling the left arm, or whichever arm is up, back in retraction as they attempt to self-stabilize. If this happens, try moving the toy closer to your baby, and even touching your baby's hand with it, so your baby forgets about everything else and playfully reaches for it, which will shift their weight forward and the momentum may cause them to continue the rolling movement.)

Baby's right upper arm pulls closer to the side of her body as her forearm rotates down toward the surface (in pronation) such that her palm is coming toward a flat supporting position.

Introducing Movements for Crawling

APPROXIMATE AGE RANGE: 5–7 MONTHS

This activity is a step up from tummy-time propping practice and an important floor skill to practice during the same stage as when your baby is also starting to work on their sitting skills. This will help to build your baby's trunk strength and hip mobility and will be beneficial with budding transitioning skills as they gain mobility with side- bending and hip cinching. These are important skills to build in prep for crawling on hands and knees as well as walking.

Before your baby is ready to crawl on hands and knees, the way you likely visualize crawling, their body will be more ready to do so with the legs a bit "froggied" out to their sides. If you're wondering, yes, this is related to physiologic flexion; and, it also gives them a wider base of support underneath their low body as they learn to balance their teetering weight as they go.

Most people presume a baby will naturally crawl sooner or later, but this is not necessarily so; some babies actually miss the crawling stage entirely. This can very simply boil down to lack of exposure to and practice of tummy time, whether due to the baby being frequently upset and resisting or caregivers being unaware of the importance of strength and mobility gained by early propping skills.

To skip crawling deprives a baby of valuable months of important strength building throughout their whole body, physical coordination building of reciprocal arm and leg movement, developing motor skills that will help them to strongly progress to more upright skills, and the independence and self-confidence that come with exploring the world on all fours.

This activity introduces babies to the leg movements they need to eventually start crawling. Once added to their repertoire, babies are likely to start playing around on their own and discovering more movement skills from here, such as propelling themselves forward, either with both legs at the same time or reciprocally, and—ideally—eventually doing so with alternating arms and legs. This will provide a great base for more advanced hands-and-knees crawling where the legs are less outwardly rotated and instead more neutrally aligned in the hip sockets.

Pictured here is a five-month-old baby boy.

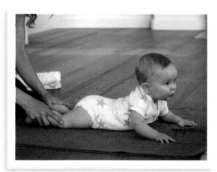

Baby is on his tummy (on top of a yoga mat with a towel mat liner). My hands encompass his ankle joints and lower legs, gently straightening his legs in a neutral alignment so that his knees and toes are straight down to the floor. I spend a good few moments there letting him observe the toy that is out of camera view, but directly in front of him at eye level. I am still, steady, and allowing my pressure to be a stabilizing force for his body as he decides how high from the surface he wants to prop up with his arms (which he is currently holding in a strong symmetrical position with his elbows slightly ahead of his shoulder joints).

Baby boy looks strong and stable with his head in a tall neutral alignment, with his chin lined up over the center of his chest, and his ears over top of his shoulders without either one leaning closer to either shoulder. His eyes are strongly out over the horizon, locked on his toy, so he has a great focus point as I prepare to introduce the movements with this activity.

Note: Because I am going to focus on introducing movements to his legs, I am not concerned with seeing him prop up all the way on extended arms with straight elbows. This will more naturally come as a baby becomes stronger in their all-fours ("quadruped") skills and more comfortable in a higher hands-and-knees style of crawling. What we are working on with this activity is more of a precursor to that advanced crawl pattern.

My right hand advances the baby's right leg forward. I don't apply pressure to the ankle joint or over the top of the knee joint, but simply guide the hip and knee to bend by helping to lift and shift the weight of the lower leg. Meanwhile my left hand remains still, keeping the baby's left leg stable.

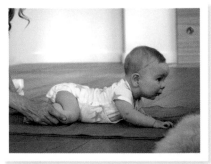

If you look at the baby boy's arms, you will note that he has dropped his weight toward his left shoulder, bringing his arm inward toward his chest; and his right arm has advanced slightly in front of him. Overall, this is actually great as his head and neck push forward, remaining in neutral alignment with his spine.

When it comes to low crawling, the arms bend like this as they advance and grab the ground to help pull the body forward as the legs push. So this little fella successfully met this challenge.

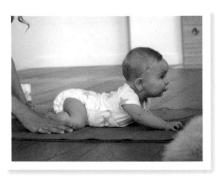

In the next photo you'll see that he shifted his gaze back upright as he acclimated to his new position, and how I shifted my hands with him to both accommodate him with stability and create a platform to encourage his pushing off with the advanced forward leg.

To further stabilize the baby, I place the index finger of my right hand along the baby's shin and my thumb flat at the base of the baby's heel. Baby responds by lifting his head and beginning to push his arms into the mat. My hands also give the baby a platform to push against as he straightens his hip and knee, propelling him into a movement akin to early crawling as his left forward arm digs down into the floor and pulls toward his torso to help advance his body (which, unfortunately, was not captured by camera during this session, but if you return to the previous chapter's section on tummy-time positioning, you can see images of six-month-old Sunny executing this during her tummy-time floor play).

As you approach this activity with your own child, it is well advised to switch sides. You see me here working with advancing the child's right leg. Within one session I would immediately follow this with advancing the left leg if the child didn't do so on their own. Spending several minutes at a time working on this, alternating back and forth between legs without removing hands, can equate to a fun play session that motivates a baby to do more independent moving. The repetition will be helpful not only for introducing the movements to the various joints and surrounding muscles, but also teaching the brain to pattern the maneuvers that string together to produce crawling.

Also note: Toys can be placed at various levels on the floor and scattered about their environment to give the baby the motivational enticement to move from one point to another within their environment.

There are other activities you can and should work on with your baby during this midyear to second half of the first year. It's such an important window of time. If you're thinking in terms of head down (cephalocaudal) development, your focus is now on their trunk, hips, and legs (more upper legs at first than lower, though the reality is the whole thing is going to move together, so you want to be mindful of all of it, as you focus first on the muscles close to the hip joints and how they direct the leg's position).

The next activities will show you some safe ways to begin to introduce your baby to such transitions as sitting to standing, sitting to all fours, and kneeling to standing.

We begin first with the transition to standing, in a few different variations, as it is often very motivating to the baby to pop upright and see the world from this new place (most babies I've encountered are agreeable and happy to do so, as compared to slightly more resistant to participating in some of the other more involved and slightly more challenging-to-coordinate positions).

As expressed, if your child has exhibited trunk strength in sitting and recovering their balance with reaching (meaning they're beyond simply propping on their arms and their hands are off the floor), these next activities are absolutely worth trying with your support and guidance.

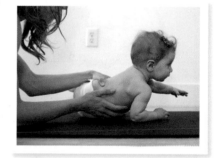

My hands continue to remain in the same places.

Baby begins to bend her right shoulder and elbow farther as she pulls herself forward on her right supporting arm and her left hand reaches for the toy ahead of her. She continues to rotate her body toward her right, her stomach coming closer to the ground here.

My left hand continues to shift with the baby and my right hand starts to slide off her back as she rolls farther, dropping toward the ground.

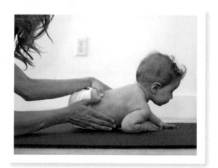

Baby girl lowers her chest and plants both her hands on the floor. Her transition to her stomach is almost complete as she works to rotate her lower trunk, hips, and legs the rest of the way.

While in this example the baby was shifted to her right, when you perform the activity multiple times you should alternate between shifting right and shifting left. This helps ensure that both of your baby's sides are exercised equally, which is important for building symmetrical muscle strength around the trunk and mobility in the hips and low back.

Once you've transitioned to the ground, your baby can, of course, work on their previously gained propping skills (in this case that might look like her reaching for the toy in her mom's lap and simply holding herself up in a propped-on-arms or propped-on-palms position).

Another area you can begin placing focus is on introducing movements to your baby's legs that will encourage crawling. This next activity will walk you through this with a five-month-old baby boy.

From Sitting
on Lap to Standing
(in "Free Space")

APPROXIMATE AGE RANGE: 5–9 MONTHS

You can certainly continue this longer, but beyond this age range most babies are likely to be pulling themselves up to stand at support surfaces more independently.

The seemingly simple act of transitioning from sitting to standing offers your baby a tremendous amount of muscular engagement, joint mobility work, proprioceptive feedback about where their body is in space, and information for patterning movements within their brain. The biggest piece to consider here is what it offers your baby in terms of muscularly connecting their core with their legs as they rise from bearing weight through their seated bottom to doing so through their legs. This gives their legs quite the "workout" and offers global strengthening of the muscles from their core to their feet.

This activity guides the caregiver to help the baby make this transition from sitting atop the caregiver's lap to standing in "free space," meaning that the baby is not standing at a support surface where they can place their hands for additional stability. Nor are they responsible for holding up their full body weight on their legs. This is safe for their hips because the caregiver is supporting a good portion of the baby's body weight; and it makes for a simple introduction to the act of standing (similar to how you previously saw nearly three-month-old Sunny standing in the first mentions of standing a few chapters back).

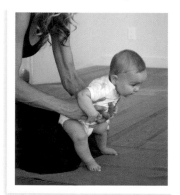

Seen here is a five-month-old baby boy.

We start out with the baby placed sitting atop my knees such that his bottom is both still and level (one side not rising above the other—keep an eye on your legs to ensure you are sitting in a way that is conducive to this). His feet are flat on the floor, and his body weight is shifted forward with his trunk hinged over his legs with shoulders roughly over his knees and knees over ankles. His legs are naturally rolled outward to a small degree (as noted by his toes pointing to the sides of his body), and you'll see him alter this on his own as he rises (which gives us a subtle clue that he is well stabilized in his trunk through this transition).

His spine is well aligned from head to tail, and his visual path is currently low to the floor ahead of him.

I'm sitting in a low kneeling position with my bottom atop my heels. My hands are in full contact with the baby's trunk, offering his body's midsection ample stability with my palms to his sides,

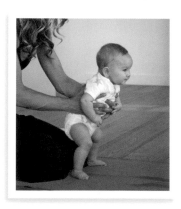

my thumbs behind his torso, and my fingers spread broadly across his abdominal muscles. Note how he grabs my hands with his own hands and arms, self-stabilizing as he goes.

A subtle lift of my arms encourages the baby to rise. I do not move where my hands are positioned, nor do I alter the pressure they exert on his body.

Baby boy extends his hips and knees and presses up through his heels and flat feet as he lifts his head and visual path. If you look closely, you can see a small smile come across his face (notable in his mouth and eyebrows); he is motivated by his nanny across the room shaking toys and cheering him on. This aspect is so important during this sort of play, especially if the caregiver is positioned behind the child as seen here. Another great motivator, in place of a toy or caregiver in front of the child, is a mirror in which they can see their reflection. (Note: Visual feedback as they execute such a maneuver offers an additional layer of information for the brain's movement center, helping them to process the action as it's occurring and adding to their ability to pattern it again in future efforts.)

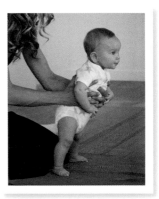

His spine remains neutral with his body weight shifted forward, trunk over legs; and his legs have strongly shifted inward to a more neutral alignment.

Neither of us shifts our hands as baby boy extends his hips and knees more to press all the way up to standing.

His spinal alignment is great; and this forward weight shift of his trunk over his pelvis helps him to engage his anterior and posterior chains effectively through his torso and legs. This is a very successful introduction to transitioning sit to stand from a lap in this manner.

Keep in mind that this baby is only five months old here and he has not yet developed solid strength in the muscles of his low back, bottom, and legs to help his body hold his alignment more upright. As your baby gains more strength and control, they will naturally stand more upright with less forward lean of their trunk.

In this example, the baby was in "free space." In the next example you'll find another version of standing practice that is similar, followed by one that places the baby in front of a couch to offer a support surface.

But first let's take a quick pause from the transitional activities to look at what a baby around the midpoint of their first year simply looks like standing, as we talk about the best ways to stabilize and support their body in this new and challenging upright position.

Here we have a six-month-old little boy. This first image in the

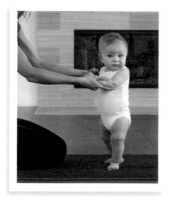

series shows what happens if you try to simply support your child by holding them by their hands or arms at this stage. Said simply—this is not enough stabilization to the core.

At this stage, a baby is still trying to coordinate their trunk with their legs and, while it may not yet look obvious that he is struggling, follow these photos and note the details to gain a better understanding of some subtle signs that can alert you to how to better support your child.

Positives here are that the alignment from his head to his tail is neutral; and he is able to rotate his neck to turn his face and view the photographer who was calling to him. His hips to his feet are holding his weight well; however, to be noted is that his left leg is rotated outward (as shown by toes pointing to his side) compared to his right. It's perfectly okay to spend time standing here; however, if he were to lose balance here and jolt excessively through the leg less neutrally aligned, he could potentially put forces through his joints and surrounding muscles that are less than beneficial. (As reinforced in the fundamentals that preceded the activities, learning movement in well-aligned postures is best for babies' brains as they are learning to pattern their own movements.)

Note: Here you see me kneeling atop my legs with my bottom resting on my heels so that I can be low to the baby's level. While my torso is decompressed here, the lever my arms are creating is long away from my body. This means that the weight of the baby is a potentially strong force on my arms and torso as he moves. In the next shots you see me come closer to the baby to provide him more stabilization as we experimented with his responses in this play session. In this position my bottom raises from my heels and my spine rounds forward. This is not a strong neutral; my spinal weaknesses are showing themselves and I point this out because, while natural for my body at that time, it's not ideal. It's super important to be very real about what our body goes through as we move and shift with the little ones in our care. Preparing for this sort of play with exercises that expand, elevate, and decompress the torso are well advised. Because I'm kneeling, a Kneeling Founder would be a great choice. And following this sort of play with similar exercises is also a great idea, especially ones that offer more extended leg positions (a Founder followed by Standing Decompression would make nice choices) to get the blood flowing after compressing down into flexed limbs as you see me doing here.

I bring my hands to the baby's torso to provide stability direct to his core. I begin first here with my hands high on his torso, starting around the level of his armpits to his rib cage and upper abdomen. I'm experimenting with a top-down approach in terms of the cephalocaudal development; bearing in mind that his upper spine developed stability first, I want to see how well he can coordinate his lower abdomen, hips, and legs from here.

Baby boy has brought his hands immediately to hold mine. His hands and arms close to his core, working to establish some stability for himself.

There is a visible improvement in his trunk posture and leg alignment. If you look closely from the previous image to this one, you can see that he has gone from his left leg being outwardly rotated to advancing it slightly and bringing it, along with his pelvis and low abdomen (as noted by his tummy now facing me), to a neutral alignment such that his toes and hip both now point ahead.

This tells us that the stabilization provided here, closer to his core as opposed to more distal from his core as it was previously out at his arms and hands, is better for him at this stage.

In the next image you'll see me shift my hands lower down his trunk to see how he does with more stability provided in that region.

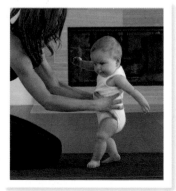

My hands are now on the low trunk, my thumbs at the bottom edge of the rib cage where the abdominal muscles attach, my palms across the front of the abdomen, and my fingers wrapping broadly around the side and back of the torso, with pinkies at the top of the pelvis at its side edges.

This is a dynamic shift for baby boy and he responds by deciding to dance! Just kidding, but this image delights me because he looks like he's busting a move.

What we see here is that he has enough sense of stability to free his hands—which is a big step—and he immediately uses everything from his head down to recruit more of his own stability. We see he brings his chin down toward his chest, losing his gaze downward as he presses his head back. His right arm raises out to his side as his left arm retracts behind his torso, seeking to add stability and balance to his position. As he does so, you can note from the crease in his onesie that his trunk has subtly rotated toward his left. We also see that he has pushed up to the ball of his right foot and his left leg has again rotated outwardly with his pelvis. If you look closely, you will also note that the toes of his left foot are clawing at the ground. Toe clawing is another sign that your baby is not feeling stable. He is literally trying to recruit the tiny muscles in his feet and toes to help him gain more stability.

Note: These efforts to find balance are not a negative, rather a learning curve for his body as we experiment. And the outward rotation of the leg is not in itself a negative either. As babies first learn to stand and walk, they are naturally going to have outwardly rotated limbs. This goes back to physiologic flexion. Time and experience weight-bearing through the legs, particularly time spent in the action of sidestepping (aka "cruising," an act we anticipate seeing once babies have developed comfort transitioning to stand and shifting their weight between their feet, around approximately months nine to eleven) at support surfaces, will help to develop the muscles in the inner and outer thighs to further control a neutral alignment with the toes pointing more ahead than outwardly.

His efforts are big here and in the next image we see them come together as he sorts out how to better find stability with my newly provided stabilization (which does not change moving forward).

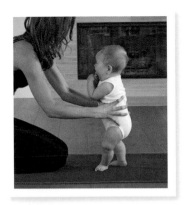

Baby boy brings his arms forward and hands together at his mouth (remember from the earliest stages of the baby's first month, the mouth is a center for them that is rich in feedback about body position). As he does so, his chin returns to neutral, his gaze returns to me, and his torso resumes a strong forward-facing position. His feet are both flat and his toes are no longer clawing.

He is now in a fairly neutral alignment with his spine well stacked. This hand placement is more ideal for him than where we started.

Here's another option with the baby facing away from the caregiver, and the caregiver positioned low to the ground.

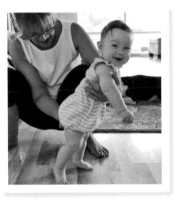

This is six-month-old Sunny, seen here standing with her grandma (who exemplifies a strong deep squat; her warm-up and recovery were FT Founders and Squats). Grandma is doing a great job of support-

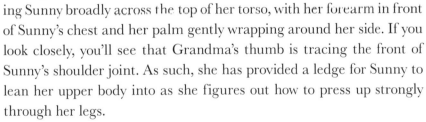

ing Sunny broadly across the top of her torso, with her forearm in front of Sunny's chest and her palm gently wrapping around her side. If you look closely, you'll see that Grandma's thumb is tracing the front of Sunny's shoulder joint. As such, she has provided a ledge for Sunny to lean her upper body into as she figures out how to press up strongly through her legs.

Grandma's other hand provides a bumper of sorts. She is both cupping Sunny's bottom with the palm of her hand, ready to catch her and provide a lift if necessary (she's not actually in contact, but a mere half inch or so away); and, the outer edge of her hand, her pinky and ring fingers, is in contact with the outer aspect of Sunny's upper thigh, providing a stabilizing force as Sunny plants her foot in a neutral alignment and bears her weight down.

Sunny is clearly ecstatic with this play, and her alignment from her head to her tail remains strong as she turns to joyfully coo to her mom (with the camera) about it.

You can see that Sunny was pressing off her right foot, preparing to advance that leg. In this supported position she naturally wanted to press up and down on her feet and take small steps.

If you refer back to the chapter on containers, you will recall that we discussed using a wheeled walker with an inner sling seat and why that was not preferable as a means of supporting babies in their first experiences of walking. In a comparative sense, what you see here with the caregiver involved is optimal in that it provides dynamic support that can change with the baby as they experience holding a portion of their body's weight and make attempts at movement.

Now back to transitions. These next few activities are powerful for building strength, coordination, and stability between the trunk, hips, and legs.

From Straddle Sitting on Your Lap to Standing

Beyond this point most babies are likely to be pulling themselves up to stand at support surfaces more independently.

This activity guides your baby in supported standing and sitting from straddle sitting on your leg. This is simply another option that involves using a caregiver's leg to provide a "safety net" that the baby can use for support or to fall onto if they lose their balance or grow tired.

Seen here is a seven-month-old baby girl.

Mom sits on the floor with one leg stretched out in front of her and her other leg is flexed along the floor in a half-ring-sitting position. Her posture is exemplary, as she sits tall on her "sitting bones," with her pelvis neutrally aligned (i.e., preserving the natural curve of her back), and her spine stacked tall over her pelvis.

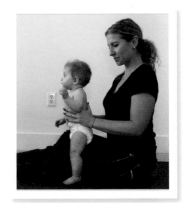

Mom places her baby in front of her, facing forward, standing with a leg on either side of (i.e., straddling) Mom's left leg; and she keeps her leg low to the ground so the baby can stand over it rather than merely sit on top of it.

Mom's hands broadly support the baby's torso with fingers to her abdomen, palms to her sides, and thumbs on her back. She is simply here for support. No pressure is being exerted in any direction as she observes how her daughter manages her own weight here as a second caregiver approaches from the front with a toy.

Baby's feet are planted flat on the floor. Her body is tall and neutrally aligned from top to bottom, her eyes looking straight ahead at the horizon level (where I'm holding a toy to capture her attention); her head and neck are stacked tall with her ears over her shoulders, her shoulders are over her hips, her hips are over her knees, and her knees are over her ankles with her weight down over her heels and dispersed well across her foot (toes not clawing). Her attention is piqued by the toy and you can see that both her hands begin to rise in her desire to reach for it.

It's a little hard to tell because the mom's pants are dark, but the baby is NOT sitting atop her leg here. She is practicing standing here and will, in a moment, work on reaching forward for a toy. Should her mom notice that her baby is off-balance, she can merely shift her hands lower or higher on the trunk to help her find more stability and either continue to stand or come down into sitting.

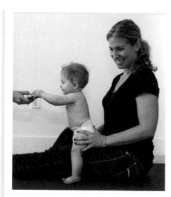

I bring part of the toy close enough for the baby to reach. Feeling secure, she reaches out both hands and grabs it.

Note: As your baby becomes more practiced with this activity, you can expand their range of motion by offering toys from farther away to encourage reaching out and recovering back to an upright position, or from their left or right sides to encourage turning or bending their torso. When you do this, take care to try to present the toy the same number of times from either side so your baby ends up working all their trunk and leg muscles fairly equally. You can refer to an activity in pages ahead called "Standing Up and Reaching Out," which is similar in nature, for more direction.

Mom responds by shifting her stabilization down to the baby's hips, bottom, and thighs. She also exerts a subtle, gentle downward pressure to encourage the baby to keep her feet flat on the floor.

You can see from this image to the next that the baby has raised her big toe and then plants it as she pulls the toy closer to her body, flexing her elbows and bringing her arms nearer her torso. Her maneuvers are subtle, but they add stability to her frame as she works to find balance from this challenging position being upright on two feet.

Baby maintains this strong standing posture as she plays with the toy. Eventually she begins to lose interest, though. Instead of ending the play session, we try to extend it by making a simple adjustment . . . as shown in the next photos.

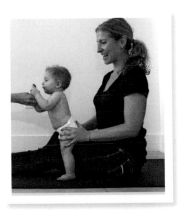

To give the baby a fresh perspective, Mom shifts her hands back up the baby's trunk and turns her around. This shift allows for direct eye contact and communication.

This can be extra helpful for the caregiver to see their baby's facial expressions and be immediately responsive to their needs (e.g., ending the session before a meltdown if the baby is sleepy or hungry).

Baby's spine is fairly well stacked over her pelvis, hips, and legs, as she looks up and makes eye contact with her mom. While this is good, a few things are notable here: (1) her right foot is rolling outward (noted by her weight landing atop her fourth and fifth toes instead of flat against the ground), (2) both her arms are flexed and held high, one of them actually in her mouth (which may be related to teething or hunger),

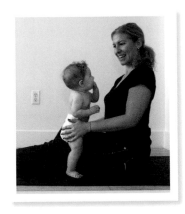

and (3) the base of her skull is hyperextending toward her back with her shoulders elevated. All these things can be signs of instability, which is quite likely due, in this case, to fatigue. We had been going for a while already in this session, so it's quite plausible that this baby was both tired and hungry.

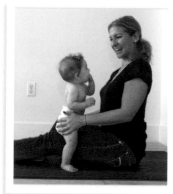

Mom moves her hands back down to the sides of her baby's low trunk, hips, and thighs.

Baby subtly leans forward with her mom's support. She no longer hyperextends her head, her right arm is less flexed with palm opening, and her right foot is now flat.

Baby's left hand is still in her mouth, though; and since she's otherwise become more relaxed, this probably means she's hungry versus teething.

We therefore act to end this session. From this image to the next you can see a subtle change in the mom's hand position.

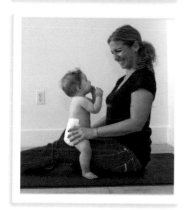

Mom moves her thumbs to the front of the baby's thighs and uses her palms to exert a gentle downward force to guide the baby's bottom down to her leg.

Baby responds by bending her hips and knees and lowering herself into a well-aligned seated position.

This smooth transition from standing was superbly done. Nonetheless, baby now has both her hands by her mouth . . . so we're pretty sure she's hungry.

Fortunately, the baby is now in an excellent position to take a nursing break.

From Sitting to Standing at a Support Surface

This activity helps your baby practice rising to stance and using a support structure to maintain balance. In this example the structure is the surface of a couch, but anything roughly the height of your baby's chest that is stable and they can easily grab onto will do. Baby planting their hands to the surface ahead of them helps to provide a sense of stability as they engage their core and legs to balance in the upright position. Focused practice can serve to strengthen the leg muscles and improve the position in which your baby holds their legs, both at work and at rest.

Including toys on the surface incorporates reach-and-grasp fine motor play as the bigger task work of standing is hidden.

Once your baby can transition to standing at a support surface, cruise along it, or take steps away from it, the act of intentionally practicing the sit to stand transition is only really necessary if you want to do focal work on your baby's leg alignment.

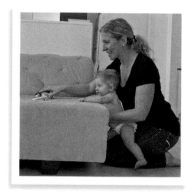

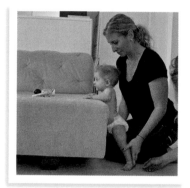

Seen here is a seven-month-old baby girl.

This activity began with the baby sitting on her mom's lap and Mom moving a toy on the couch to entice the baby to stand and reach out for it. Instructions had not been given at this stage to guide the mother in precisely how to position the baby, and what resulted here offers a few great pearls of guidance since this is real life, real time, and realistic to happen to just about any baby/caregiver duo.

Baby responds well by placing both arms on the couch's surface, showing she is engaged as she starts reaching. While that's a good start, there are several hurdles to overcome.

Mom's left arm starts out across the baby's lower chest and upper abdomen. That's not working out very well, as the baby's legs are straddling her whole lap and neither foot is in contact with the ground. It's too wide an area for her tiny hips and the baby is therefore falling forward, leaning her upper trunk into the surface. She cannot physically shift herself into standing from here.

In the second image we see Mom try to help the baby shift into standing. Mom shifts her hands to the baby's lower legs as she tries to guide her feet to the floor.

The baby doesn't plant her heels and rises on her toes as she presses more of her chest and abdomen into the couch. Note: Tiptoe stance is not necessarily terrible for a baby to spend some time in, but it should not be their go-to or habitual posture. It provides deep pressure to the joints of the toes, which does help a baby to feel where they are in space as it lifts them closer to interesting items that might otherwise be out of view or reach. However, it's also likely to make them lean forward—as is the case here.

Another problem with this position is it does not promote the same engagement of the baby's core. If you look carefully, you'll see a crease across her lower back. This indicates she is overextending her back as she leans forward and juts upward. This can potentially put excessive pressure on joints in the low back and hips.

So we want to replace this posture with one of the baby standing tall, engaging her core more with less leaning, while pressing up through flat feet.

With some guidance, Mom and the baby scoot back a bit from the couch to create more space for repositioning. Mom's hands are back to the sides of the baby's low trunk, hips, and upper thighs, with her thumbs to the baby's back.

The baby is now sitting on her mom's lap, straddling one leg, with her feet flat on the floor and parallel to each other.

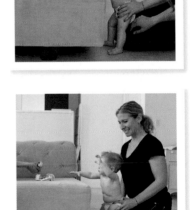

Her body, from head downward, is in a nice neutral alignment; and her torso is hinged at the hips, with her chest starting to come over her feet as she readies to shift her weight.

Baby's hands are in front of her, resting on the couch. She's gazing at the toys and her face shows she's excited to go after them.

In the second image on this page, Mom's hands remain, providing stability and a gentle downward force as baby flexes her knees and ankles to relax into a stronger seated position.

With baby better aligned, I begin moving toys in front of her to try to motivate her to stand. Baby's arms reaching out for the toys show this is working.

Note the crease in the baby's tummy (abdominal muscles) at the base of her rib cage, indicating she's engaging her core as she raises her arms in excitement. This is a great sign of her growing trunk strength.

Between the previous two images there is a very subtle, almost imperceptible, shift of the baby's weight into her bottom, hips, and down through her heels as she loads her weight and prepares to rise. You might notice, if you look closely, that the mom has shifted her hands ever so slightly toward the backsides of the baby's thighs and hips. And the baby has rocked her weight in such a way that her toes and forefoot lift up from the ground.

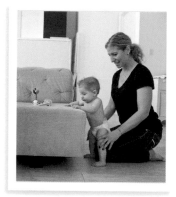

Next we see baby lean her trunk and body weight forward as she extends her hips and knees to stand and reaches forward with both hands pressing on the couch to help maintain balance. Her alignment from her head to her tail and down her legs to her flat feet looks great, but she is still directly (straddling) above her mom's leg and cannot currently reach the toys.

As her baby moves, Mom's hands slide down her thighs to just above and below her knee joints. She is in minimal contact and ready to provide more stability should it be necessary.

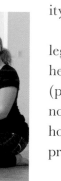

Baby next steps her right leg forward first. Her left leg did not advance quite as symmetrically and is seen here with knee and toes slightly externally rotated (pointing out to her side). This is okay, as long as it's not habitual; so it's pointed out as a cue to you to watch how your baby postures during similar transitioning practice.

Closer to the couch now, the baby extends her trunk and pelvis over her legs, bringing her head, neck, and back more upright along with her visual path. She manages to grab one of the toys as she leans her chest, upper abdomen, and elbows on the couch for more stability.

In response, Mom shifts her hands up to the baby's torso to provide more stability at her core. At first, she is not in direct contact, just ready to be if her daughter were to lose balance. She pauses, giving her daughter a moment to enjoy having successfully reached the toy. (Note: Moments of success are important as they keep the baby motivated and engaged in play. Think about it; if we are constantly moving the item of interest and they never actually get to make contact, that can be hugely frustrating and lead to meltdown and refusal of participation.)

What the camera can't quite capture is that the baby girl grew tired of the first toy, threw it, and was making sounds indicating she wanted the second toy.

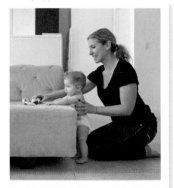

Because she is observing her daughter's responses and dynamically flowing with her, Mom shifts her left hand farther up the baby's torso and uses her right hand to move the red toy just a little closer to see if her baby will reach for it.

Thanks to the higher level of support from her mom, which is given with a broad hand spanning the baby's torso, baby girl shifts her left leg and now stands with her hips squared and toes pointed at the surface ahead, as she reaches both hands toward the toy.

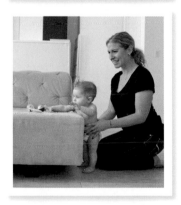

In the middle image here, to reach farther to the toy, the baby rotates her torso and opens her left hip and leg to her left. While her posture is mostly solid, you may note that she's curling her toes to grip the floor. This, like leaning into the surface, helps her body find more stability and balance as she goes.

Mom responds by shifting both hands lower down her baby's torso, encompassing the top of her pelvis.

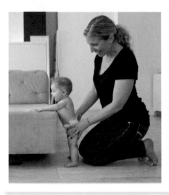

In the final image, we see baby throw the toy across the couch as she rotates her torso, hip, and leg back toward the surface. (Note: At this age the baby's grasp and release are fine-tuning, not yet a fully developed and refined skill. You can refer to the supplement

"Notes from a Pediatric OT," at the back of the book for more details on fine motor skill development.)

Mom continues to flow with the baby's actions and shifts her hands farther down her baby's hips to her upper thighs. She has wrapped her three middle fingers from the front of the hip joints to around the sides of her upper thighs, her thumbs on the baby's lower back and upper glutes, and her pinky fingers along baby's hamstrings for broad stabilization.

Baby responds with a beautifully aligned standing posture. Her hands are on the couch level with her chest, and her chest barely touches the couch. Her hips are stacked well over her knees, ankles, and flattened feet.

Caregivers, beware—this activity is yet another that can lead to your neck leaning forward and put compressive force on the blood vessels in your legs. Performing an FT warm-up before starting and a cool down/recovery postactivity could be beneficial for your body (see Part III).

Note: It is important to pay attention to the height of the support surface you are utilizing with your baby during this activity. Simply put, a surface that is too high is likely to cause your baby to extend their upper body and arms to reach, whereas a surface that is too low is likely to cause your baby to hinge forward.

Standing Up and Reaching Out

APPROXIMATE AGE RANGE: 6–9 MONTHS

This activity helps your baby practice their sitting-to-standing transition, and it layers in the act of reaching out for objects while standing. This helps build leg strength and control between the torso and the legs, as it also adds in additional trunk mobility work and challenges to maintaining stability while reaching out of a balanced center of gravity.

Note: Mom is seen in this activity tailor sitting. Caregivers need to pay attention to the alignment of their legs, what their lap creates for a sitting platform for the baby, and how the baby sits atop that platform. Ensure that one hip is not hiking above the other by looking for postural asymmetry in the foot placement, legs, hips, shoulders, and neck.

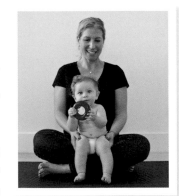

Seen here is a seven-month-old baby girl.

Baby starts out sitting on her mom's lap. Baby's feet aren't flat on the floor, but the mom helps correct for this by gently pushing the baby's bottom forward as

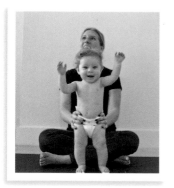

she subtly lifts upward. Her hands cup the baby's bottom and upper thighs with her thumbs to the tops of her legs. In doing so, she encourages the baby's feet to flatten as they take on the weight she transfers forward.

As the baby stands, the mom shifts with her, placing her thumbs behind the baby's pelvis and her fingers to the fronts and sides of it.

Baby's hands are raised to the sky. While this looks like a cool victory pose, it's actually the baby's way of adding stability and balancing herself, known as a "high guard position."

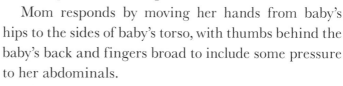

GUARDING BALANCE WITH THE ARMS...

One common strategy babies often exhibit with early stance and walking is called "guarding." This refers to their arms. In this activity we see a baby exhibiting a "high guard," which is the arms being held up, hands above shoulders. It offers the most stability for the baby. The next step down, and a sign your baby is developing more muscular control in their core and limbs for stability and relying less on their arms being raised, is the "mid guard," which is when babies' hands are at their chest to abdomen level. A "low guard" is when their hands come below their hips but are not yet moving freely such as in reciprocal arm swinging.

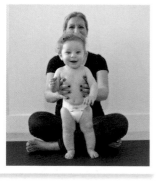

Mom's adapted hand placement has afforded the baby enough additional stability to correct her foot placement as she shifted, but not quite enough to feel as though she didn't need to raise her arms for more help with balancing.

Mom responds by moving her hands from baby's hips to the sides of baby's torso, with thumbs behind the baby's back and fingers broad to include some pressure to her abdominals.

The higher hand placement adds the stability that the baby needed and her posture noticeably improves. Baby's shoulders become level, and her arms lower to a mid guard because she's feeling balanced.

With the baby more balanced, Mom shifts her hands back to her baby's hips. Baby girl drops both of her arms farther, and her hands are now to the level of her hips in a low guard.

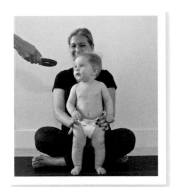

This activity is best performed with two caregivers, so I now step in from baby's right side to present a toy at roughly eye level. I want to challenge her to turn her head and neck, and see what she does with her upper body if she attempts to reach for the toy.

If a second caregiver isn't available, you can offer the toy yourself, allowing one of your hands to leave your baby so it can hold and enticingly move the toy around. Alternatively, you can place the toy on a nearby elevated surface (e.g., a couch or coffee table). If your baby has not yet developed adequate trunk stability and leg strength, though, this may be too advanced an activity for them.

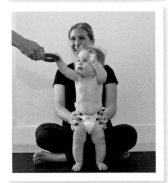

Baby rotates her upper body to her right and reaches for the toy with both hands. Her abdomen is visibly engaged, as shown by her abdominal muscles contracting at the base of her rib cage.

Baby subtly rotates her torso, pelvis, and hips, shifting her left foot back slightly to keep her balance, as she grabs the toy and begins to pull it to her chest and open mouth.

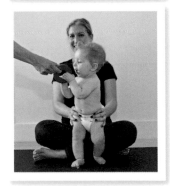

I keep my hand on the toy for a subtle amount of resistance as baby pulls it nearer, letting go as she begins to rotate her torso back to neutral (facing forward).

Baby rotates back to neutral and leans ever so slightly to her right limb as she advances her left leg back to parallel with her right.

She transfers the toy to her left hand and releases her right, which she is seen here starting to lower back down, as she victoriously raises the toy to show it off.

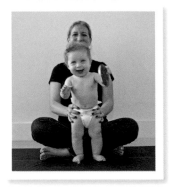

Note: This is a great show of fine motor skills to transfer the toy hand to hand.

For a seven-month-old little one, this was a highly successful standing activity.

Now that you have a few ways to practice gaining leg and trunk strength with the sit-to-stand transition, let's take our focus to another age-appropriate skill that will put your baby into the next level of advancing their skills in the prone position—being on all fours.

From Sitting on Lap to All Fours

APPROXIMATE AGE RANGE: 7–10 MONTHS

This activity, while unplanned during the play session in which it was captured, offers a great way to help your baby to gain comfort with transitioning forward from sitting to four points of contact with the ground, atop their hands and knees (also known as quadruped). The transitional shift guided here helps the little body to gain strength, mobility, and control in coordinating the shift of their weight over their seated base and helps prepare them for crawling on hands and knees.

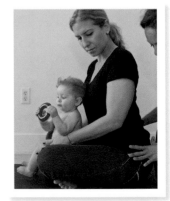

Reminder: In the previous chapters on tummy-time positioning, there was one activity that guided you in how to position your child in all fours over your leg. Practicing that prior to introducing this transition will be beneficial in helping your child to gain comfort with the position.

Seen here is a seven-month-old baby girl.

Mom sits cross-legged on the floor, and the baby sits

atop her mom's lap while playing with a toy ring. Mom is positioned on her "sitting bones," creating a solid base upon which her spine can align.

Mom's hands are on the sides of the baby's hips and thighs. Her index fingers are draped along the sides of the baby's knees, guiding the knees to point straight ahead as baby's feet rest on the floor. The feet should ideally be just below the knees, which helps the baby support her own weight into her heels.

Mom uses the base of her palms, wrists, and forearms on the sides of the baby's torso as "guardrails" keeping the baby from leaning over too much on either side.

Baby's bottom cheeks are level, which is good (indications of un-evenness include wrinkling in the sides of the baby's torso or hips, or one shoulder appearing higher than the other); however, she is lean-ing back too much toward Mom, as indicated by her toes and forefeet

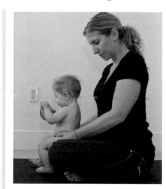

rocking up into the air. This posture will improve in a few moments.

Mom's palms supportively press into baby's lower torso, and the sides of baby's thighs and hips.

Thanks to the guidance of her mom's hands, the baby has shifted her trunk forward over her pelvis; and her leg alignment also improves, with her feet becom-ing more flat to the ground.

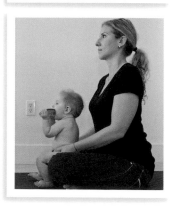

Baby brings the toy to her mouth and continues to maintain the same posture as the previous image. The biggest shift in this picture is actually with regard to the mom's neck, which she now holds tall with her ears over her shoulders.

Tip: If you're in the habit of making forward head movements to check on your baby but tend to forget to check in and self-correct, consider sitting in front of a mirror. You'll continually see what your baby is doing without having to look down. In addition, you'll instantly notice if you slip into poor posture habits.

This frontal view shows more clearly how Mom is supporting baby's leg alignment.

Notice that the baby's bottom is sitting with hips level.

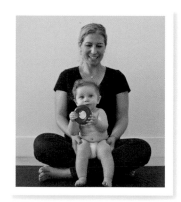

On the downside, the baby's feet are no longer flat on the floor. Mom could solve this by shifting the baby directly forward, so that the weight of the baby's torso hinges forward over her pelvis. This would encourage the baby's feet to flatten as they take on the additional weight.

Another issue is that the baby's torso is leaning a little more toward her right side, as indicated by the creasing in her belly. To address this and promote a more neutral posture, Mom could move her forearms inward to directly contact the sides of the baby's torso for more external stabilization; and if more help were still needed, she could shift her hands up to the baby's abdomen to encourage her to engage the muscles of her core more.

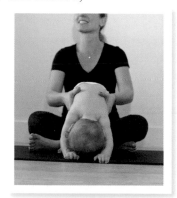

The plan at this point was to bring the baby to a standing position by the mom providing gentle upward force with her hands; however, her baby girl took the help and went a different route.

Becoming fatigued with sitting, and having only her feet in contact with the ground, the baby bends forward and brings her hands down so they're also touching the floor.

While this is entirely unexpected, it's not bad for a baby. In fact, it's just like a yoga pose (called a downward-facing dog) and provides a nice stretch for the baby's hips, back, and shoulders.

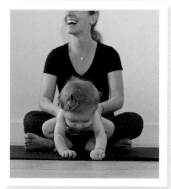

Mom therefore plays along, keeping her hands in steady supportive contact with the baby's trunk as the baby does some great weight-bearing through her hands and arms.

Mom's hands remain the same, steady in their support.

Baby brings her head up in line with her spine; bends her shoulders, hips, knees (which are in the air), and ankles; and brings her weight back into her bottom on Mom's lap.

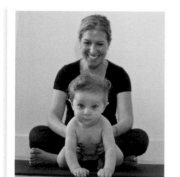

Mom gently exerts a small forward push to encourage the baby to shift off her lap.

Baby extends her neck to lift her head and look forward as she shifts her weight toward supporting herself on her hands and knees. This is great precrawling practice.

If your baby achieves this position but isn't ready to move farther, you can try keeping your hands steady and shifting your baby's body forward/backward and side to side subtly to see how your little one responds. These are great precrawling activities as the rocking introduces subtle movement to the joints of the hips and shoulders while in the supported all-fours position. Simply put, this prepares the joints for more independent moving to crawl in the all-fours position.

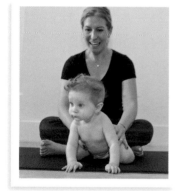

In addition, you can place a toy before the baby, or have your partner offer a toy in the hope the baby can be enticed to reach for the toy. This will challenge their trunk stability as well as their ability to hold their weight on three points of contact as they shift and reach.

In this case the baby has grown tired, and she is unwilling to reach for anything from this position. Since she's still interested in looking at toys, we simply switch the play to visual tracking.

Mom's hands remain in the same place as I move the toy in an arc around the front of the baby. While this camera angle doesn't capture me doing this, it does give a good view of the mom's hands.

The baby responds to this play by subtly shifting her arms apart and opening her right hand. She maintains strong posture and balanced alignment as she turns her upper body and face to view the toy being presented from her right.

This session demonstrates the value of being prepared for anything and adaptable in your play.

There are more activities to come in later chapters showing how to practice all fours over a prop (specifically a Boppy pillow) and then, later (with this same baby when she is a little older and more developed), you'll find guidance on more independently practicing the active transition from sitting on the floor to all fours.

In addition to all fours, sitting, and standing, a baby at this age and stage can also be introduced to transitioning from a kneeling position to standing.

Kneeling and Standing Using Parent for Support

Achieving a kneeling position is a big deal, a landmark milestone in the progression your child makes from the days of low-to-the-floor skills to more upright skills on their way to walking. It marks the shift from being on four points of contact up to two points of contact. Before most babies are comfortable shifting to kneeling at a support structure of some sort, they will often do so using a parent or caregiver for support.

This activity guides you in assisting your baby to practice finding balance in kneeling and to make the transition from kneeling to standing while using your body, both on the floor and, more optimally for the caregiver's body, up on furniture.

The kneeling position in itself offers your child's body a great deal in terms of core and hip girdle muscle strengthening. The trunk and pelvis work together, at first hinging as a unit until the baby develops more of their lumbar lordosis (spinal curve in their low back) and their pelvis gains more ability to tilt forward and backward. To extend the trunk and pelvis over the legs, the posterior chain muscles of the low trunk and bottom (gluteals and hamstrings) are strongly called upon; and, the core and muscles in the thighs help to provide stability and counterbalance the rise onto two points of contact as the hands are removed from the floor.

Even though the trunk and pelvis move together, it is still beneficial to pay attention to how your child transitions and holds their body weight so that healthy habits and movement patterns are being initiated in their brain and body. Practicing this work, paying attention to ensure that your child alternates which leg is leading the transition and exercising both symmetrically, will help to introduce the same forces across the pelvis and low back. These forces contribute to how muscles will pull the pelvis and low trunk, and therefore how they are aligned. Healthy alignment without tilting to either side, forward, or backward is your focus before your child begins moving more on their legs and adding additional forces.

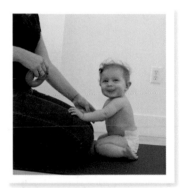

Seen here is a seven-month-old baby girl (as she is being introduced to the activity for the first time).

This activity starts with Mom in a low kneeling position on the floor (her bottom atop her heels) and she places her baby in front of her on her knees with hands to her lap. Baby has four points of contact, also essentially in low kneeling; however, her bottom is not sitting atop her heels, rather it falls between her legs creating a mini w-sit position. This isn't ideal, because it puts pressure into her developing knee joints. While enticing baby to move with a toy, Mom uses a gentle stabilizing touch and light pull with just one hand, to encourage the baby to shift upward.

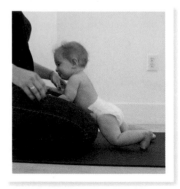

Baby cooperates by extending her hips and knees,

pushing through her feet, and thrusting her abdomen forward onto her mom's legs.

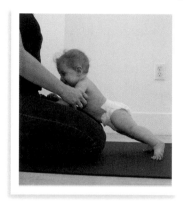

Mom offers more stability by holding the baby's upper arms. The gentle pressure Mom's providing to the muscles above and behind the elbows encourages the baby to extend her elbows and press down more into her hands.

Baby begins pushing up from her toes and extending her hips and knees with more symmetrically aligned legs. She's not exactly kneeling or standing here, though she has achieved a strong plank position. Since this provides a new perspective that still offers strengthening benefits for the baby's arms, core, posterior chain, legs, and feet, and baby has made effort to get here, Mom lets her stay and explore the toy for a moment.

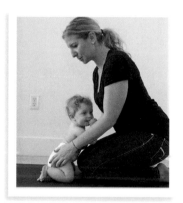

Next, she aims to guide her baby to a more upright kneeling posture.

Sensing that baby is tiring, her mom acts to maintain her interest by switching positions with her. This is a quick and easy way to keep a play session going, because the new visual perspective created by the switch provides fresh stimulus to the baby's brain.

Baby begins on her knees again, but this time leaning forward on Mom's thighs with her elbows and with her bottom touching her feet.

Mom places her hands on both sides of the baby's thighs and gently cups her bottom to provide symmetrical stability.

Mom also takes care of her own body, assuming a low kneeling posture with strong spinal alignment. She is hinged closer to her baby in this round and, as she begins, her bottom is not actually in contact with her feet. This position requires strength and stability; a great warm-up for this is the FT Kneeling Founder. (As a reset after, an exercise that promotes the legs decompressing more would be beneficial, such as a Founder or Standing Decompression.)

Mom spreads all her fingers to encompass the span from baby's pelvis to her knees as she strongly extends her arms.

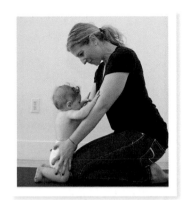

Bringing her hands up and pushing into Mom's arms, the baby engages her upper posterior chain, as she extends and aligns her head, neck, and upper back. At the same time she extends her hips, engaging her gluteal muscles of her lower posterior chain as she brings her trunk vertical from the forward flexed position it was in previously.

The result is a tall kneeling posture, with excellent spinal alignment, bottom lifted off heels, and pelvis vertical.

Less ideal is that the mom has lost her own spinal alignment, flexing her neck far forward. While this is a natural and loving movement that can easily result from her current position, she'll take care to address it postactivity.

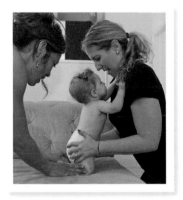

This is a big shift for the baby and a new posture to learn, so we spend a minute here with the mom lovingly engaging her baby before progressing. Since the baby was not interested in standing from here, what you see next was how we modified the play position to try another way.

To facilitate better posture for Mom, less pressure on the baby's legs, and more closeness for comfort and encouragement, we place the baby on an elevated, softer surface—in this case, a couch.

We go right back to where we left off, and begin by placing the baby in a kneeling position facing her mom (who is now in a tall kneeling position at the edge of the couch).

Baby takes immediate interest in her mom's necklace, which places her head, neck, and torso all in an extended alignment.

Mom places her hands broadly around the baby's hips and upper thighs and cups her bottom. Her thumbs are wrapping around the sides of the baby's pelvis toward her lower back.

I step in and gently guide the baby's lower legs to alignment with my fingers as my thumbs provide stable pressure to her heels to give her a sense of where her body is, as well as a platform into which she can push.

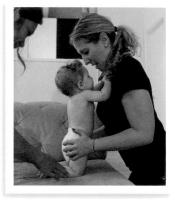

Baby supports her weight with her toes and knees; and also partly with her elbows and forearms, as her hands play with her mom's necklace. The baby's current posture isn't terrible; but it noticeably improves when she engages her posterior chain and extends her hips to rise up in the next photo.

I remove my hands as the baby transitions to a more vertical position.

As the baby rises, she also tucks her chin down a little more toward her chest and decreases the extension of her neck. At the same time she elevates her shoulders to achieve a bit more stability.

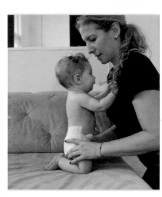

Despite this shoulder elevation, she is nicely aligned through her spine.

I'm no longer needed, so I step away.

Mom subtly hinges her torso and hips, bringing her face and chest closer to the baby and improving her neck alignment.

Baby responds by dropping her bottom to her heels. As she does so, her chin also drops farther and her shoulders lower back down.

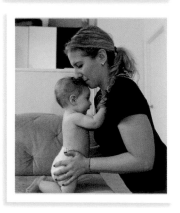

Mom's hands shift with the baby, maintaining contact with her pelvis and upper thighs, but moving her thumbs to the front of the hips. She'll give her daughter a moment to rest and just be in this position before encouraging another lift to take pressure off her knees.

Mom shifts her hands back to their previous placement and exerts gentle upward pressure.

This results in a stronger posture for the baby, who

responds by extending her hips and bringing up her bottom. This time the baby's head is not hyperextending on her neck, nor are her shoulders rising for extra stability.

Mom hinges her hips just a little more and leans in closer. Her kiss is providing comfort and an additional source of pressure that her baby's body can register as an external source of stability.

Baby has been interested in her mom's necklace since getting on the couch, so Mom rewards baby's success at achieving eye level with it by letting baby play with the necklace.

This pause in the activity gives the baby a chance to sense her body's new position. It also aids her strength and stability as it challenges her endurance to sustain the position.

Before baby fully fatigues and since she is still so motivated by her mom's necklace, we decide to attempt to escalate the activity to work on the transition from kneeling to standing.

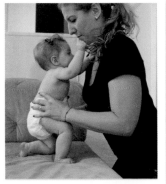

Mom shifts her hands up the baby's torso, with her thumbs now at the bottom edge of the baby's rib cage. She continues to exert a subtle lift that encourages her baby to rise upward.

Baby responds by lifting her right leg and planting her foot forward. Her weight is now supported by it, her left knee, and the top of her left foot. She has achieved a position referred to as half kneeling.

Mom continues to gently encourage her baby to rise upward.

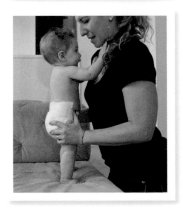

Baby responds by pressing into the couch with her right foot and extending her right hip and knee as she lifts her left leg, advances her left foot forward, and aligns it with her right leg. Success! Baby stands!

Mom's hands shift back down to her baby's bottom, hips, upper thigh, and lower abdomen, flowing with the baby's movements.

Both the baby and Mom look tall and strong in their relative positions. (And the little one is still enthralled with her mom's necklace.) This was a job well done for this first introduction to rising up to two points of contact.

As you introduce this with your own baby, remember to take it slow and provide ample support as they gain their comfort, confidence, strength, and stability.

In the pages ahead, you'll encounter more ways to not only strengthen the torso and mobility your child has in their hips, but you'll be introduced to several helpful ways to functionally tie together the strength gains in their legs and trunk. Developing strength and control with how one shifts the body's weight between positions is beneficial groundwork for more independent and advanced upright movement skills with the body well aligned. First we return the focus back to seated skills. There are many ways to build your baby's strength and comfort with moving more independently on the floor, and this next series of activities provides some great options.

Floor Play with a Pillow Prop for Stability

APPROXIMATE AGE RANGE: 6–8 MONTHS

During this mid to latter half of the first year, another way you can practice skills and work toward the same goals of building trunk strength and hip mobility—in a less hands-on manner—incorporates the use of an external prop, such as a Boppy pillow, to help your baby find balance and stability. These next activities provide additional variations from which to practice sitting and reaching and other floor-play skills like all fours and kneeling that you can add to your repertoire.

Seated Practice with Boppy Prop

These activities incorporate the use of a Boppy pillow to provide an external source of stability and, basically, a cushioned bumper pad to help protect your baby as they learn to shift their weight over their seated base. This not only offers them protection, but it promotes a sense of independence with their budding skills (which can also be extremely helpful in mitigating frustration some babies have with being touched or held at times).

A Boppy pillow is a C-shaped pillow with an opening at its front. In addition to use for nursing and feeding, it can be used to surround the back, hips and bottom while sitting, providing a supportive structure that makes it easy for your baby to reach out and interact with whatever's in front of them. It can also go under their torso for prone or all-fours propping or can be positioned under the side of their torso to help with practicing a side prop.

Note: If you don't own a Boppy, feel free to substitute anything that provides comparable stability offering padding—for example, rolling a long, thick towel and tucking it similarly around your baby.

These activities are most suitable for ages six months and up, after your baby has spent some time practicing prop sitting and sitting and reaching activities. Beyond about nine months your baby should exhibit independence with transitioning in and out of sitting to other positions (prone, all fours, and possibly kneeling and standing), as well as have developed their protective extension skills to their sides and perhaps even to their backside (as discussed in "Baby Fundamentals," this reflex should be present to the sides by month seven or eight; and to their backside by month nine or ten).

To determine whether your baby is ready for this type of play setup, check to see if they can keep their head, neck, and torso upright and well aligned over their seated base on their own with one or both hands self-propping. If your baby rounds their spine, loses midline alignment of their head-neck-torso, excessively tucks their pelvis underneath them, or loses their balance, then this activity is probably a bit premature. You'd do better to practice hands-on prop sitting and other activities that will help your baby to build trunk strength to support a stronger alignment when your hands are removed.

If your baby appears ready, give this a try with both your hands supporting the situation at first, then with just one hand, and then with no hands and careful supervision as you guide the play session. When you know your baby is in a safe environment, this seated play setup can allow a parent some hands-free time so long as they can still supervise for safety and be close enough to get to their baby should the need arise.

Sitting and reaching is the first activity we've included here. Depending on the degree of trunk extension your child has and their comfort, you may also endeavor into safely practicing all-fours propping, kneeling, or side propping using the Boppy. In the activity ahead you will see play-by-play images captured from our session that provide guidance as to how to flow from one position to the next. The activities are with a seven-month-old and we'd like to note that our own daughter was not keen to practice kneeling or all fours until closer to month eight. Every child is different, so approach these activities with ample support and playful encouragement.

In these first four photos you see our daughter, Sunny, in her first Boppy-seated play experience at nearly six months old. Pay close attention to the play-by-play notes ahead and then look onward to activity modifications you'll see with the seven-month-old girl in the next photo sequences. These will help guide you in practical ways when approaching these activities with your own baby.

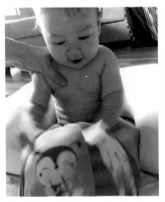

The Boppy was placed first and then Sunny was placed to sit within it, the C wrapped around her seated base with the opening to the front and her legs placed in a long-sitting position. You can see my hand at the top of her torso providing a gentle but encompassing grip with my thumb to her chest, palm to top of her shoulder, and fingers wrapped behind her back. I gave just enough pressure to help guide her trunk to fully upright sitting.

She immediately shifted her legs back to a wider base of support, rolling them outward to create a ring-sitting position. This is not atypical for this stage, and it will be more visible in photos ahead.

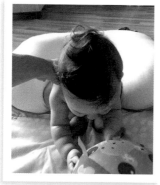

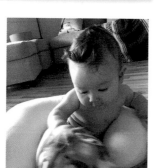

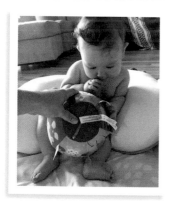

A colorful ball was presented directly in front of her, within a distance she could comfortably reach while remaining upright sitting.

Despite my hand placement, when the ball rolled forward, Sunny reaching forward with her arms resulted in her trunk weakly hinging forward over her legs.

I removed my hand from her shoulder as I wanted to see what she would be able to do in terms of correcting her trunk alignment if I were to move the ball back close to her.

In the second image here, the ball is brought closer to her and she attempts to pull her trunk upright.

This results in her beginning to lean to her left side, which she compensates for by pulling her neck to her right, cinching her side (note cute tummy rolls in middle picture) and flexing her right hip upward (note right shin/foot in third picture). As her balance was being lost toward her left side, we see here that her left arm and hand are extending out over top of the Boppy. She is effectively utilizing her Protective Extension Reflex.

This was not the intent of this practice, but it gives a very real image of how practice with a little one can go. If I had simply thrown in the towel when she crumpled over or forcefully put her back into upright sitting, then she would have missed what turned out to be valuable practice of these important reflexes.

This goes to show there is value in allowing your child to experience positions, to feel their body, to attempt to problem solve and simply move with the skills they have.

Note: We went on to practice using her other arm in the same way (not pictured), which I guided by rolling the ball forward to me with her hands, leading her to lean forward. To guide her back upright, I rolled the ball back and used the same grip on her left shoulder that you saw in the first picture. As she sat up, I gently pushed toward her right to set her off-balance in that direction. Key word being *GENTLY*. Small pushes, or "perturbations" as they are called in the movement world, can be usefully hidden in play to challenge your baby's balance. I was looking to see her protectively extend her right arm as she had her left.

And now here is the same activity approached with our seven-month-old girl model.

Baby girl is sitting upright and facing forward in a Boppy pillow. A toy is placed a few feet away, elevated on a different pillow to prevent her rounding her spine downward as might happen if looking at a toy on the floor (as we saw Sunny do in the previous images). I keep my hands on her legs, seen here in ring sitting, until I'm sure she's sufficiently stable in her upright posture to play in the Boppy on her own.

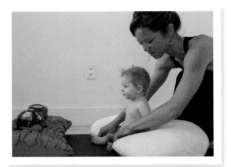

When I remove my hands, she moves forward toward the toy but doesn't reach for it, instead choosing to plant both her hands on the floor to maintain her balance. She extends her head and neck farther to view the toy but doesn't bring her hands or trunk upright to go for the toy. A modification is therefore in order.

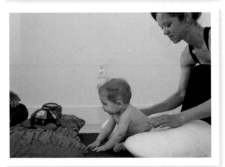

I move the toy close enough for the baby to access while remaining in the Boppy pillow. Baby now reaches for it right away.

She remains in fine alignment; her posture and seated balance are both excellent.

Tips: You can play around with placing the toy at various distances and heights from your

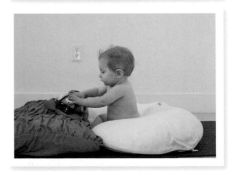

baby to get different responses. The higher the toy, the more trunk extension it will likely elicit for them to elevate their eyes-head-neck-torso to view the item of interest.

Try shifting the toy more to the left or the right instead of being directly in front of your baby to see how they handle these subtle variations. Each position brings different challenges to your baby's developing torso muscles.

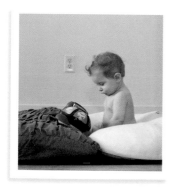

As the baby plays with it, the toy slides down; and she bends her neck to continue watching it. It's fine for her to experience this downward gaze and resultant neck position, but she shouldn't stick with it for too long (e.g., an entire play session) because it's a rather short-ened position for the muscles at the front of her neck and a lengthened position for those at the back of her neck. Ideally, in a play session the muscles are all being worked in a relatively neutral alignment with shifts out of neutral, through various ranges of motion, and back to neutral. This will help the muscles to strengthen more symmetrically and in such a way that your child is gaining the ability to find and maintain neutral on their own, in whatever position their body should be in at the time.

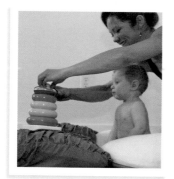

Tip: Toys will inevitably slip and slide. The best way to deal with this is to supervise your baby's playtime closely to observe how they respond and reposition. There's definitely a balance to be found between allow-ing them independence to explore movement and making necessary adjustments to their posture and/or the toy placement.

I gave baby girl a few moments on her own, observing her posture and to see if she would shift the toy and self-correct. Likely because she was a bit tired in this play session, she did not. So I simply came in from behind the baby's line of sight and replaced the toy with a taller one, which made it easier for her to play with it at her eye level.

With her head lifted again, baby was back to a solid alignment of her neck and torso.

I lay out the rings of the toy for baby's play. Baby reaches for and takes hold of the red one. She then returns to a healthy upright sitting posture while exploring the ring with her eyes and hands.

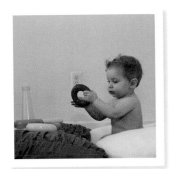

Kneeling and All-Fours Practice with Boppy Prop

These next images are a continuation from the same play session with the seven-month-old little girl seen in the previous activity. She was fatiguing with sitting so I flowed forward in our session with these next positions as simple attempts with the next set of age-appropriate challenges (all-fours play and two points of contact in kneeling) to see how she'd respond with the engagement and props utilized. She did great! And this series just reinforces how valuable it can be to go with the flow to maximize your baby's energy and efforts in any given session.

Note: You will find more guidance on all-fours position and kneeling in activities ahead. The ways you see them practiced here serve as a great early form of introduction to these positions as they involve substantial stabilization and support by the caregiver and a prop. As your baby gains more core strength via practicing their sitting skills and continuing to roll and shift while playing on the floor, they will naturally become more ready for the more advanced activities to come.

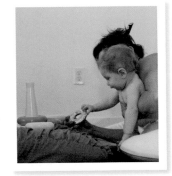

First I decide to vary her play by transitioning her to a kneeling position as it will require a simple shift of her torso forward over her legs. This requires lifting the baby up and leaning her body weight toward the front of her body as I bring her to her knees (which, as you'll see in the next images, she does very well on her own as she feels her torso supported and her legs find the space to clear the floor). To prepare for this, I kneel behind the baby, lean forward, and wrap my arm around her torso. At the same time, I use my other elbow and forearm to support myself as my hand guides her attention forward via shifting the toy in her hand.

Tip: Lifting a baby in this manner can put a lot of force on your spine and challenge your muscles in ways that might physically compress and irritate your nerves. A great exercise to prepare your body for this stress is Foundation Training's Kneeling Founder as it will engage the portions of your posterior chain you most need to rely on to leverage the child's weight and protect your own body (see Part III).

As I lift the baby more upright while enticing her to bring her

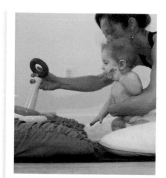

visual path, head, neck, and torso up by tracking the red ring, she starts adjusting the position of her knees. At the same time, the baby is shifting her upper body and arms from their low position as she begins to reach for the ring.

Baby's mom steps in and takes the ring tower, holding it first at eye level to motivate her little one for more play with stacking. This frees up my hand to now have both of them on the baby.

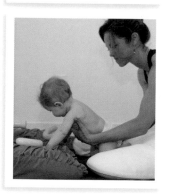

I shift my left hand more centrally on the baby's abdomen, using less forearm to her front and now wrapping it toward her low torso and hip. My right hand is now at the outer aspect of her right lower trunk and hip, providing additional support as the baby finds an all-fours position.

Baby's spine is in a nice straight line from her head to her tail (bottom), well aligned, with her legs sandwiched within the Boppy and her feet pressing into the back curve of the pillow (this gives her a sense of external stabilization and cues as to where her body is in space, feedback that can help her muscles learn to sustain this position). She has one hand planted flat on the pillow and the other is to the surface, but gripping a green ring.

This is success already as she is so engaged in play that she is unaware of the work she is doing.

Note: My back is not in frame, but it was rounding as I created a longer lever with my arms to continue to support baby girl. This is noted because (1) this is normal given the position the baby is in and where my body is in relation to her; and (2) because this could be a gnarly force to a body if one doesn't adequately prepare and recover with smart body work. A Kneeling Founder, a Founder, and an 8-Point Plank would be a great series for the caregiver replicating this.

Taking it up a notch, Mom elevates the toy, encouraging the baby to extend her torso farther to view it.

I flow with this, feeling for the baby's response and modifying my touch along with her movements. This means I keep my hands in the same position and apply slightly more pressure to provide stability and encourage her to engage her muscles to self-stabilize as she rises.

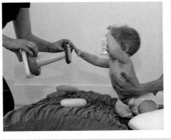

Baby responds phenomenally, lifting her hands up to reach the toy when Mom shifts closer. Her core and posterior chain have engaged enough for her arms to not only feel confidence leaving the ground and rising to reach for the ring, but she shows accuracy with the stacking of the toy!

She has nailed a kneeling position! This is a wonderful moment of success that should definitely be noted, regardless of the short endurance our already fatigued baby model had to hold the kneeling position.

Note: To build upon this sort of play, if your child has the energy to do so, you would do well to encourage reaching with either hand.

Keep in mind that ambidexterity is a skill your baby should most certainly still have at this age and stage.

Baby drops her hands back down, now interested in another colored ring.

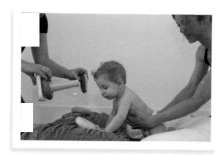

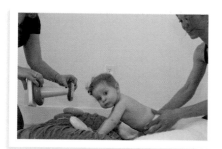

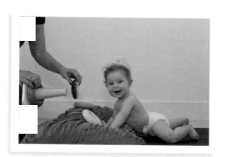

Because I want her to learn to stabilize herself more, I begin to shift my left hand from her abdomen and chest toward her left hip, matching my right hand on her other hip.

Baby shifts her torso lower and brings her weight back toward her bottom and heels. My hands follow her movement and shift lower to symmetrically encompass her low trunk, hips, and bottom at their sides and slightly to the front and back.

She is again in a solid all-fours position with her spine neutrally aligned. Spending a moment here is not a bad play strategy to hide endurance-building muscle work, especially if your baby is fatiguing of doing more movement.

Here we hide this work by having the photographer call out to her, attracting her attention to turn her head and neck to her side, effectively working her neck range of motion while maintaining the position. Baby girl does beautifully for a moment.

Baby handled the challenges so well and I knew she was pretty tired, so I wanted to phase into something different while she was still happily engaging with the photographer. Look at that smile!

So I fully remove my hands and pull away the Boppy pillow to see how she responds.

Baby responds by dropping down from all fours to a propped tummy-time position. Her upper body and torso are still strong, but without the Boppy she has lost the on-knees position. Not a call for worry, just noted and, because she's smiling and happy, we keep going.

I place the Boppy pillow around the baby again, but this time reposition a closed section in front of her so she can prop her arms over it with a little assistance to keep her torso upright. I wanted to see what her response with her legs would be.

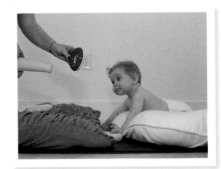

While you can't tell from the photo, she's on all fours again, with her knees directly below her hips, which is great.

In an activity like this, your baby's hands should ideally be either reaching down to the floor or up for a toy. In this case, because of her fatigue, the baby girl is simply leaning her arms into the pillow.

Side Propping with Boppy Prop

Despite Mom's efforts to entice the baby more with the rings, her baby girl has grown tired of them and starts wondering where I am. Baby instead rotates her neck, upper torso, and hips to roll onto her side, where she can see me behind her.

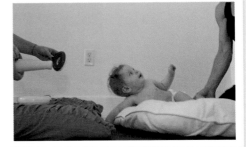

Baby is supporting herself with an arm to her side, propping through her hand on the ground, which is good; however, she's doing so with limited strength because her arm isn't in ideal alignment (notice the angle of her arm versus being stacked vertically such that her arm is more directly over her palm.

I adjust the Boppy pillow to get baby's arm in a better position for practicing side propping.

We shift to an overhead shot of the baby in the Boppy pillow. Because she has grown tired, I've taken things down a notch by

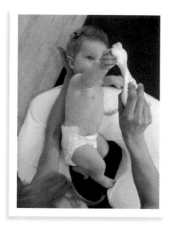

switching her to a position in which she props herself on her elbow and forearm (which requires less energy and coordination than doing so on a taller propped arm with elbow extended).

My left arm supports her along her back, from the base of her head to her pelvis, as she is actively supporting herself with her arm propping into the floor.

Meanwhile, my right hand tries to interest her in a new toy . . . which she visually tracks, reaches for, and grasps. We've now woven some excellent neck range of motion and fine motor play into our session, keeping things fun and the work hidden, as her smile continues to show through these images.

You can see that her lower (left) leg is flexed, supporting her weight through the outer aspect of her upper thigh and hip; and her upper (right) leg has shifted from simply being stacked over the lower leg to now propping her foot into the floor.

This position allows the baby to work on building strength and coordination through the arm that is propping while keeping her core stable. From here the caregiver could assist the baby to extend the lower elbow and prop through the palm, which would then push the body more upright. This would serve to give the arm practice toward the skill of pushing up from side-lying on the floor to sitting.

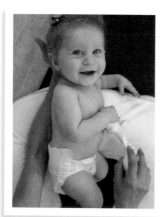

As seen here, the addition of reaching for the toy and allowing the baby to experience success with bringing it back to her body also challenges the arm, core, and pelvic muscles to keep the body still as opposed to rocking and rolling over.

Baby grabs the toy and holds it to her chest in triumph. Still propping herself up with her left elbow and forearm, she smiles and engages with me.

From here we switched to her other side and practiced propping and reaching in the same way so that her body received symmetrical challenges and forces.

The photos might not capture it, but this has been a long session. We decided to cap things here and shift baby girl from floor play while she was still in a happy mood.

In this activity, the baby's varied movements—transitioning from sitting to kneeling to being on all fours, and then on her sides—were great for strengthening her muscles, helping her find more control in each of these positions, and challenging her in ways that provided support in positions that were appropriate for her age and stage of development.

There is more on building seated strength and hip range of motion for transitioning from sitting to other more advanced positions to come. But first a quick pearl related to protecting your baby while helping them build safety and confidence as they transition from sitting with your support to more independent floor play.

No Hands!

APPROXIMATE AGE RANGE: 4–9 MONTHS

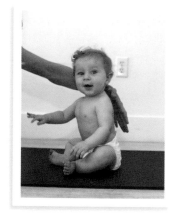

In this stand-alone photo, I'm keeping my hand close behind this seven-month-old baby girl. This is here as a simple call to attention since the image just happened to be captured during our play session and baby girl looked adorably proud of herself as she showed off her skills. The image offers a tiny reality-based pearl from my clinical experience; simply put, control is not there until it is. And even when you think your baby has mastered sitting and is safe alone, an excited baby who is distracted by a toy (or literally anything else in their environment) and lacks protective extension skills (using the arms to catch themself from losing balance) may very easily topple over.

You'll note that my hand isn't touching her but is near enough to quickly catch her and prevent a tumble if she loses her balance backward, which could easily happen to any baby who is new to sitting upright and hasn't yet developed protective arm extension skills in the direction behind them.

This hands-off but ready-to-be-applied external stability is especially helpful if caregivers want to provide babies with a certain degree of independence so they build confidence, but also provide them the protective security they trust caregivers to provide. As you go, also remember that not all tumbles are bad. You do actually want your child to experience the full result of what the shifts in their weight can do; and, in truth, falls will happen and bumps can add pressure that helps build bone density. This also helps them to learn the effects and consequences of their movements in this gravity-laden world. Of course, you'll still want to be sure your child isn't going to smash their head on hard tile or rocks; so there is a level of judgment you'll need to steadily utilize with their safety forefront in mind.

Also, notice that the baby's arms are up. She's just turned her head to look at the photographer, which challenges her seated balance, so she's elevating her arms to add stability to her trunk. She looks strong and adorable as she keeps both balance and alignment.

As she went, my hand was essentially sending the message, *Don't worry. I've got your back.*

To clarify, this is not the level of protection I'd always provide, but I knew the baby was fatiguing from a long session, that she hadn't yet fully developed Protective Extension Reflexes to her sides (and she definitely didn't yet have the reflex toward her back). Because I had a few more activities planned and wanted to avoid a meltdown, I simply prevented a possible tumble from throwing a monkey wrench in our play plans.

It's for the newer sitter who may have success with propping forward but has not yet developed protective extension to their backside (anticipated around months nine or ten) and may still be prone to inadvertently flinging themself off-balance with the excitement of play.

As your baby's trunk and hip muscles grow stronger, to help support their independent sitting you can put time and energy into improving upon the seated base your child assumes with their leg positioning. The way they align their legs creates a different platform from which to sit, reach out of their base of support, and recover back to upright sitting. This poses different challenges to the muscles in the surrounding area. The next activity will cover this further.

Optimizing Sitting

APPROXIMATE AGE RANGE: 6–9 MONTHS

This activity guides your little one to sit in different positions, from ring sitting to long sitting, essentially creating varied bases of support underneath them. Shifting their weight over their seated base becomes more focal in play now that their trunk has strengthened, their protective arm propping is present forward and to their sides, their hips are more mobile, and their legs are stronger. This opens the floor play to more reaching/recovering work and further prepares them for transitioning to other positions.

Seen here is a nine-month-old baby girl.

Baby is sitting on the floor in a ring position, legs forming a circle with feet together. Her base of support is as big as her legs are wide, and in this moment she did not feel stable or confident enough to reach out for the toy her mom was presenting. Instead, her gaze is on the ground.

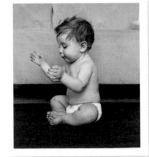

On the upside, the baby exhibits a strong spinal alignment; and she's holding her arms up in an attempt to become more stable.

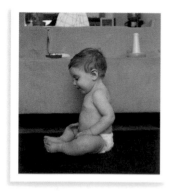

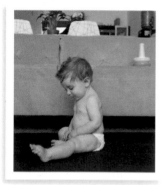

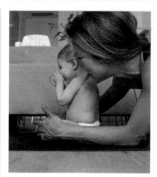

Here we see how the baby begins to self-correct her posture.

She first extends her knees, shifting her feet forward and giving herself a broader base of support. She then lowers her hands onto her legs, which shows she is feeling more stable.

Still experimenting with how to sit, the baby pulls her right foot closer to her body, as she rotates her left leg and extends her knee. This achieves a position that is half ring sitting and half long sitting. She continues to gaze at the floor to maintain her balance, keeping her hands close to her body.

This is definitely a great position for your baby to spend time playing in; however, in this session our little one was growing tired, fussy, and hungry (note her hands to her mouth in the next image).

Keeping the baby's visual path clear to see her mom and the toys she's presenting, I move in behind her to provide some guidance to her legs. I'm in an all-fours position with my weight balanced between my elbows, upper forearms, knees, and shins.

As I get close to her and bring my hands in contact with her body, I verbally engage her (so as not to startle her, rather, to playfully motivate her) by saying, "Yay, Sage! Let's play! Let's see what toys Mama has for you!" (Note: Using your baby's name can help them feel comfortable and connected as they learn to attach understanding to it being their own in their mind. Attention to details like this and the tone and pace at which you speak with your baby are important as behavioral responses can be stimulating or hindering to their willingness to move and participate.)

I guide her legs back into a broad and symmetrical base of ring sitting (clearly visible in the next photo) that provides greater stability.

Baby responds by smiling and starting to look up toward the toys.

I place my hands on baby's pelvis and upper thighs. This extra stability gives her enough comfort to not only look at the toy, but she also starts clapping in excitement for what her mom is holding.

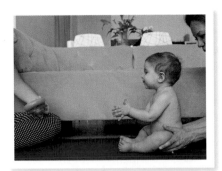

Note, caregivers: My position here continues to be a low kneel. As described in other activities, this can be hard on your body. Prepare and reset with Kneeling Founders, Founders, and Standing Decompression. Another solid choice to follow this would be an 8-Point Plank.

I separate the baby's feet to begin taking her out of ring sitting and toward long sitting (legs straight out in front of her).

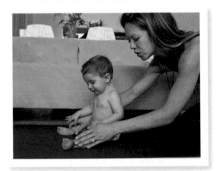

This move is just a first step, though, as the baby's legs are still externally rotated—as shown by her knees and toes still pointing outward. Baby brings her hands down to mine to add a little more stability to her posture as we shift.

I then slide my palms above the baby's knee joints, with my fingers on her lower legs— surrounding her knee joints but not putting any pressure directly through them. I gently maneuver to rotate her legs inward as I also widen them at her hip joints; and, at the same time, I straighten her knees.

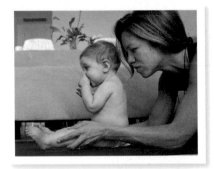

She makes progress, but her knees aren't yet fully extended, and her legs aren't yet flat on the ground. Her hands have returned to her mouth, which could mean she is not feeling 100 percent stable here or could simply be an indicator she is growing tired and hungry or bothered by teething.

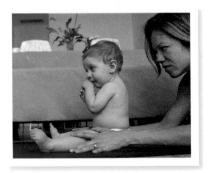

In the final image on the previous page, I shift my fingers out from behind her legs and apply a gentle downward pressure through the tops of her thighs and shins. Baby's legs straighten out, now flat against the ground. She has successfully achieved a long-sitting position and my hands can now shift back to see how she sustains this.

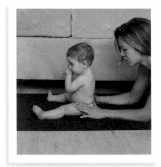

I move my hands to the top of the baby's thighs, and encompass the front, sides, and back of her pelvis. This photo provides an angle that allows you to see how we have widened her legs (and therefore created a bigger base of support), creating even more stability in this long-sitting posture.

Giving your baby more options for how they sit on the floor is likely to increase their comfort and confidence with how they hold and move their weight, which should result in them experimenting more and more with how they move in and through each position. The activities to practice in sitting remain similar to all you've thus far been introduced to—visual and auditory tracking, reaching for and grasping toys, and then, of course, recovering back to upright sitting. In the next activity you'll see this put to action with more advanced sitting and reaching play.

Advanced Sitting and Reaching

APPROXIMATE AGE RANGE: 8–11 MONTHS

These next several images show older babies practicing sitting and reaching as they shift their seated base through more advanced positions—long sitting, half-ring sitting, and side sitting.

This simple activity enhances the strength, range of motion and coordination of your baby's low trunk, core, and hips. It also helps prepare them to more smoothly transition from one position to another, such as from sitting to all fours and from all fours to kneeling.

Your baby is probably ready for this activity if they can sit independently on the floor and, if necessary, extend an arm to either side to keep from falling over.

Seen here is a ten-month-old baby girl.

This session began with the baby being placed on the floor in long sitting (with her legs a little more than hip distance apart and both knees and toes pointing up toward the ceiling). She was handed the lid of the bucket of this shape-sorting toy as I showed her, just outside her reach, one of the blocks from within the bucket.

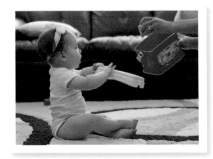

Almost immediately the baby begins to shift the lid into her right hand as she crosses her right leg over her left, with her legs still stretched out ahead of her in a variant of long sitting.

This might have been a precarious position for her at a younger age, potentially resulting in her toppling over. At ten months old, though, she shows strong seated balance as she sits with her torso tall over her seated base. In a moment, as she reaches farther, she naturally corrects this on her own.

Note: Should your child do something similar, take a moment to observe how they balance and if they can self-correct and maintain their balance with further challenges imposed; that is, reaching outside their base of support. Crossing the legs as such would be considered problematic if the child habitually assumed the position with the same leg steadily elevated, as this could lend to asymmetrical muscle usage patterns and resultant imbalances across various joints. It would also be considered problematic if it consistently caused them to lose balance and fall.

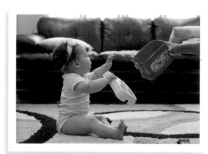

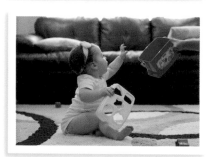

I place the toy block in the bucket, which further piques baby's interest. Her left hand lets go of the lid to reach up and out for the block.

Baby girl uncrosses her right leg as she reaches; and with her left leg she creates a wider base of support under her by rotating her hip outward as her knee flexes (similar to ring sitting). Her right hip has rotated inward until it's in a neutral long-sitting position. All this occurs as she shifts her body weight forward, biased toward her left.

Baby continues advancing her left hand to reach into the bucket for the toy block.

At the same time, she also externally rotates her left hip, internally rotates her right hip, and flexes both knees to transition into side sitting. Her weight has shifted up and over her lap and is supported more in her left outer hip at this point.

Directly following this photo, I moved the bucket closer to let the baby reach into it and retrieve the toy block so she could experience the success for her strong efforts.

She then reverted to her long-sitting position and played with the toy.

Now here are three images, similar in nature, that show our daughter, at eight months, playing seated between my legs. She reaches outside her base of support but doesn't maintain her trunk upright as the previous baby did. What she instead exhibits we can consider pre–all fours, and it shows how a child further builds independence in their skills with floor maneuvering and transitioning skills.

As we started out here, I was in long sitting and I had placed my baby girl in ring sitting between my legs, facing me. She had a maraca toy in one hand and I had placed a pop-up toy on the other side of my leg, just outside her reach.

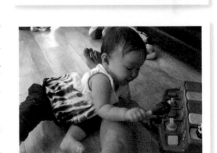

Before I could even get my camera ready, she had reached up and over her side, over my leg, and planted her left arm to the floor as she reached across her body's midline with her right arm to bang the maraca on the toy.

I called her name in the act and she turned to look at me with a massive smile while supporting her weight between her left hand and the outer edge of her left thigh (which was somewhere between a half-ring sit and a side sit). Her right leg was off the surface, counterbalancing her reach with her foot planted to the floor.

From here she could have continued to rotate her right leg inward and shift her weight forward to achieve an all-fours position.

Instead we see her start to pull her right arm back and rotate her right leg outwardly.

While the act itself wasn't pictured, pushing through her downward-positioned left arm resulted in her dropping her right leg and bottom back to the ground as she brought her trunk upright over her seated base.

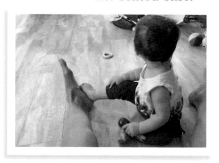

Baby brought herself back to sitting tall and pivoted on her bottom with her right leg outstretched.

I turned my left foot inward to give her a stable surface to push her right foot as she brought herself more upright, moving toward a long-sitting position with her right leg and a ring-sitting position with her left leg.

These babies' moves have been shown to highlight that skill building is incremental. Your baby's flow from one seated posture to another, and the resulting core strength and range of motion that they gain, will end up helping them learn to get around more smoothly and independently with floor skills and transitions. Your task of focus, as caregiver, is on setting up play environments that involve more transitions with less support so that the work of making these shifts is hidden for your baby within fun play activities.

A Few More Examples of an Older Baby Sitting

These next several images are being included simply because the baby's movements exhibit exemplary indications of her increases in strength, stability, and mobility. As your child grows and progresses, sometimes the small gains might be hard to notice. This section is here to help you note a few subtle signs of improvement.

These two images show Sunny at nine months (just a month older than she was in the previous activity) playing on the floor in a ring-sitting position.

She is lifting a rather heavy shape-sorting toy over her head, challenging her trunk strength nicely as she extends her arms and torso over her seated base. From one image to the next you can see her

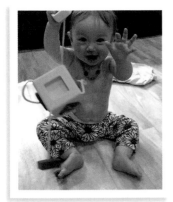 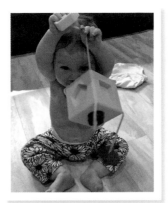

tummy muscles contract as she works to lift the toy. Her grip with each hand is also notable. At first she is using just a palmar grasp with her right hand; then, she brings her left hand to the small rope attached to the yellow shape to help lift the toy using a pincer grasp. As she executes this triumphant raise of her toy, she maintains her head, neck, and torso in excellent midline alignment. You can also see that she has brought her feet slightly closer together and dropped her knees toward the ground, giving herself a stable ring as her base.

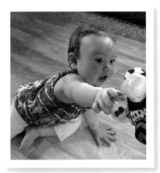

Here we see Sunny go from ring sitting to side sitting, propping through her (left) arm to her side to reach across her midline with her opposite (right) arm extending high above her head. At the same time she extends her head and neck and keeps her spine head to tail in a strong neutral alignment as she goes.

Reaching across midline like this is a great way to challenge your baby from six months onward (as discussed earlier in other floor-play skills) and you can take things up a notch by challenging them to reach farther and higher.

Here's another image of nine-month-old Sunny having shifted from ring sitting to side sitting to reach a

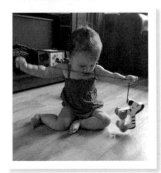

wheeled pull toy. Her head and neck rotate and flex downward to gaze at the rope and toy as she experiments with fully stretching out the length of the rope, using a pincer grasp with both hands. The alignment of her spine from head to tail remains solid and stable during this play.

This image serves as a great example for using simple but age-appropriate toys for your baby to explore in their environment. With adequate "play station" setup (in terms of safety and appropriate toys), by this age and stage most babies can self-entertain and self-challenge at the same time.

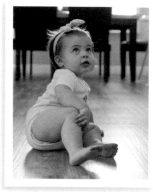

Next are a few images captured in a play session with an even older baby, aged between eleven and twelve months. These are a bit ahead of some of the activities to follow in terms of age and skill set; but, for the sake of visually comparing the advancements of seated stability and mobility, they are being presented here.

The baby is seen here exhibiting her ability to catch her balance with her arm toward her backside as she moved about on the floor. Something across the room caught her attention as she was midtransition between long sitting and all fours. As these reactions develop, coupled with trunk strength and hip mobility, the ease with which your child moves from one position to the next will increase, becoming more fluid and faster. Notice her hand to her right leg as she pauses to watch, her right heel acting as a rudder on the ground to help her pause and control her body.

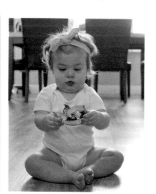

These next two images provide a good example for strong seated posture versus weaker, less engaged seated posture. The shifts from one image to the next are subtle and worth noting so you have this on your radar when playing with your own baby.

First we see the baby seated tall atop her sitz bones, legs in a closed ring, with her spine and pelvis in a solid, strong, neutral alignment head to tail. Encourage this.

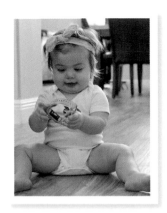

Next we see a very subtle shift in baby's seated posture. She has widened her legs from a ring to this externally rotated version of a wide long-sitting posture, and she also rocked her pelvis backward. As a result she is no longer tall on her sitz bones, and her abdominal muscles are allowed to slacken in her midsection. This is less ideal as her body weight is now putting pressure through her lower back versus her bottom. Realign your baby if they don't self-correct from this sort of posture.

Once your child gains comfort with their floor skills and their arms are strong and stable holding their weight, you're likely to see them reaching farther and farther out of their seated base of support and planting their hands on the ground to self-support as they reach farther still. Shifting their torso over their lap fully and changing their leg alignment should begin to result in propping up on hands and knees. Time spent in this position offers a child so much that you truly don't want them to skip it.

Simply bearing weight on hands and knees first and later taking that a step further by gaining confidence, strength, and increasingly greater control while shifting weight on all fours are important steps in your baby's transition toward crawling. For that reason, the next several activities and images you'll encounter center around helping you to guide your child to experience and enjoy time in this position as well as build their ability to transition into it on their own.

From Sitting on Floor to All Fours No. 1

APPROXIMATE AGE RANGE: 8–10 MONTHS

This activity guides your baby in transitioning from sitting on the floor to getting on their hands and knees, aka "on all fours" or "quadruped."

In this position a baby experiences the pressure of their body's weight through the segments of their body in contact with the ground as well as a reaction force from that contact transmitted upward through their limbs, meaning not only do their hands feel pressure, but so do the muscles of their forearms, upper arms, shoulders, and even into their upper back and shoulder blades. And the joints throughout that region all garnish information from the experience as well. Similarly, their knees, legs, bottom, pelvis, and low back also benefit. The experienced sensations teach your baby's brain about their position in space and give information about how to further contract and control their body in and through this position. This experience and information is helpful for their budding mobility on the floor in crawling, and it also carries over to later skills. The hips, pelvis, and low spine experience movements that will later translate beyond just crawling to rising to two limbs for kneeling and walking skills. The hands-and-arms experiences build strength and mobility that can be considered fundamental for more finely tuned gripping and grasping functional tasks such as throwing a ball, finger feeding, using utensils, cutting with scissors, and even handwriting.

WARNING—DON'T SKIP ALL-FOURS PLAYTIME

Quadruped is a powerhouse position that can all too easily be skipped over if (1) a baby is not spending ample time first propping up in tummy time, because fundamental strength and mobility are established here first that have direct benefit to the arms' and legs' ability to prop in quadruped; or (2) they're in a rush to be upright. Well-meaning parents might inadvertently add to this by placing their baby in stance too early and too often, either with their own support or with the support of containers such as a jumper, stander, or walker with saddle seat.

In this example our baby model happens to start out as an unwilling participant, so the session also addresses one way to calm and engage a baby who is less than enthusiastic about participating in these movements that may be outside their comfort zone.

Seen here is a nine-month-old baby girl.

This activity began by placing the baby in ring sitting with her mom positioned to her side with toys to entice the baby to move. The hope was to see our model shift her trunk up and over her seated base, over her right thigh, and plant her hands to the floor in the direction of the toy.

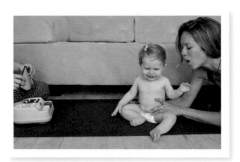

I come in beside the baby (I'm in a modified quadruped position myself, supported by my knees and elbows) and cheerfully ask her what toys her mama has and if she is ready to play. I am playful but also slowly and intentionally ask her to do precisely what I am about to guide her to do: "Let's lean over and move to hands and knees"

(this can give the baby additional feedback to tie together the actions, to pair meaning to movement).

My right hand is broadly cupped over her right lower back and pelvis. My left hand provides an encompassing grip around the baby's left low trunk and hip. My thumb is behind her pelvis, the web space of my hand traces the side ridge of this bone, and my middle finger comes to the front of it. My index finger traces the lower edge of her rib cage and my ring finger and pinky fall to the top of her left thigh. As I approach her, my position is deliberate and I hold it steady and still, providing support so she can feel stable and safe as she cognitively prepares for the movements I'm about to nudge her toward.

I tell the baby that we're going to start moving ("Ready? Let's go see Mama!"), and I then push gently with my left hand toward her right to encourage her to shift her weight toward her right hip and hand. My push is combined with an attempt to subtly lift and rotate her left hip inward as her trunk rotates to her right, and my right hand remains still to provide stability for her to lean into as we go.

Baby girl isn't used to moving this way and she resists. The expression on her face (in the first image on the previous page) shows she's less than thrilled about this new learning experience. Seeking to feel more balanced, this next image captures her as she starts moving her right hand to the floor and raising her left hand in the air to counterbalance the weight shift. Both these arm maneuvers are steps in the direction we want to head, so we continue on, sensitive to the baby's reactions but still encouraging more movement.

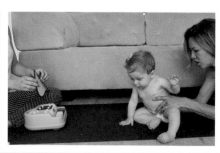

Baby rotates her head, neck, and torso toward her right as she plants her right palm to the floor and her left arm begins to rotate inwardly. Her left hip begins to inwardly rotate and her left foot is coming toward being flat on the floor.

Her visual path being directed to the floor ahead of her is encouraging that her left arm will follow in this direction; from there she would need to continue to rotate her left leg inward for her hip and low trunk to follow to achieve the shift to all fours.

Baby flattens her left foot to the floor and puts on the brakes. Her left hip begins to rotate outwardly once again (it's subtle, but if you look at the position of her knee and lower leg, you can see them starting to point more toward me than inward toward her mom and the toy). Her left arm also subtly begins to pull back outward, extending her elbow and bringing her hand closer toward me versus across her body toward the ground, the toy, and all fours.

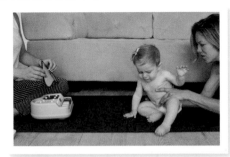

Continuing to be apprehensive, she now has begun to protest with a furrowed brow and less than happy eyes.

I see this isn't going to get us where we need to go, so I decide on a different approach before a meltdown occurs.

To distract the baby from her upset and persuade her to feel differently, I first completely remove my hands so she no longer feels any sense of force applied. I then move my body very close to her, providing her with

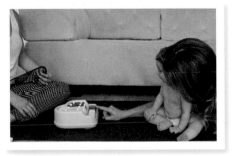

the comfort of nearby external stability in this previously challenging open space where I'd asked her to move. In addition, I try to draw her attention to the toy piano by making sounds on it. If you look closely, you can see her expression begin to change as her attention is piqued.

The nuances of how to calm your little one will surely vary, with factors including their individual personality and temperament at any given moment. Fortunately, in this case the baby perked up when I moved in warmly and produced some fun sounds on the toy piano, as shown by her relaxed right arm, her lowered left arm, and her unhappy expression changing to one of pleased interest. Baby is sitting with her spine upright and weight centered. She's in an optimal position and interested, so we are good to go for another try.

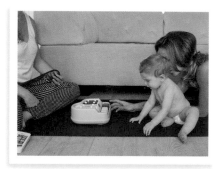

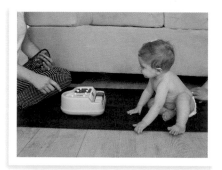

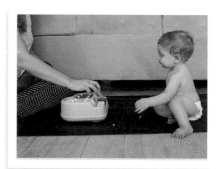

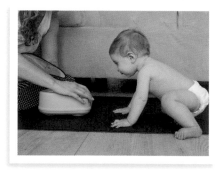

I stop playing the piano. If she wants to hear more, she'll have to move to it and play with the toy herself. I encourage her by saying "Yay, music! Your turn! Play music!"

With a furrowed brow indicating she's a bit disgruntled about the music stopping, she begins turning her body toward the piano. Baby girl first plants her right palm ahead of her as she starts to shift her body weight over her right hip and rotate her left hip inwardly.

She next places her left hand on the floor ahead of her legs, rotating her chest and abdomen farther over her right leg as her left leg rotates inward and her foot moves toward the floor.

To spur her baby on, her mom reaches toward the piano and verbally encourages her to play with it as I move back so as not to distract from the situation.

Baby responds by turning more fully to the piano and gazing directly at it with an interested expression and smile resuming.

While this activity got off to a rocky start, some gentle persuasion is leading baby to transition to all fours.

In the third image we see baby move closer, rotating her torso so that it is now fully facing her mom and the toy and it's stacked in a neutral, more vertical alignment from head to bottom. Her left leg has rotated farther inward and her left hand has lifted from the surface and is reaching toward the toy.

Mom presses different keys on the piano to entice her baby further; and baby responds with more interest and moves closer to the toy.

In the final image of this series, she is seen planting both hands as she internally rotates her left leg, shifting her body weight up and over her hips and rotating her torso to fully face the ground. Her spine and pelvis are in a strong, neutral alignment, with the top of her head pointing ahead of her body, her ears in line with her shoulders, and her shoulders in line with her hips.

From here we would like to see the baby press her weight farther forward still and bring her knees down to the surface so that her weight is held through vertical thighs; but she was tired and that didn't occur.

Regardless, it was still a fruitful session, rich in practice experience.

From Sitting on Floor to All Fours No. 2

APPROXIMATE AGE RANGE: 8–10 MONTHS

As in the previous activity, this provides a visual example of guiding your baby in transitioning from sitting on the floor to being on all fours. This one is fully hands-off. In the previous example the baby began as uncooperative, but in this session she's happy to play along.

For a variety of reasons, a baby may be more comfortable moving over one side of their body than the other. This is not atypical, though it is also not something you want to persist. This particular baby model happened to prefer moving over her left hip. If your baby

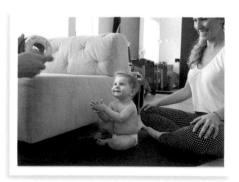

also favors one side over the other, this activity will help you work with that. Your goal as caregiver is to introduce similar movement forces to both sides of your baby's body. Strategic setup of your play areas can be helpful with this.

Seen here is a nine-month-old baby girl.

This session begins with the mom placing the baby in a ring-sitting position.

Because of her individual preference, the baby immediately shifts her weight to her left hip. This can be seen by her right leg inwardly rotating toward her left.

Because we previously worked on shifting over her right side and I want to work her body symmetrically, I hold toys up in front of her biased to her left side (instead of straight ahead).

I bang the two toys together, and ask her if she'd like to try doing the same thing. (Banging items together requires fine motor skills from hands and arms while maintaining balance, and at nine months this baby is ready for it.)

Baby girl sits tall with her eyes locked on the toys as she claps her hands in cheerfully engaged reply.

Note: The mom is sitting tall, strong, and well aligned in a cross-legged "tailor sitting" position. She is present and supportive without distracting the baby, but at the same time providing a beautiful physical example for her baby to follow with regard to healthy sitting. To help decompress her flexed legs and promote unimpeded blood flow following this position a Founder and a Standing Decompression would be great choices (see Part III).

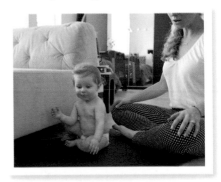

I place the toys down on the ground and to the left of the baby and move away to avoid distracting her.

Baby locks her eyes on the toys and starts lowering her hands to the floor in anticipation of moving.

Baby rotates her right leg inward to the ground, while at the same time shifting her body weight forward over her left hip and lap to place both hands on the floor.

Just like that, the baby transitions to being on all fours!

Baby continues shifting her upper body forward, using her left arm pressing down on the

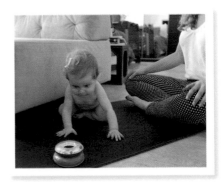

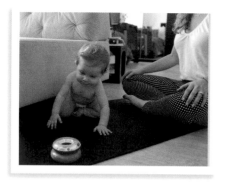

floor to support herself as she lifts her right arm to advance forward toward the toys.

While it's not shown here, the baby proceeded to further rotate her left hip inward until her left leg sat neutrally in its socket (with knee pointing ahead) with her weight evenly distributed between both legs. She planted her right hand and repeated the same forward weight shift with her left hand reaching toward the toys.

This went very well and completed the practice session with having worked the baby's muscles to practice the transition over both sides of her body.

With your own baby, be sure you aim to practice the same amount of time or repetitions both ways. This ensures that force distribution is even across the pelvis and low back, and it reduces the risk of asymmetries in musculature and across joints.

The shifts of arms, legs, and body weight as your baby moves from sitting to all fours provide excellent preparation for reciprocal arm and leg movement in the all-fours position—otherwise known as crawling. And before your baby is ready to actually crawl and advance their body, don't be surprised to see them experiment with rocking forward/backward and side to side. Back in the tummy-time activities, you were introduced to a great way to help them practice exactly that over the top of your leg, and that play is very much still beneficial to your child as they age, advance, and prepare to move more independently.

Remember to also consider and switch up the actual environment in which your child practices, more specifically, the type of surface (texture, firmness, and flat versus slope) upon which they experience weight-bearing and weight shifting. It may seem simplistic, but time and experience in various environments affords their muscles added challenges. Practice is essential in the process of building strength, stability, and coordination.

Other skills that will develop en route from being on all fours to standing are kneeling (bearing weight through the knees with the trunk extended) and half kneeling (bearing weight through one knee while the other leg flexes at the hip and knee to bear weight through the foot).

You were previously introduced to ways to practice kneeling using the Boppy pillow as well as the supportive caregiver; and, because this will naturally be worked through the process of transitioning to stand, we are not including additional activities that focus specifically on sustained play in either of these transitional, in-between postures. That is not to say such play does not offer strengthening, mobility, and control-increasing benefits to your child's body. Should your child assume these postures and sustain them for play, they can very much be beneficial. They can also run the risk of putting a great deal of pressure into your child's knee joints, hips, and back; and, as such, the alignment of their legs, pelvis, and spine should be monitored as you've been learning to do thus far.

From All Fours to Standing

This activity helps your baby use a support structure (in this case, a couch) to practice transitioning from being on all fours to kneeling, from kneeling to half kneeling, and from half kneeling to standing. In doing so your baby gets practice contracting muscles all the way around their torso, through their pelvic girdle and legs, to maintain stability, control, alignment, and balance as they transition from four points of contact on the floor to an upright stance on two points of contact.

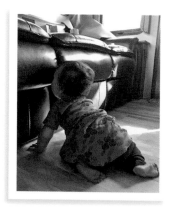

Be encouraged to pay attention to each step of the process as your baby works to extend their head, neck, upper back, arms, and torso, creating a wave of motion. You can actually observe how the baby transfers their energy, that wave of motion, through their muscles as they shift their torso over their hips and load their legs with weight. You'll see the wave continue as they press into the floor and coordinate rising to stand.

Pictured is an eight-month-old baby girl.

Baby is placed on all fours before a couch. She

extends her head and neck to view the colorful toys on the couch's surface.

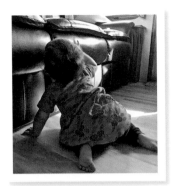

Baby leans her weight into her left side, pressing her left hand and knee into the floor. At the same time, she lifts her right arm toward the toys. As the baby reaches, her head and neck extend, her chest elevates, and her back extends in a wave of motion that lifts her torso more upright.

The next image is an overhead view in which we see baby's right hand grasping the edge of the couch, and her torso leaning to her left as she elongates her right side. Baby subtly bends her left elbow to help push her palm off the floor and engage her left hand in reaching for the surface first (and then the toys!) . . .

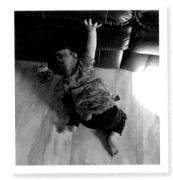

Baby looks up ahead of her as she brings both hands toward the surface of the couch. Her torso extends and rises as she works to bring her legs more directly underneath her. This asks a lot of the core muscles around her torso both above and below her pelvis. Her tummy and back muscles are all firing, and the muscles in her pelvic girdle, especially those between her legs that pull her thighs inward (her adductors), are all called upon in this seemingly haphazard fling upward.

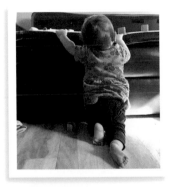

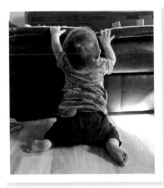

The next several images show baby transition herself vertically as she goes after the toys on the surface above her. As she seeks to go higher, she narrows her legs to kneel, bearing weight through her knees and feet.

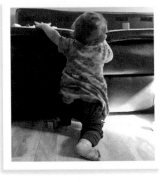

Here we see her reach her left hand toward a nearby toy, as she plants her left foot flatly on the floor, switching to a half-kneeling posture.

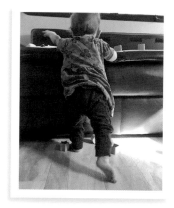

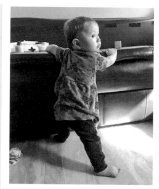

She then extends her hips and knees, pushing off the ball of her right foot to stand upright! She uses a wide stance for greater balance as she explores at this relatively high surface. Still motivated by the toys, we see her lean forward as she reaches with her left arm.

Baby turns to look behind her as her mom cheers her on. To give her more stability, she hooks her left arm onto the couch's surface and lowers her right heel. With this she can distribute her weight more evenly between her right and left sides.

As your baby practices this activity and develops greater strength and coordination between their arms, torso, and legs, over time you'll see better balance, smoother movements, and standing with less leaning of their body into the support surface for additional stability. You can also anticipate seeing their legs in a narrower base of support.

To work a broader range of your baby's muscles, you should vary the height of the support structure they are using to pull up. For example, you might start this activity by placing your baby in front of a relatively low piece of furniture such as an ottoman or even an overturned laundry basket (which is well stabilized by something so it won't slip or topple over on or with your baby), and later progress to using a higher structure such as a couch or coffee table, or even the wall. The next few images will help you to see the difference between one and the next. And in each of these images, the baby has preceded her stance position by crawling on all fours to the toy and pulling to stand as seen in the previous activity. This is pointed out to help you tie activities together so that you can create robust playtime experiences that are rich in exer-play (exercise + play) with the work well hidden and layered together so it doesn't feel like a big undertaking of different skills to practice or a long, daunting task for you or baby.

Next you see our Sunny girl at a low support surface, her toy music table, which is at the level of her hips (and is an example of a commonly seen standing toy out there for babies). To bring her face closer to the surface to play, in this example she has hinged her hips, bringing her trunk forward as she brought her bottom behind her to counterbalance her reach for the toy. She is resting atop her elbows and forearms as she activates the toy with her hands, and her feet and legs are a little greater than hip distance apart without rigid hyperextension at her knees, making this a pretty solid stance position. To those of you familiar with Foundation Training, this may look a little like a Founder. While there is nothing wrong with this hinge, the baby is still notably leaning into her arms for support, and the goal of standing is to do so with the muscles providing the body's stability as opposed to leaning into some external source of stability. That said, it is not uncommon for children to do this as they build their strength and skills.

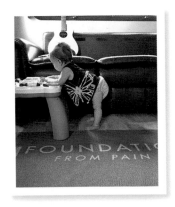

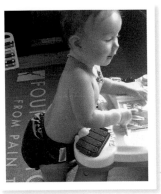

Here she is at the same age, using the same toy to practice standing. This time we see her with a narrower stance, leaning her abdomen into the surface as she is activating the toy with her hands *without leaning on her forearms*. This is another balance strategy children might exhibit and would be considered a progression if compared to how we saw another model standing at seven months, just a few activities back, leaning her chest and upper abdomen into the surface with a very wide stance. If you find that your baby habitually leans each time they play, you can try helping them to find more stability and better balance by widening their stance to give them a broader base of support.

On the next page we see the same baby, same toy, same play session, different view. I moved behind her and called her name to see if she could comfortably turn to look behind her without losing her balance. She did great. This shows how the same principles from earlier days carry over and apply—you can very simply guide your baby to

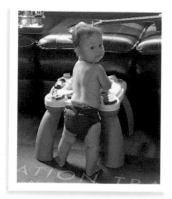

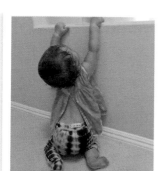

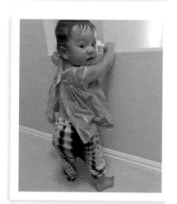

work on visual/auditory tracking to build stability and challenge their balance in this new upright position.

A wall can also be used as the support surface for transitioning to stand.

The next two images show the same baby, two months later at eleven months old, using a (low) wall to transition to stand. These were captured after she crawled to the wall and pushed through her legs, extended her head, neck, and trunk, and reached her arms up to plant her hands at the top of the wall (which happened to be well above her shoulder level).

This first image shows her starting to transition from kneeling on two limbs to initiating the forward advancement of her right leg to plant the foot to achieve a half-kneeling position. The in-between steps of the transition, pressing up from half kneeling and advancing her left leg, are not shown here.

Next we see her completed transition to standing. She is holding on with her hands, but not leaning any portion of her trunk into the surface. Her alignment from head to feet is strong as she looks over her shoulder and behind her at her mom who was calling her name.

While these images show the baby's hands at the top of this low wall, you can encourage your baby to transition similarly with their palms reaching forward and pressing flat into a wall.

At support surfaces and with caregivers, focal practice during this window of time remains centered around transitioning from the floor to more upright bipedal postures. As strength, control, and confidence continue to develop, expect to see your little one experimenting with how they hold and shift their weight.

Shifting weight from one foot to the other helps babies prepare their bodies for the next milestone task of "cruising," which is taking side steps at a support surface while holding on to the top of the surface. Cruising is a precursor skill to taking steps between nearby surfaces, which prepares babies for taking steps away from surfaces and walking.

Before we dive into guiding your baby in weight shifting, we first return to a few more activities that will help build necessary leg strength to better prepare your baby's body for those skills to come.

From Sitting to Standing, and Optimizing Standing

This activity helps your baby transition from sitting to standing with focus on their leg alignment throughout the transition and once in standing. It guides you to focus on their best posture for maximum stability and is a great activity for strengthening their legs while promoting their independence with standing using a support structure.

Seen here is a nine-month-old baby girl.

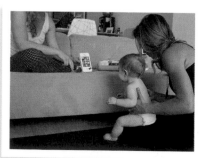

Note: You previously encountered a similar transition from sitting to standing activity with the same model when she was two months younger. This version is a progression and there are notable advances in her skill set that will be highlighted.

This activity begins with me placing the baby in a seated position atop my knees (as I sit in a low kneeling position in front of the couch). My hands are broad around the sides of her trunk with fingers gently pressing into her abdominal muscles and thumbs supporting along the backside of her torso.

I hold her with ample trunk stability and gently guide her to place her bottom firmly while also leaning her trunk forward so she hinges at her hips and brings her body weight forward. My hope is to position the baby slowly in a way that encourages her to place her feet flat on the floor below the weight of her upper body.

The baby starts out with her legs fairly well aligned, though subtly externally rotated, as shown by her knees pointing out to her sides, and her feet pressing more on their outer edges than sitting flat.

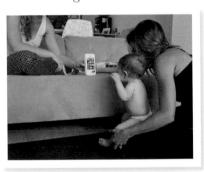

She's feeling a bit unstable and insecure in this position, as indicated by her arms being flexed close to her body and raised up for balance (as opposed to reaching for toys).

Mom sits cross-legged atop the couch. She's holding up a toy to entice her baby to stand and reach out toward the couch's surface.

I begin to address the baby's alignment from the ground upward, and I move in even closer to her to help her feel more secure. I encompass her feet from close to her ankle joints, with my pointer fingers to the top of her feet and my middle fingers around their sides, as my thumbs contour her lower legs from just below her knees. From here I'm ready to assist in rotating her legs inward and her feet standing flatly on the ground.

Baby girl keeps her elbows close to her torso as she begins to raise her hands toward the surface of the couch.

Sometimes less is more. I'm providing subtle, gentle guidance and giving her time to respond instead of rushing her into standing.

Baby is not 100 percent solid in her stability, though, and she changes her mind about reaching for the toys almost straightaway. She is seen next dropping her hands back down toward her lap with her elbows still flexed and upper arms held close to her torso. At this point she continues to keep her gaze on the toys at the couch's surface, so I think she is still tolerating this activity well and I continue onward.

I gently guide the rotation of the baby's legs inward, so that her knees point straight ahead and her feet follow, pointing more directly ahead as they sit flatly on the ground. As I do so, my forearms come higher up along the sides of her legs and torso. Despite how the image looks, I'm not actually in contact with those portions of her body; however, I remain close enough to lean in and provide more stability should the baby grow wobbly and show signs she

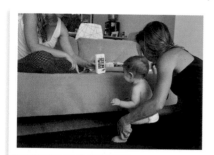

needs more contact for external stabilization and balance.

Believing the baby is ready for the next phase of this activity, I move my hands up her legs to her pelvis as I prepare to gently lift her bottom, while biasing her weight forward over her feet, to encourage her to press through her legs to stand.

Baby doesn't respond well to these changes, though, as shown by the unhappy expression on her face; her looking down at the floor instead of up at her mom and the toys; her arms swinging up again and retracting back to attain balance; her left leg rotating outward again; and her toes clawing at the ground. In addition, baby has started to move backward, away from the couch and up my leg.

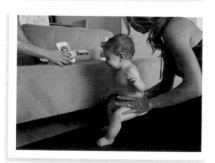

I respond to baby's anxiety by moving in closely again to offer comfort, stability, and more guidance.

This time I place my left arm across the baby's abdomen, and press my upper arm and shoulder against her shoulder, upper back, and provide a resting place for her to lean into with her head.

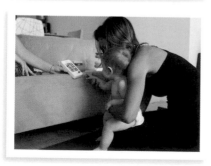

This "sandwiching" of the baby's core provides pressure higher up her chain and still affords me the ability to subtly guide her to hinge her torso forward at her hips so that her weight can press through her legs.

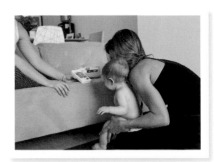

In response, her facial expression calms; she looks up with interest at her mom and the toys; she relaxes her arms; and her toes stop clawing at the ground. These are all indications that the baby feels more stable, comfortable, and confident.

As seen in the final image on the previous page, once my left arm is in place, I take the baby's right hand and guide it to reach for the toy her mom presents. This is actually a first step toward getting the baby to place both her hands on the couch.

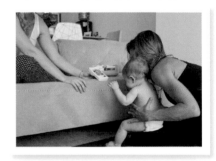

With the baby once again engaged and motivated by the toys, I move my hands back to her legs to improve upon their alignment—which I'm now able to more easily guide to a neutral position facing the couch.

As I transition to a broad grip on the baby's lower torso, with my pinky acting as a bumper to prevent her thighs from rolling back outwardly, the baby begins to reach for the couch's surface (and the toy).

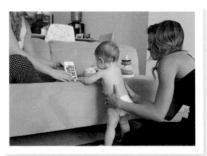

Baby extends her hips and knees, pushing herself up to standing as she plants her hands and forearms on top of the couch.

Mom pulls the toy back from the edge to draw the baby's attention forward. Baby responds by reaching her arms farther onto the couch to pursue the toy.

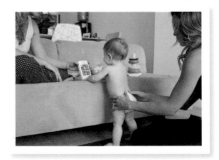

To encourage the baby to stand independently, I shift my hands down to her pelvis, with my

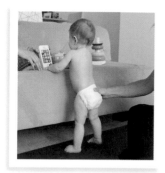

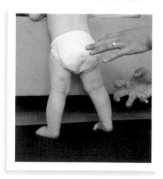

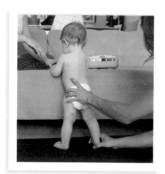

thumbs resting near the middle of her lower back. This reduces the level of support I'm providing.

The baby is fine with my hand shift, and she pulls her chest and shoulders back to stand up straighter. (In contrast, if she were feeling unsteady, she'd probably lean forward into the couch with her chest, abdomen, and/or hips.)

Having persuaded the baby to stand, and seeing that her torso is well aligned without leaning, I now refocus on her leg and foot alignment to improve her independence and balance in this position.

I decrease the support I'm providing at the pelvis to just one hand. Baby doesn't overtly protest, remaining engaged with a toy on the couch. However, her body provides subtle signs that she is less stable without my other hand. She starts leaning to her right; she brings her left elbow closer to her side; and she is elevating her shoulders—all in an effort to achieve greater balance. Also, it's hard to tell from the camera angle, but her right foot's big toe has started to claw at the ground in an effort to add stability. I remove my hands and prepare to switch the stability. (The middle shot on this page gives a view of this with my right hand representing the clawing action).

Still seeking stability, the baby leans her chest into the couch. She also continues to claw into the floor with her right foot.

I place my left hand across the baby's pelvis in a broad grip, with my thumb and middle finger gently compressing her hip joints on both sides, to help her feel more stable.

In an effort to help her flatten her foot without clawing, my right hand presses down on the top of her right foot, with my index and middle fingers gently straightening her big toe, and my thumb pushing down at the back base of her heel. My hand is steady and stable, moving with her as she wiggles and shifts her weight to find a place of balance and stability.

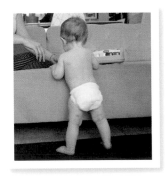

I remove both hands to see how the baby reacts. She responds better than before, no longer clawing at the ground. However, she continues leaning her chest into the couch.

This different camera angle makes it clear that the baby's feeling unbalanced enough to lean her chest into the couch as she tries to play with the toy. Her left hip is slightly rotated away from the couch compared to her right hip, as indicated by her left knee and foot pointing more outward than her right knee and foot.

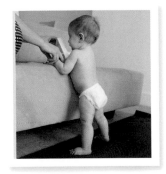

That said, overall, her current position isn't terrible. Her legs are just wider than hip distance apart with her hips over her knees over her ankles, and her feet are flat. This is a common occurance for new standers and those moving about, but next I'll make some adjustments to help the baby shift into a more neutral standing posture to optimize her play position for strengthening both sides of her body more equivalently.

Baby's hips should ideally be facing straight ahead, squared off with the surface before her. To help guide her to a more symmetrical position, I cup my right hand around her right hip, with my index finger in front of her hip bone and my thumb behind it, to provide her stability as I prepare to shift her left leg from its outwardly rotated position. I place my left hand around

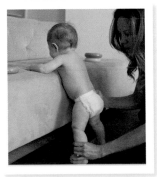

the baby's left ankle, with my pinky finger running along the edge of her foot to guide it to point ahead as it presses flat against the ground, and I guide her leg to step forward, inwardly rotating as it goes.

This results in less outward rotation of the whole left side of her body and her weight being more centrally distributed across both her upper and lower body.

I keep still for a few moments to let the baby feel these changes before I reposition my left hand, as shown in the next photo.

Note: Working in a low squatting position, as you see me do here, provides leverage for working with your low-to-the-ground baby, but the position will put compressive force on the blood vessels within your legs. FT Standing Decompression, a Founder, and/or Prone Decompression will help take pressure off the blood vessels and improve your alignment postactivity.

I place the two middle fingers of my left hand on the side of the baby's left hip, exerting gentle pressure that is countered by the same

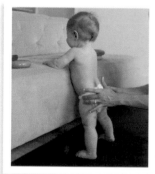

pressure of my right palm to her right hip, to help her maintain stability.

Baby responds with a posture that's ideal! Her posterior chain of muscles is activating superbly, helping her to pull up and back. Her head, neck, and back are beautifully aligned. Her hips and legs are facing forward with each joint well stacked and her weight split between both her feet, which are flat on the floor.

Since the baby has achieved stability with her stance, I now aim to challenge her slightly while at the same time making her feel increasingly more comfortable in this position.

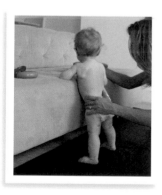

I remove my right hand from the baby's hip to grab a toy and move it around on the couch to the right of her position. My intent is to encourage her to track and potentially reach for it. At the same time, I increase the contact of my left hand across the baby's left hip, holding from the front to the back of her low torso and hip, to keep her feeling stable.

She responds by subtly rotating her body to the right and locking her eyes on the toy.

As this activity continues, I'll use one hand to provide an external source of stability for the baby, and the other to move the toy around and keep her engaged as she works on adapting her standing posture and maintaining balance while tracking and reaching to both sides. As you work on this with your child, the natural progression is to alternate which side of their body you provide stabilization from and eventually to remove any of your stabilization, periodically, to see how they respond (of course, stay near for safety).

As your baby develops greater strength, mobility, control, and balance via the experiences you provide and challenge them with, you can make this sort of activity more advanced—for example, by guiding your baby to widen their stance, shift their weight from side to side, and eventually use side steps to move from one side of the support surface to the other. To help your baby advance to that place, there are other ways you can help them strengthen their legs while standing at the support surface; that is, lowering from standing to squatting or sitting and then pressing through their legs back to standing. You'll find these activities in pages to come.

Before we progress to more advanced upright mobility skills, let's first take another look at the floor-to-stand transitioning activity with a slightly older baby.

Mature Floor-to-Stand Transitioning

This is included to show a baby who is close to one full year old moving with increased strength, control, and stability as she transitions to standing and prepares to move along the support surface. A few notable signs of her progress will be highlighted here to help you better track your baby's progression.

Pictured is an eleven-month-old baby girl.

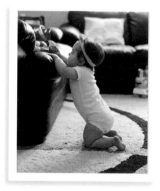

Baby has crawled to the couch and gone through a strong contraction of her posterior chain to rise up from all fours to kneeling with her hands to the support surface.

Her head, neck, and spine are in a neutral alignment with her trunk and pelvis hinged forward at her hips, subtly leaning forward over her legs with her weight supported through her knees. As she gazes at the toys on top of the couch, she is motivated to move and is seen here beginning to shift her right foot as she flexes her hip to advance her leg. She has subtly shifted her weight into her left knee so that she can unweight and swing her right leg up.

Baby brings her right leg forward, foot ahead of her, flat on the floor with knee and hip both bent about ninety degrees. She has effectively switched to half kneeling, with her weight now split between her right foot, her left knee, and her left foot's toes. Still well balanced, she keeps her left hand in place, pressing down more with her left forearm as she turns her neck and trunk subtly to her right, and reaches forward with her right hand to grab a toy block.

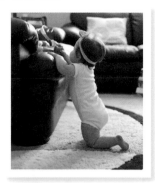

While continuing to get support from her hands pressing into the couch, the baby extends her hips and knees to rise to an upright stance. And not only has she risen, but she has also pivoted on her lead (right) foot farther to her right and she is pressing off the toes of her back foot to reach the toy in her right hand closer toward the other toys.

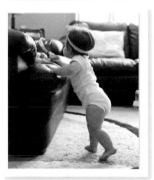

When she was younger, she needed help stabilizing her body to transition from kneeling to standing with strong posture. Now she manages to quickly stand on her own, without leaning her chest or abdomen into the surface for any extra stability. With this simple act she shows that she has developed sufficient strength, balance, and upright skills to no longer need such help (when transitioning between solidly stable environments such as the carpeted floor and the couch).

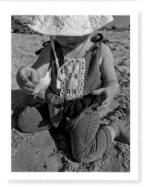

Note: This skill might absolutely present differently if she were transitioning between loose sand and a less stable item like a beach chair. This next image of Sunny at nearly twelve months exemplifies this to a degree.

At this stage Sunny had already developed the ability to transition from kneeling to standing at surfaces with great alignment; but here the fairly loose packed sand presented more challenge to her kneeling skills. We see she has her hands up passing a shell back and forth between them and, to give herself more stability, she has widened her seated base from kneeling into what is nearly a w-sit.

Since this one photo is not a full expression of her skills and she moved through this position into other positions quickly, it was not seen as a reason for concern.

This offers the gentle reminder to keep switching up the play environments and steadily observing skills as you go. Not everything needs immediate correction or redirection.

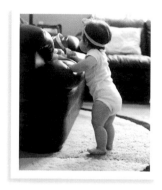

Baby steps her left leg forward, bringing it parallel with her right leg, and in a narrower stance. This narrow stance might have created instability at an earlier age, but now she has no trouble staying upright.

She extends her trunk and pelvis on her hips to stand tall, with her ears over shoulders over hips over knees over ankles over flat feet. She maintains both hands to the surface for support as she goes and she does not elevate her shoulders excessively (which is one form of compensatory muscle usage babies sometimes exhibit to create more stability when their core and legs are not giving them enough). What she's exhibiting here is excellent posture.

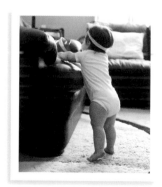

To be able to reach farther onto the couch, the baby pushes off the ball of her left foot, with her right foot flat on the floor and right hand on the couch giving her stability as she transfers her weight toward her right side.

At the same time, she lifts her left arm from the couch and reaches across the midline of her body for more toys. Crossing the body's midline is an advanced skill; and the baby's actions not only indicate that her core is strong and stable enough for her limbs to freely move and shift her body's weight, but also that her brain has developed sufficient coordination of her limbs to allow her to pursue an object with either hand.

When your baby can maneuver like this, celebrate! It means

they've successfully integrated numerous skills and strengths. Your baby is now in a great position to begin shifting their weight even more, to endeavor into cruising along the couch.

Before we review how to practice weight shifting and cruising with your baby, you'll find activities to help strengthen little legs and core, and build balance and coordination even further. Some activities work the muscles in the front and back of the legs more (such as this transitioning to stand activity) where other activities work the inner and outer legs more (side-stepping). Keeping such play variations in your baby's mix helps prepare them for the upcoming challenges that will rely on one leg holding their shifting weight.

From Standing to Squatting

APPROXIMATE AGE RANGE: 9–12 MONTHS

This activity encourages babies to stand before a support structure and lower their bodies into a squatting position, and then rise from the squat to stand again. This is great for strengthening the core and legs, increasing coordination and control of balancing the torso atop the legs, and bolstering the range of motion of all joints from the spine to the feet—all of which helps prepare the body for walking.

As you go, expect your baby's legs to gradually build strength to control both their descent and their rise back to stance. Until that strength and control are present, your baby will naturally lack the ability to control their body as they lower and will likely "plop" on their bottom at the lower end of their squat. You can encourage them to rise back to a support surface with strategic toy placement, or take the play a different direction and entice them to shift gears into practicing crawling by placing toys on the floor or another nearby surface in their environment.

Seen here is an eleven-month-old girl.

Note: We are capping the age range at the one-year mark simply because that is the focus of this book; however, the act of squatting is hugely beneficial for bodies of all ages. As your child's balance and stability increase, you'll progress this activity by challenging them to squat away from support structures, in "free space."

Baby stands before a couch with toys on it. She already has a green block in her right hand but is reaching into a red bucket to grab a second block with her left hand.

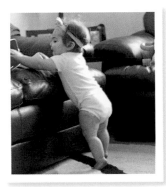

She has good alignment and balance overall. It wouldn't be ideal for her to spend extended playtime on her toes or for her chest to remain leaning into the couch, but in this case these aren't signs of instability, simply the result of her need to reach forward to grab the toy she's after at the bottom of the bucket.

Baby successfully retrieves a yellow block.

Now that she has a colorful prize in each hand, with her mom's (off-camera) encouragement asking her to "tap tap tap the toys together," the little girl has decided to remove all her support from the couch and lower herself to play.

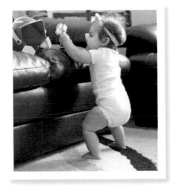

She retracts her left arm as she resumes flat feet and shifts her bottom back and down, aligning her torso and pelvis upright over her legs. She then bends her hips, knees, and ankles and lowers into a squat.

She achieves a beautiful low squat position.

Her alignment from head to feet is strong and steady, her raised arms adding stability to her descent.

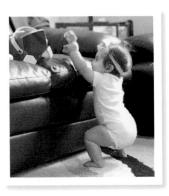

Baby's spine is showing the solid start of her lower back's curve (called lumbar lordosis). The mobility that comes with this curve will continue to develop strength and control over the coming months and this is important because of what it contributes to lower body movements, including walking.

Her feet remain flat against the ground and her knees are at a roughly ninety-degree angle, tracking over her feet, which is great.

Note: As a general rule, your baby's knees shouldn't go far forward beyond their feet, or go widely out to their sides. You can use your hands to adjust your baby's positioning anywhere from their trunk to their hips to their legs, just as you have practiced with the sit-to-stand transitioning.

Though not shown here, the baby can't maintain the squatting position for very long and soon plops down on her bottom to inspect her successfully captured treasures. We encourage this playtime so she feels successful, having reached and grabbed what she was after. Not only does her body benefit from the task of transitioning her weight, but also reaching, grasping, and manipulating tiny objects in her hands provides fantastic fine motor–boosting benefits as well.

After she's had a chance to play with her toys, her mom places new toys on the couch and encourages the baby to stand back up. There are many toys and games you can creatively engage with to encourage more squatting play. Nature allows for a wonderful opportunity for squatting to inspect flowers, animals, bugs, rocks, and so much more. The idea is to get your tot moving into, out of, and through their squats.

The act of lowering into a squatting posture and then rising to standing serves to contract and lengthen various muscles in the lower portion of the body, making them stronger . . . and ultimately helping better prepare the body for other skills such as shifting weight, side-stepping (aka "cruising"), and walking.

From Standing to Sitting

This activity is one step beyond the previous activity of squatting but requires a bit more control that babies develop as they gain more strength. This activity encourages your baby to transition from standing before a support structure to sitting. Lowering their body with slow control challenges and strengthens their muscles further, which helps carry over more strength and control to skills from crawling to walking.

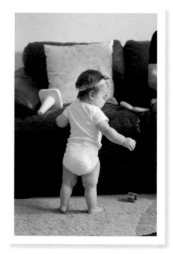

Seen here is an eleven-month-old girl.

While standing in front of a couch, she spots a toy on the floor. Her attention is piqued and she is motivated to move. *Hello, purple star. I see you down there, and I want you!*

As her left hand presses into the couch giving her support, her right hand begins to reach for the toy.

Her hips and knees flex and lower, with her feet planted flat on the ground.

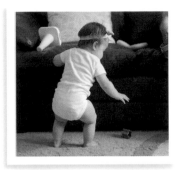

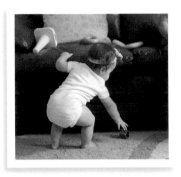

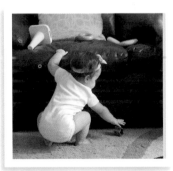

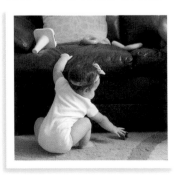

She hinges her torso forward as she bends her hips and knees to further lower herself. In doing so, she pushes her bottom farther behind her, which serves to counterbalance reaching toward the toy.

As she continues her descent into squatting, hinging her torso over her legs and driving her bottom behind her, we see her begin to widen the position of her legs (as seen in the third photo on this page with her knees starting to point subtly out to her sides and her torso beginning to dip between them).

In the final image on this page we see her bottom is almost on the floor and her right hand is nearly touching the toy. Her torso is farther between her legs, and she'll need to shift it more to her right to finally grab the toy.

On the next page we see her lean her weight over her right thigh and drop to the floor in a ring-sitting position with her left thigh elevated.

This move finally brings the baby close enough to grasp the purple star.

Success! With the star securely in her right hand, the baby removes her left hand from the couch and fully settles onto the floor, extending her trunk to sit upright atop her strong ring-sitting base.

She then starts to play with transferring the star between her hands, as she rotates her head, neck, and torso to her right to triumphantly engage with her mom and show her what she's got.

Note: In this example, the baby was enticed to move to her right. However, your baby should ideally spend relatively equal amounts of time playing on either side of their body, so be sure to strategically arrange your play to encourage movement in both directions. This will challenge different muscles and provide different visual perspectives.

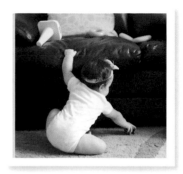

This was a great show of skills from this baby, and, from where she is last pictured, her mom would do well to encourage any one of a number of different complementary ongoing movements in this play session.

She could encourage the baby to move toward her (off-camera to baby's right), which would entail the baby shifting her trunk and body weight farther over her right leg to achieve all fours and crawling.

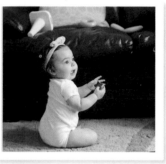

The mom also could encourage the baby to rotate her head, neck, and trunk to her left and shift her weight over her left leg in the same manner.

Or she could encourage the baby to return to an upright stance at the couch, which would entail shifting her trunk and body weight forward over her lap and then transitioning through kneeling, half kneeling, and up to standing.

From Standing to Half Kneeling

APPROXIMATE AGE RANGE: 10–12 MONTHS

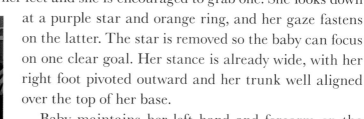

his activity shows a baby transitioning from standing before a support structure to lowering her body into a half-kneeling position. This is another, slightly more mature, way to strengthen babies' legs and bolster the control and range of motion of their cores and legs to help prepare their bodies for walking.

Seen here is an eleven-month-old baby girl.

Baby stands with both hands pressing into a couch. Two toys are placed by her feet and she is encouraged to grab one. She looks down

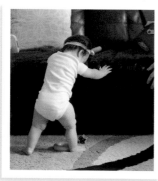

at a purple star and orange ring, and her gaze fastens on the latter. The star is removed so the baby can focus on one clear goal. Her stance is already wide, with her right foot pivoted outward and her trunk well aligned over the top of her base.

Baby maintains her left hand and forearm on the couch for stability as she begins to flex her hips, knees, and ankles to lower. She drops her right hand between her legs as she lowers, widening her stance by slightly abducting her hips while subtly flexing her spine as she curves her neck to look down at the target toy.

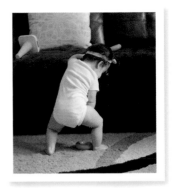

Bending her right hip and knee to get lower still, the baby balances herself using her left hand pressing the couch and her right foot planted flatly on the floor, as she drops her left knee to the ground and props on her lower leg and toes. This half-kneeling position lets the baby reach the toy, but she is unable to grasp it without making a few last adjustments.

Baby extends her right knee to shift her bottom back and create space to shift her arm, raking with her hand and grasping the toy. She counterbalances this move by subtly leaning her weight more into her left hip and toes.

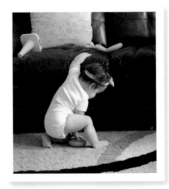

This activity may strike you as very similar to the two previous; however, the half-kneeling position works your baby's muscles differently than squatting or sitting down. These variations provide important practice for a wide range of your baby's developing muscles and help better prepare them for balancing the weight of their trunk over two legs as well as biasing it over one.

Before we progress into activities that further challenge this concept of biasing the body's weight over one leg (which is a major leap toward taking steps and walking), let's first consider one more skill that entails multiple points of contact to balance and move the body's weight.

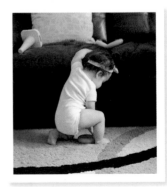

Crawling/Climbing Up Stairs

APPROXIMATE AGE RANGE: 12–18 MONTHS

Crawling up stairs is similar to crawling but with a vertical component that makes it a bit like rising from the floor to an upright posture. A series of pulling and pushing with the arms and legs occurs to advance the body.

This skill is typically one that babies will attempt if their environments include stairs and the movement is encouraged. Walking up and down stairs isn't a skill they develop and refine until well into their second year, though, so it's not going to be focal in this book. Nor will descending stairs be presented, except to mention that the skill can present differently from kiddo to kiddo. Some babies will look over their shoulders and cautiously back down (as our Sunny girl did, which you can see her debating doing in the first image), and others will turn around, sit on their bottoms, and scoot down the stairs using their hands and feet.

If crawling up and over items and/or ascending stairs is something your child endeavors during their first year, it offers their limbs yet another opportunity to strengthen and enhance their movement control.

Pictured here is an eleven-month-old baby girl.

The hands advance together to the next step, followed by one knee, as the other leg extends to push the body forward.

In the next image, the previously seen back (right) leg flexes, advances to the next step, and slides to the front of the step where the baby presses it into the surface for stability as she advances her arms and begins to extend her now rear (left) leg.

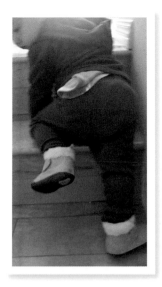

Alternating legs is the goal, but as a baby first starts applying crawling skills to ascending stairs, it's not uncommon for a child to repeatedly lead with the same leg. So, if you're going to encourage them to try this skill, you can certainly guide them toward symmetry (think here: with your hands to your baby's trunk to provide stability, similar to how you have done during all-fours-related activities) as you keep a close position to protect their safety.

As they go up the stairs, be sure to position yourself behind them so that you are close enough to catch them should they lose balance. As they go down the stairs, you want to be in front of them. You should always be on the lower step to prevent any tumbling down the stairs.

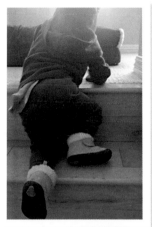

To help your child advance their crawling and climbing skills in prep for stairs, you can play with creating obstacles around the floor at home to encourage them to climb up and over things, such as couch cushions, pillows, or weighted laundry baskets (and if you're seeking more options, you can even order foam climbing and crawling play sets complete with wedge-shaped ramps, cylindrical bolsters, elevated blocks, and arches). Essentially, create a baby obstacle course to add more structure to their floor play.

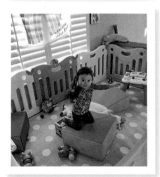

Practice of this nature will serve to further enhance a child's core to hip to leg strength, mobility, stability, and control as well as increase their independent movement within their environment.

Shifting Weight While Standing

APPROXIMATE AGE RANGE: 9–12 MONTHS

This activity helps your baby practice shifting their weight from one foot to the other, as they move their center of gravity over their feet while remaining balanced in an upright stance at a support surface. It's performed by encouraging them to keep one hand on the surface for stability while reaching out with their other hand for toys.

This enhances your baby's balance while standing, strengthens their coordination between their core and legs, and helps prepare them for subsequent activities such as cruising and taking steps away from a support surface.

Seen here is an eleven-month-old baby girl.

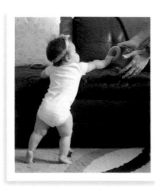

Baby stands in front of a couch and reaches to place a toy ring into a bucket, pushing herself up and forward by pressing her toes and the balls of her feet into the ground.

As she does so, her torso leans forward, with her weight biased toward her right leg and subtly hinging over her hip joints. Her head and neck are extended, pulling slightly backward to counterbalance some of her body weight during this weight shift.

She is seen pressing against the couch with her left

hand and forearm. This gives her extra stability as she reaches beyond her base of support.

Baby's right hand releases the ring, her arm still fully outstretched.

Her weight remains biased to her right, but she's advanced her left foot forward (her legs now more parallel in their hip sockets).

Baby's right arm pulls back as she begins shifting her torso more upright, centering her weight more evenly between her left and right legs.

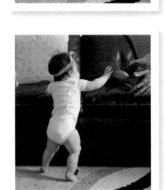

After this photo was taken, her dad moved to the other side of the couch to offer toys from her left side. This led her to shift her reach, and her weight, over to the opposite side, thereby ensuring the activity worked both sides of her body.

For your baby to master weight shifting, they need more strength and coordination in and between their legs and their core to figure out their balance. This must happen before they can coordinate becoming mobile (cruising). If your baby is not freely engaging in this play by ten to eleven months, work on helping them to build more comfort and confidence as you mindfully provide stability to their torso while they stand at a surface like the couch or a coffee table. Revisit the hand placement and stabilization used with sit to stand transitions. Engross them in a play task that involves reaching for toys as you can naturally encourage shifting weight with reaching.

To take their movement skills to the next step, cruising, they will need this seemingly simple skill of weight shifting to be performed on repeat. The difference is the addition of actually lifting one leg while solidly holding their weight on the other leg (with hand support), and then abducting (stepping to the side, leg moving away from the body's midline) the lifted leg to create a wider stance. From there, the leg that has stepped outward has the body's weight shifted over top of it so that the previous weight-bearing leg can now lift and step closer (adducting, moving closer to the body's midline). Repeating this sequence results in cruising, which is the next activity presented.

Cruising

This activity leads your baby to take side steps while using a support structure to remain balanced, which is called cruising. This is a big leap in their independent mobility, and an important one that strengthens the muscles of your baby's hips, improves the coordination between your baby's core and legs, and bolsters their ability to stay balanced while moving on their feet, all of which helps prepare them for independent walking.

Your baby will be ready to tackle this progression of skills once they've developed strength with the previous several activities, especially "Shifting Weight While Standing."

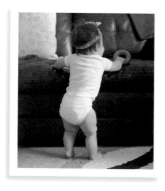

Seen here is an eleven-month-old baby girl.

Baby begins at a couch with her hands and forearms pressing into it. This gives her the external stability she needs to successfully step from side to side.

Her legs are close together, providing a relatively narrow base of support. Her torso is subtly hinging forward at her hips as she leans into the surface, a toy ring in her right hand, observing the bucket her dad is presenting off to her right.

Dad encourages the baby to "come place the ring into the bucket."

In response, she keeps her left foot planted flat on the floor, but starts her right foot rolling toward its outer edge (as shown by her big toe rising, on the previous page). She begins opening her torso and hips to her right as she prepares to step her right leg outward toward the bucket.

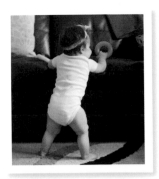

Keeping her left hand and right forearm on the couch, the baby steps her right leg toward the bucket, creating a wide stance.

Stabilizing herself with her right leg and forearms, she raises her left foot and draws it closer to her right leg.

Baby plants her left foot flatly next to her right, resuming a narrow base of support. She takes a still moment to gaze at the bucket. As she does so, her brain is subconsciously processing where she is in relation to the bucket and what she needs to do to reach it.

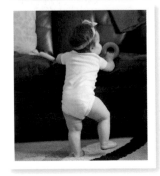

Baby shifts her weight into her left hip and flexes her right hip and knee to step closer toward the bucket.

During this phase of single leg balance, she has both forearms on the surface for extra stability; and her right hand is seen beginning to lift the ring.

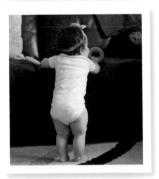

On the next page, baby plants her right foot flatly on the floor, with her toes pointed toward the bucket. She begins to shift her weight to her right leg again as she lifts the ring farther and her dad brings the bucket closer.

Baby pushes off the ball of her left foot and toes of her right (her left forearm still in contact with the couch for stability as she goes) to propel her outstretched right hand. In a moment she'll achieve her goal and drop the ring into the bucket.

As with every other activity, be diligent to perform this with your baby toward both sides to challenge the

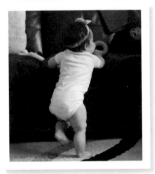

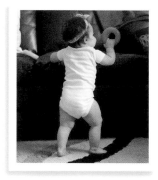

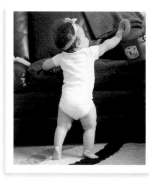

muscles on both sides of your baby's body. This will help prepare your baby for the challenge of walking with balance in any direction.

Once your baby becomes skilled at sidestepping, they'll increase their speed and free their arms more for increased reaching for toys as they cruise along a single support structure. This means they are ready to graduate to stepping from one support structure to another, which requires lifting a hand from one surface and planting it on an adjacent surface. To help prepare them for that leap, you may find it helpful to practice cruising along surfaces that offer an L shape (such as a sectional couch or a couch with an ottoman pushed up next to it, or even a playpen that has its walls at right angles) as that closeness is less daunting than a wide step, say, between a couch and a table.

Stepping Between Support Structures

This activity encourages your baby to step from one support structure to another (in this case, an end table and a couch). It builds muscle strength, balance, and coordination; and, because it gets your baby moving from one spot to another, it is excellent preparation for walking. It employs the same skills as cruising but adds the ability to pivot and change directions.

Seen here is an eleven-month-old baby girl.

Baby stands facing an end table, her hips squared with the surface ahead of her. She grips the table with both hands for support and plants her feet flatly on the floor in a wide stance for additional stability.

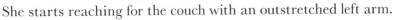

Dad (off-camera) encourages the baby to move over to the nearby couch on her left (which is on the right side of the photo). Baby rotates her head, shoulders, torso, and hips as she begins opening her stance toward her left in preparation for more weight shifting.

She starts reaching for the couch with an outstretched left arm.

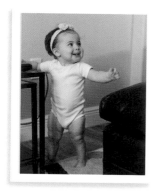

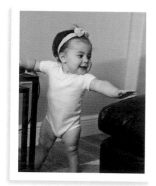

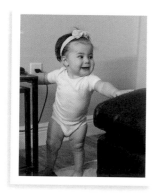

While keeping her right hand on the end table to maintain balance, the baby shifts her weight to her left leg and reaches farther. Her left hand is now nearly in contact with the couch.

Baby's right foot takes a small sideways step to join her left leg on the rug. While still keeping her right hand on the end table for balance, she lands her left hand on the couch. She's now in a great position to shift her weight more toward her left, let go of the end table, and step fully to the couch.

This session shows just one of many ways to perform this activity. It can be done from a variety of positions and using a variety of support structures.

For example, instead of positioning your baby directly in front of the furniture, start your baby off across the room from it. Place a small toy on the furniture, and encourage your baby to crawl to it, transition from crawling to standing, and then reach for the toy. Once your baby has the toy in hand, place a toy bucket or a bowl on an adjacent piece of furniture (close enough to reach it with a wide step), and encourage your baby to cruise to it with successive side steps until they're able to drop the toy into the bucket.

As another example, instead of having your baby use pieces of furniture as support structures, try getting your baby to cruise along the wall of a room. For instance, you could position your baby to stand on one wall and press their hands into it for stability. You could then hold a toy at their eye level at a neighboring wall (visualize a right angle) and encourage them to step to you while using each wall for support.

Be creative and have fun with this activity, which offers your baby numerous ways to develop the strength, balance, and confidence that will eventually ready them to take steps away from support structures.

Introducing a Toy Walker

Once your baby has mastered cruising and stepping between adjacent support surfaces, introducing a toy walker into your child's repertoire can offer another form of assistance—a sort of mobile stability—to help them transition to the immensely important stage of walking independently.

This form of play may be introduced before your child is willing to take steps from a surface to you or between caregivers. Taking steps forward as opposed to sideways, like when cruising, uses different muscles and is a new challenge to baby's strength and balance.

The walker-related activities are being included because these sorts of toys have grown very popular and common, so we feel a sense of duty to include a little guidance.

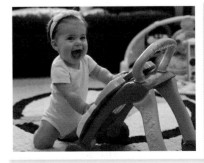

This activity introduces your baby to a walker, which we encourage you to think of as an assistive development tool. These colorful toys are something your baby is likely to have fun pushing around, and they can also be used to play in a variety of positions that serve to strengthen their body for walking; that is, kneeling and squatting down to play and grab objects from the floor.

To clarify, the walker utilized in these activities is NOT the kind that sits your baby in a saddle in the center of it. Rather, it is an upright, four-wheeled walker with a push bar for your baby's hands and, ideally, a wheel-control feature that allows you to put on some resistance or stop their roll.

Note: Some walkers have wheels that always roll freely. Other versions, such as this one, include controllers (notice the inner side of the rightmost wheel) to optionally adjust the speed of the rolling so the toy doesn't move faster than the baby can handle, or to set whether the toy can roll backward, or whether it can roll at all. These extra tools allow you to adjust the walker's mobility to match your baby's walking skills. In addition, different walkers have varying heights and angles to their handlebars, so feel encouraged to shop around and test out different walkers before you settle on the one that's the best fit for your child.

Most simply stated: I wouldn't advise a lightweight, freely rolling walker for a child who is only just starting to endeavor to take steps. This is because their body weight leaning into the toy, without resistance, could result in them catapulting forward and putting excessive stress on various muscles, joints, and ligaments, or experiencing an upsetting fall.

These seemingly basic beginnings allow your baby's body to learn the physical details of the walker, and to develop muscle memory for how to most effectively hold it, lean against it, and stand with it. These learned skills help your baby to develop a sense of being strong and in control of the walker, bolstering their self-confidence. This will be of great use to them when they're ready to play with an unrestrained walker that rolls when they put their weight into it.

Seen here is a nearly twelve-month-old baby girl.

For the baby's first intro to her walker, she is placed kneeling in front of it, as seen in the first photo on the next page. She's clearly very excited by this new addition to her world and uses her hands to explore its colorful surface.

This is time well spent, letting her develop a level of comfort with her new toy; and, because she is also practicing tall kneeling, her core and glutes get some good work (small example of a way to sneak beneficial muscle challenges into your baby's daily play).

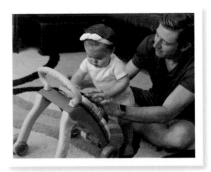

Dad sits with the baby to get her more comfortable with the walker, taking her through a sit-to-stand transition from his lap (not pictured) and then helping her explore the various play options built into its front face panel. His body forms a ring around her to make her feel safe while she focuses all her attention on exploring the details of the walker.

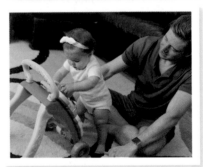

The shift from the first to the second image is subtle, but significant. Dad leans back and leaves baby girl to it. Her posture is tall and strong as she further explores the toy independently.

Another subtle shift is seen here to create a play setup that can help to take the baby closer toward being confident playing with the walker on her own. The wheel lock is on and the walker is pushed into the back of the couch so that any pressure exerted by the baby's leaning doesn't result in it moving.

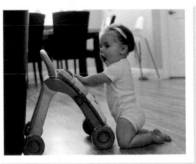

Baby has crawled up to the walker and assumed a tall kneeling position in front of it (once again hiding other exercise-play into the mix by strategically placing the item of interest in such a way that motivates the baby to move to it and explore).

If you're wondering if proceeding this slowly and carefully to acclimate your baby to a walker is overly cautious, keep in mind that your baby is used to getting support from relatively stable objects such as tables, couches, beds, and your body. Because the walker is on rolling wheels, it will obviously provide your baby with more unstable challenges than they've previously experienced, so it makes sense to approach it with (cheesy pun acknowledged) baby steps.

Starting in front of the walker with the toy panel can serve to intrigue your baby with this new and challenging apparatus—and ready them for standing behind it, holding the push bar, and eventually walking.

These next images capture some simple ways to help nudge them along.

The walker's wheels are locked and the baby is placed in standing behind the walker, with both her hands on the handlebar.

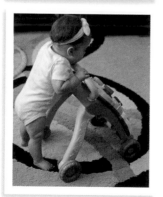

The dad then steps away to give the baby some independence, and she looks across the room at him, almost unsure of what to do.

Dad suggests to her: "Look at the fun toys!" . . . and she does so . . . by leaning forward with a subtle hinge of her hips. At the same time she subtly elevates her shoulders toward her ears.

While not definitive, this elevation (produced by the recruitment of accessory muscles, potentially to add more stability) could be a sign she's not feeling completely stable standing this way.

In an effort to steadily bolster her comfort and stability, the walker is moved to the middle of the room . . . where the baby's mother sits cross-legged on the floor. It's now Mom who keeps the walker from rolling.

Mom lovingly encourages her baby to come over and see the toy, to play with her. Her face is joyful as she verbally addresses her daughter and cheers her on.

Baby quickly complies by crawling over and beginning to transition to an upright stance from the other side of the toy.

Note: With this, her mom has nicely layered in some additional exercise-play by enticing her daughter to crawl and then rise to stance, which she does through a solid tall kneeling to half kneeling to standing transition at the toy.

As this play continues, the baby grows increasingly confident standing behind the walker.

After receiving lots of encouragement from her parents and supportive play exposure, the baby grows increasingly confident standing behind the walker, and she seems more ready to start playing with the walker on her own again.

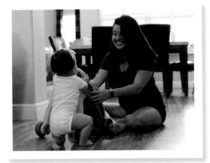

As you approach this next big stage in your baby's physical progression, it's a good idea to also spend some time initiating walking with your baby as you stabilize their torso, shoulders, arms, or hands (both at first, progressing to one). You can look ahead to the activity "Walking with You" for more guidance.

Starting to Use the Walker

This activity leads your baby to start using the walker to actually take steps to walk.

Your baby is ready for this if they've demonstrated stability with previous floor-to-standing activities (which developed greater strength and control in the fronts and backs of their legs), cruising (which bolstered the inner and outer muscles of their hips), and the previous activity (which built familiarity with the walker).

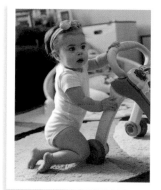

Seen here is a nearly twelve-month-old baby girl.

Baby crawls over and kneels by the walker, which has been placed in the middle of the room and positioned to roll freely. Because it's on a carpeted floor, there's naturally more traction to slow its rolling (as opposed to, say, a tiled or bare wood floor), making it easier for the baby to manage the toy.

Baby holds on with both hands and transitions to half kneeling as she gets ready to rise and start pushing the walker.

With her mom's encouragement, she presses up through her right leg and starts to extend and pull her left leg forward to advance it as she rises. In addition, the baby presses her hands into the walker to create additional stability for her shifting weight.

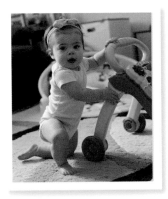

These well-coordinated moves occurring simultaneously in multiple planes of motion—rotating, flexing, extending, pressing forward—are signs of the baby's maturing movement skills. She has refined them and moves with increasing balance, control, and purpose, as opposed to just flinging herself upright without control (as a younger baby would). This is typically the result of a baby spending months building adequate strength up and down the spine, in the core, neck, arms, and legs; and developing the ability to more smoothly coordinate the different parts of their body. These mature movements show that a baby is ready to start the next challenge of moving with the walker . . . which is what our model here does next.

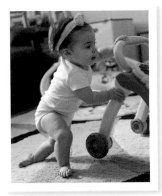

Pure joy! Baby has a wide beaming smile of excitement and pride as she successfully rises to full stance, placing both hands atop the push bar, and begins to shift her weight forward.

She leans her weight ahead of her in a way that essentially causes her to fall forward. As the walker provides stability that "catches" her, rolling forward slowly thanks to the traction of the carpet, the baby finds balance and begins to advance her legs to continue moving forward.

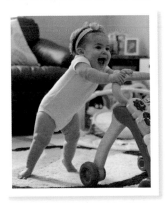

Baby's walking skills will advance as she practices using the walker, gains more strength, and more effectively engages and coordinates her muscles—especially those in her posterior chain, the extensor muscles in her back and hips.

Caregivers and parents should expect to see their baby develop an increasingly upright posture and a more stable core from which they are more controlled and freely move their arms and legs.

Continuing on with practice of walker use, let's focus on the baby's "gait" (manner of walking) as she works to coordinate steps.

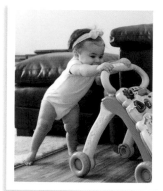

After starting off on a carpeted surface, the baby pushes the walker forward onto the bare wood floor. Because this surface is harder, more slippery, and provides less traction for the walker's wheels, she proceeds more cautiously on it. Fully stretching her arms ahead of her, she grips the push bar with both hands. She then begins what looks like a bit of an awkward gait but is common for new walkers.

As adults we perform reciprocal walking by moving our legs and arms at the same time in opposite directions. In contrast, we see this baby step forward with her left leg, then advance her right leg to meet the left. It's not until her two legs are side by side that she steps forward with her left leg again.

As for her arms, they're fixed in an elevated position with her hands gripping the walker. She has no arm swing at all, let alone the reciprocal swing adults use. (Note: What she does have, though, is pressure through her arms into her upper back, giving her muscles feedback that helps her find more stability in her trunk over top of her mobile, advancing legs.)

If your baby starts off similarly, please feel assured that this is normal. It's just a temporary phase until your baby figures out how to achieve the control and coordination necessary for advancing steps and reciprocal walking.

Their self-initiated play practice will ideally include periods where one leg is the lead and periods where the other leg advances first. As they progress, all their efforts are giving their trunk feedback as well as their legs, with strength being built as the baby plays, adding to their coordination, control, and balance.

Parents should be encouraged to layer in playful challenges by placing toys along the floor and other low surfaces that can be within their baby's reach.

The seemingly simple act of pausing their walk to squat, reach for a toy (don't expect them to remove both hands from the walker at first), and then recover their balance and return to standing, before resuming walking, provides even more dynamic learning potential. And this sort of play can absolutely help to keep the baby engaged for longer periods of play, allowing for more endurance-building potential.

Continuing to look down, as if checking on her footing as she scans the floor ahead of her steps, the baby advances her left leg forward again.

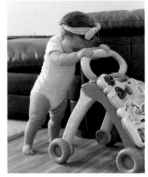

At the same time, she pivots and opens her right hip as she prepares to swing that leg forward.

As she goes, the baby is leaning a portion of her body weight forward into the walker, which is helping her to learn to grade her movement as it keeps her from falling.

Note: Keeping her eyes down may add additional stability for how the baby feels moving over her legs.

This is not a conscious/cognitive plan for her to check her footing; she's simply taking in the whole scene as she moves toward a specific toy across the room that is serving to excite her to keep moving however she can. And she's basically figuring out how she can be on the go, with the push toy helping her by taking some of the weight and forward momentum out of the equation.

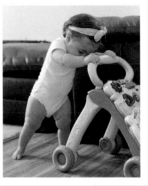

Also worth noting: When a baby is looking down, their visual path, eye muscles, head, and neck all orient downward as opposed to being more vertically upright and looking out at the path ahead of them.

Watch how your baby progresses with this. As they gain more strength and control of their body atop their legs, expect that they will begin to extend their neck more strongly and maintain a more vertical alignment of their neck and head atop their strong torso—with their eyes out over the horizon instead of diverted down. This will build to their learning to scan the room around them instead of just the floor right ahead of them.

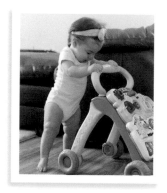

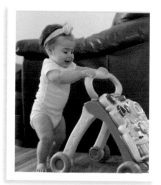

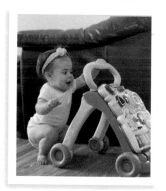

Baby advances her right leg again, bringing it beside her left. She's not yet ready to perform the more mature movement of placing her right leg a step ahead of her left; but she continues to look down, studiously watching her body, the floor, her toy, and she is steadily taking in lots of sensory-rich feedback that will help her to get there.

Another promising sign is she's not falling forward as much. Instead of fully stretching out her arms, she's now bending her elbows, holding her walker closer to her body, and standing more upright.

Her dynamic learning and improvements are becoming visible. And they'll become increasingly obvious as she continues practicing walking.

Now that she's had some time to practice, she's standing closer to the walker and holding herself relatively straight and tall, with solid head-to-foot alignment and more relaxed shoulders and arms.

She's still checking her footing but has replaced her previous intense staring at the floor with a more casual and self-assured downward glance.

Baby shows off her increasing control by going into a deep squat to closely inspect her toy. This image captures one of the perks of this sort of toy—the built-in strengthening potential it holds by enticing a baby to lower down to play with its colorful built-in features.

She exhibits a strong squat with her feet flat, thighs almost parallel to the floor, trunk tall, shoulders level, head upright and neutrally aligned, AND she is only using one hand to steady herself.

Note: This hand release is a sign that your baby is ready for you to make play more dynamic and challenging by strategically placing toys around their environment on surfaces of varying heights to encourage rising up on toes as well as lowering down to the floor and rising back up to standing with the walker.

Baby rises from her squat, using strong legs extending straight down from her hips. At the same time, she fully stretches her arms out to grasp the handlebar and push the walker forward.

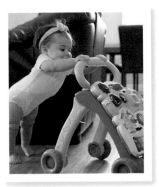

These are a great few images showing the progression of her weight shift and work toward finding herself upright with her center of gravity balanced over her feet without the walker going too far ahead.

The walker rolls more quickly on the hard wood surface than it did on the carpet. We can see the contours of the baby's abdominal muscles and the base of her ribs jut out as she works to gain stability while the walker and momentum are taking her forward. She continues her efforts, learning dynamically as she goes, and is seen here starting to push off the ball and big toe of her left foot, preparing to swing her left leg forward in an effort to keep up with the walker.

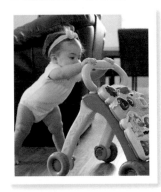

Baby advances her left leg, planting her left foot flat ahead of her, and gets ready to advance her right leg. On the surface, this doesn't look very different from what she did previously.

In a moment, though, she is going to show a huge leap in her walking skills.

Baby shifts position, bending her elbows to get closer to the walker and stand with a taller posture, with shoulders stacked over hips, knees, and feet.

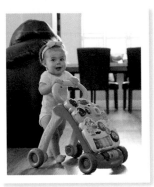

Instead of placing her right leg directly beside her left one, as she did previously, this time she moves her right leg a full step past her left.

This is huge. Baby has found enough stability in her core to trust her center to be balanced as she steadily advances her limbs—one beyond the other—in reciprocally alternating fashion.

When your baby achieves this moment, celebrate it! They are so close to walking independently!

Walking with You

Congrats!!! You've reached the activity we are choosing to mark the end of the first year. This might seem a surprising final activity as the obvious assumption might be to culminate with independent walking. We are leaving you with a caregiver-involved activity because not all babies are on the same timeline with reaching this point; and while the approximate age range for this one is eleven-plus months, some will begin closer to nine months and others closer to fifteen months. Providing your baby this guidance can help their skills develop.

For the sake of strength, stability, coordination, balance, and building a solid foundation in which to move forth beyond your baby's first year, independent walking is not something you should rush. Taking steps with support is a wonderful leap closer toward walking independently that allows for more bonding as you provide security and help your baby build the confidence and readiness to take steps away from any support into free space . . . and then continue those steps to walk.

Like everything else you've learned thus far, this is not an exclusive skill to work on by itself once you reach a certain point. Rather, at just about the same time your baby is developing skills using a toy walker, they should also be encouraged to begin taking steps with you, as well as continue to practice cruising and transitioning from floor and sitting to standing. Depending on the strength and coordination of your baby's core and legs, you can provide additional stability, security, and confidence by holding them at their torso, shoulders, arms, or hands. As a general rule, holding closer to their core (i.e., shoulders or ribcage as seen here) gives more stability and further from their core (i.e., hands) provides less.

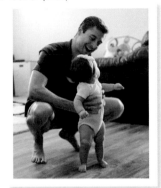

Seen here are a nearly twelve-month-old girl and our daughter on her first birthday.

Note: For the sake of transparency, and in supportive solidarity with any of you out there who may be stressing that your child is not walking before they turn one, we'd like to share that both these darling models celebrated achieving independence with walking at fourteen months.

Dad, in a low squat, provides his daughter stability by placing his hands broadly along the sides of her midtorso with his thumbs to her back and his fingers splayed to encourage her engagement of her tummy muscles.

He encourages his girl, asking if she's ready to walk. She turns her head, neck, and upper torso to look at him while her hips, legs, and feet remain pointing straight ahead in the direction she's ready to begin walking. (Her ability to manage turning her head this way while maintaining excellent balance is a great sign that she's strong, steady, and ready for more.)

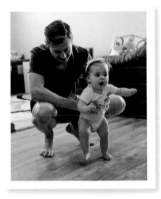

Baby shifts her weight to her left leg as she flexes her right hip and knee to lift her foot and begin stepping forward. At the same time, she raises both arms in a high guard position (for added stability) and her left arm presses slightly forward.

Note: Reciprocal arm swinging is a skill that will develop later, once the baby has managed to take steps independently and no longer holds her arms up, guarding.

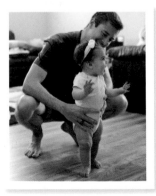

Baby advances her right foot a step past her left! At

the same time, she drops both her arms from shoulder to chest level, indicating she's feeling more comfortable and balanced.

Dad notices this and responds by dropping his hands from high on her torso to a lower area encompassing her hips and portions of her low abdomen. This is a great example of a parent instantly responding to his baby's movements, and backing off as she demonstrates less need for his externally provided stability. He is still providing supportive touch, but also encouraging her to rely more on herself.

Her brows high, smile big, and hands up and open all show she is pleasantly engaged by her mom who she was stepping toward.

She makes it to Mom and the play continues.

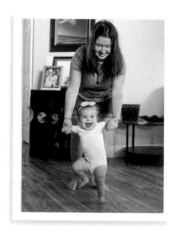

This time her mom switches the level of stabilization provided, supporting the baby by her arms, farther away from her core (which puts more responsibility on the baby girl to self-stabilize). Mom's hands are at the distal end of her upper arms encompassing her elbow joints, with her thumbs to the top of baby's forearms and her fingers creating a broad shelf or platform below her arms on both sides of the joint. With this placement she provides a place for her baby to press her arms down and also prevents her from pulling her elbows back behind her body (which would cause the baby to retract her shoulders and use the wrong muscles for self-stabilization). This encourages her to stabilize using the muscles in her tummy and back as she moves her legs.

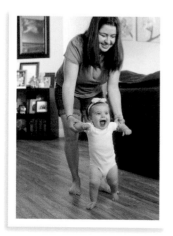

This works well and the baby is seen here exhibiting bigger, more exaggerated steps.

In the first image, she has just stepped forward with her left foot, which is pointing straight ahead. Her right foot is high off the ground, with her knee and hip flexed and outwardly rotated, as the baby prepares to advance this leg.

As for Mom, she's hinging at her hips to bring her

torso forward so she can reach her hands low enough to support her daughter. (This approach is far better for a mom's body than rounding her spine or tucking her pelvis under.)

In the second image on the previous page, Dad is across the room, encouraging the baby and making her excited to walk over to him.

Baby swings the whole right side of her body forward, placing her right leg a full step ahead of her left.

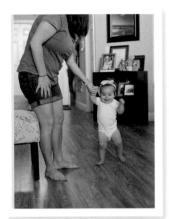

In a steady flow, without pause, the baby's left leg begins to push off the floor. Her big toe presses into the ground as her heel rises and her hip begins to rotate open (indicated by her knee starting to point outward).

She is absolutely beaming with excited energy and doing such a great job, her mom decides to decrease her support further still and see how baby girl does.

In this third example, Mom provides much less support, holding the baby only by her right hand (so now she is not only one less arm, but that arm is held much farther away from her body's core). Baby creates additional stability for herself by pulling her raised left arm closer to her body as she tucks her chin and takes her visual path down to the ground.

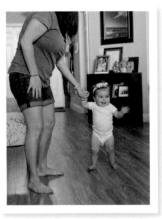

Baby feels less balanced than before, though, and she reverts to smaller steps, merely stepping her back foot forward a tiny bit closer to her front foot.

Her physical response indicates that she is not quite ready for this transition; nonetheless, it was a valiant effort she didn't shy away from or protest.

How much or how little stability to offer can vary with your baby's energy level and from surface to surface. As you balance providing your baby with support and building their independence, pay close attention to their body language and behavioral signals, and do your best to respond in positive, supportive flow.

Last is our cover photo. Here you see my husband, Eric, and our daughter, Sunny, celebrating her first birthday at the beach.

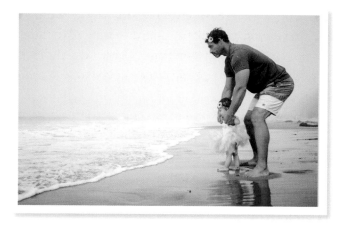

This photo demonstrates the beauty of walking with your child beyond your home. Aside from the sheer pleasure of sharing nature with your little one, being outside allows your fledgling toddler to walk on many fascinating and uneven surfaces. Sand, mud, grass, leaves, mulch, pebbles, boulders, and all the various "floors" of nature offer a wealth of physical and sensory experiences for your baby's feet, ankles, legs, hips, and all the other body parts involved with walking. Each new surface presents its own special challenges for finding balance and coordination.

Eric is holding Sunny's hands with his thumb and fingers wrapped around her wrists and forearms. His hands give her a level shelf of support into which she can press her arms at any time to generate more stability. In addition, his hands prevent her from retracting her arms to activate less optimal muscles to add stability. This allows her body to instead focus on engaging muscles in her abs, back, glutes, and legs.

As for Sunny's posture, her trunk is tall, well aligned, and subtly but strongly hinging forward at her hips. Her arms are in a "high guard," which gives her trunk a little added stability. Her legs are hip distance apart in a steady stance with her feet facing ahead, as opposed to a wide stance with toes outward (which was seen as a strategy for more stability in her younger days).

All this indicates increasingly solid stability in Sunny's core and that she is developing excellent coordination of her legs moving strongly as extensions from her core. These are the achievements you want to see in your baby before they begin toddling into walking independently.

Last, notice that all the parents in this activity are bending their bodies to accommodate the height of their children. This bending can lead to physical problems if posture is not focal.

Eric is handling this challenge by assuming a subtle hinge with his back expansively decompressed as he bends his hips and knees to lower enough to provide the support Sunny needs.

Be sure to take care of your own body before, during, and especially after walking with your little one. Our preferred and recommended ways to optimally do this are by performing Foundation Training exercises like the Founder, Standing Decompression, and Woodpecker or Lunge Decompression. Much more about these exercises appears in Part III.

Before we begin a dive into helping you strengthen and protect your own physical foundation, let's first take a look at independent walking and strengthening the legs and core for continued skill development.

Steps Beyond the First Year

It is so important to remember that *not all babies are on the same path*. Some will walk independently before they reach age one; others will not begin until well after their first birthday.

I feel it important to share that I've worked with some kids who were referred for intervention for "delayed motor skill acquision" because they were fifteen to eighteen months old and not yet walking. *And each eventually got there with dedicated strengthening and/or sensory work.* (Some kids are avoidant of pressure and other sensations in their feet, which can limit their willingness to put weight through their legs. Without this, standing and walking can be limited.) I share this to express that a delay in walking is sometimes just that—a delay— and not necessarily indicative of an underlying problem or condition. It can simply boil down to lack of exposure and opportunities to build some of the necessary baseline strength and precursor skills. I also want to share that when a kiddo first begins walking, it is not un- common to see things like a little belly protruding to lead the way, knees hyperextending, or toes turned inward or outward. Your child is working to coordinate their whole body and skills may seem er- ratic at first. Like everything else, time and practice are needed for muscles to strengthen and patterns to improve. Monitor your child and consider discussing such patterns with your child's pediatrician if they do not appear to be improving or are causing frequent tumbles and falls after a solid two months of independent walking.

As a reminder, there is a box discussing shoe recommendations in "Baby Fundamentals" in Part I.

In this chapter we will take a look at some more organically captured images of two of our toddler models as they take their skills up a few notches. Our hope is that this cuteness and commentary will inspire your play and offer more insight for what you see with your own little one. This chapter will not cover specifics for how to guide running, walking up and down stairs, or jumping, as they are more advanced maneuvers of toddlerhood that necessitate weeks and months of additional strengthening and coordination between the core and the legs. (Jumping isn't anticipated until somewhere around the second year, roughly months twenty to twenty-four.) We absolutely find each of these skills important within the bigger picture of development, but the focused content of this book is to help you strengthen your little one in their transition from being primarily horizontal to stepping forward on two feet, vertically. That said, what you see in these next few pages will certainly help your toddler in building the strength to get to those next skills.

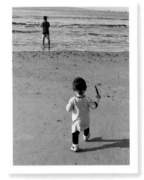

Our own daughter, who lived and practiced the concepts in this book from her first moments landside, began walking independently at fourteen months. And within mere days of her first solo steps in the comfort of our home, she was walking two to three blocks at a time with us through our neighborhood, on sidewalks and grass; AND taking steps fearlessly toward the water at the beach. Here she is seen first toddling across the firmly packed sand with her arms held in a high guard.

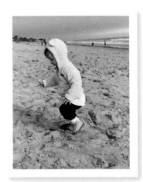

And less than three months later she was running uphill in loose sand at the beach, with her arms in a low to mid guard position and swinging reciprocally. (Note: Reciprocal arm swing means that the opposite arm and leg advance at the same time and this is typically anticipated somewhere between fifteen and eighteen months of age. Running is typically anticipated between eighteen and twenty-four months.) *This is 100 percent proof positive that taking the play to various environments helps to bolster babies' skills. Don't be surprised to see rapid progression as your baby's confidence builds.*

SUNNY'S PROGRESSION...

A few extra notes about our girl, for a base of reference, since she basically lived the program of this book.

By twenty to twenty-one months, she was starting to walk up and down hills with pretty solid balance. Trips and falls occasionally occurred but did not deter her.

By twenty-one to twenty-two months, she was walking backward on flat surfaces as well as downhill, looking over her shoulder and not losing balance. At this age she also began to hop and jump in place, finally clearing feet from the floor at almost twenty-three months, hopping forward two to four inches and hopping down from a two-inch step with one hand held for safety and down from a ten-inch step with two hands held for safety. She could likely have made these jumps solo, but we elected to continue with hands held to reinforce safety awareness since this tends to be absent in most kids at this age. We also wanted to be sure that her landings were controlled to protect the integrity of the ligaments surrounding and within the ankle, knee, and hip joints. Those structures have much less blood supply than the muscles. The unfortunate reality there is: if an injury occurs or the ligaments are overstretched, torn, or damaged, they lack the ability to heal and tighten back up to support the joints as the muscles can. This can predispose the body for reinjury and potentially impact motor skills.

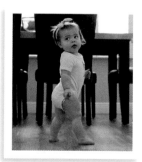

In these next few images you see another sweet fifteen-month-old girl taking her bipedal skills to the next levels. Note the variations in the alignment of her legs as she grows more stable, balanced, and confident over two limbs.

She's seen first with her hands in a low guard position and head-to-foot neutral alignment as she casually looks back over her shoulder at a caregiver calling her name from across the room. This is a simple show of increased strength and stability, noted by her visually tracking behind her while her body continues to advance forward.

We next see her pause while walking and put her hands to her head. She shows fantastic alignment and stability as she reaches her arms up high, into a position that promotes her torso extending. This was a great show of increased balance skills in this more mature, upright posture; and too cute not to include!

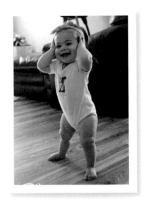

The following two images show her stability challenged even further as her caregiver elevates the toy she is interested in, causing her head and neck to extend even further than in the previous image.

First we see her left arm reach for the toy as her right arm extends out to her side to offer her some counterbalance, with her legs a little wider than hip distance apart for stability.

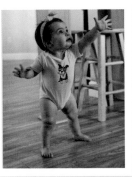

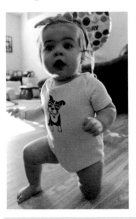

Then we see her drop her hands and widen her stance as she looks straight up. Her alignment is solid as she holds her balance steady and strong.

These next few images offer glimpses at her advancing floor transitioning skills. Practice of maneuvers such as these will benefit your little one's developing strength and coordination, which will add to their balance and confidence. All things that will help them to take their walking skills toward running and advancing abilities to do things like pivot and change directions.

First we see her pause in a half-kneeling position while she is mid transition from floor to standing. She is steady atop one knee and one foot with her hands at a low to mid-guard. This is an advancement as she no longer needs a support surface to hold as she splits her stance and transitions her weight in this way. Before this image was taken, she went from crawling on all fours to lifting her hands and kneeling on two knees, then to this. This progression strengthens a baby's control of their torso over their hips and their legs as a whole, which will help advance their walking skills.

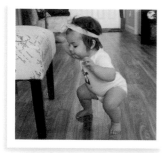

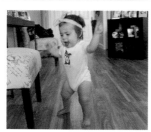

The next two images show part of the transition from standing to squatting and back to standing (in free space), which will do a great job of continuing to strengthen your baby's legs and core. She began standing near a chair, looking for a toy that fell nearby, and is captured here exemplifying a solid squat. She then rises to stance, with her hands in a high guard, via strongly pushing both legs to extend at the knees and hips.

Next she exhibits a modified version of all fours as she reaches one hand forward to grab the string at the base of the balloons. She's got her bottom high in the air in a position referred to as "bear crawl." Some kiddos will use this as a position they shift through while changing positions (as we see her go on to do); others will actually crawl in this position. From there, her hips and knees flex until she eventually drops to a seated position to explore this treasure she's successfully reached.

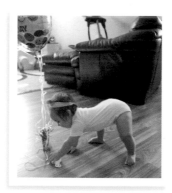
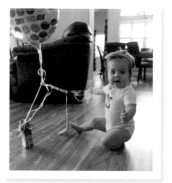

In the next three images we see Sunny (age sixteen months) squatting and reaching for a toy with arms widely outstretching. Grabbing like this creates a challenge to her stability and helps drive the progression of her movement skills. Here we see her rise, pivot, and

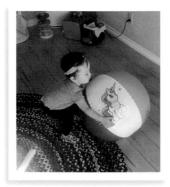 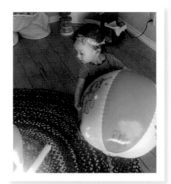 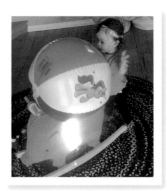

throw her ball on her piggy's back, completely unaware of the work she's actually doing as she has fun "sharing with her piggy."

Here, in the same play session, Sunny squats strongly to attempt to pull apart her colorful ball-spinning tower. Squatting-to-standing transitions were the "practice" I was trying to encourage within her play. Reality is, there are many, many ways to inspire this type of play. These examples include additional challenges to core stability, strength, and balance as the children incorporate reaching, grasping, pulling, and pushing fine motor tasks. Other ideas not pictured can include magnets on your refrigerator or stickers on a wall to encourage your child to look and reach upward as they work on standing balance and reaching, and begin to explore pressing up on their toes to reach higher and higher. *Dynamic play distracts them from the muscle-strengthening "work" they are actually doing.*

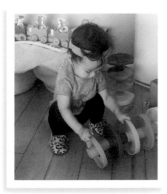 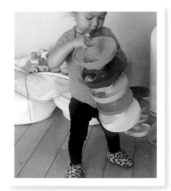

Here we see Sunny (seventeen months) approaching her ride-on balance bike. First she's in a very Founder-like hinge as she eyeballs the seat and makes her approach. Then, lowering toward a seated position, she strongly plants her heels and engages all the way through her core and legs. Her profile shows excellent spinal alignment and curves (proud mom and dad moment!).

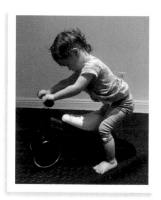 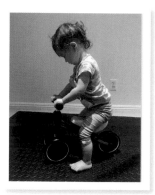

Let these next images be your motivating reminder that nature provides some of the very best "toys" to intrigue little minds and drive their movement. Here we see Sunny exploring a flower bloom in a beautiful deep squat before then rising to stance. If you look closely at her feet you should notice a slight elevation of her toes and forefeet as she pushes strongly through her heels, extending her hips and knees to rise.

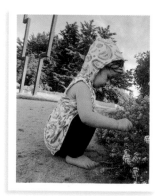 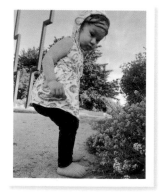

The next five images show Sunny enjoying the robust playground that the beach offers. (1) She is seen squatting to fill her bucket with sand and shells. (2) The heavier her bucket becomes, the more work and challenge it is for her little body. (3) When a rest from the work was needed, taking things down a notch to sit in the sand and fill the bucket provided seated trunk-strengthening work as she rotated about her base to scoop and transfer sand. This was fantastic sensory and fine motor play for her hands. (4) Of course we couldn't leave the beach without exploring some of the amazing driftwood, which provided a great jungle gym to practice climbing skills. (5) And someone's artistic creation of beach wood provided a great zone for a power-charging snack, while also providing some additional leg work trekking through the loosely packed sand to get there and back. This terrain offers so much play potential, no toys or tools are truly necessary.

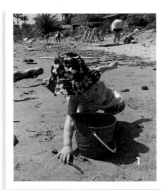

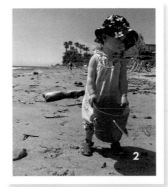

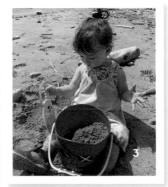

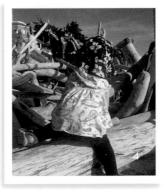

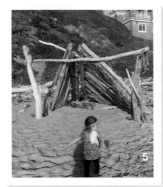

We hope this chapter has given you playful inspiration for motivating the young one in your care as they take their strong foundation forward in bipedal exploration of the world around them. These images are just a few examples, and the options are limitless.

Definitely let your children be little; play offers their developing minds and bodies so much. As you go, aim to make the most of all the ways you can engage and guide their physical development. Try to remain mindful of your word choices and to avoid getting in the habit of simply saying things like "good job," "be careful," or "no" when it comes to observing your kiddo in action. Those words don't offer any teaching potential, and can easily get blocked out by the child who hears the same thing parroted over and over. Let the power of your words enrich the learning experience. Instead of a generalized "good job," try "Way to go—up to stand! You're so big, so tall. Your legs are so strong. Well done!" And instead of "no" or "be careful," give more details that allow your child to begin to make sense of why you're concerned. For example, "The ground is wet and you could slip, so watch your steps," or "Hold a hand, bumpy, bumpy ground, I'll help you balance." Your language and demeanor will add shape and color to their experiences.

There are infinite ways you can guide and shape your little one's play sessions at this delightful age and stage; and we wish you joy, patience, and many happy days as you move onward into toddlerhood.

Before we can feel good calling this book complete, we first want to offer you more instruction for the Foundation Training exercises we've been suggesting throughout. They truly can be a game changer. And you don't want to miss the pages ahead that show practical ways to layer these moves seamlessly into your days' movements and play with your kiddo. We hope you enjoy the process of growing strong together!

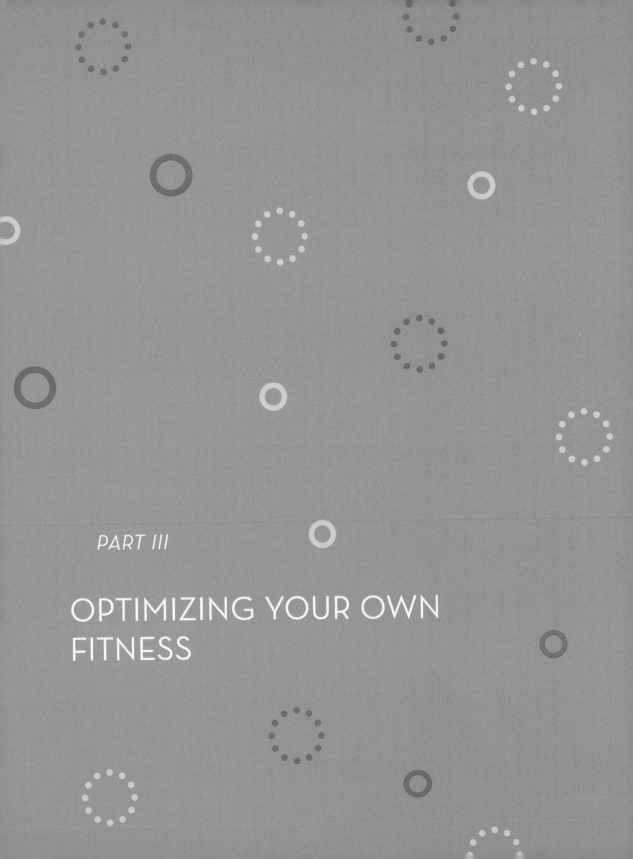

PART III

OPTIMIZING YOUR OWN FITNESS

Foundation Training
Exercises for Parents

This book has primarily focused on helping your baby develop with optimal physical health and fitness. However, the chapters in this part are devoted to helping you protect and enhance your own fitness. The Foundation Training exercises included in the next chapter are highly effective at preventing and/or healing the kinds of physical damage you're most at risk of suffering as a parent, such as muscle strains and nerve irritation.

If you're new to childcare, the wear and tear your body is experiencing daily might not be immediately obvious to you. But caring for a new baby can lead you to operate without adequate rest/sleep, put your body in positions that are less than comfortable, and place repetitive demands on your body the likes of which you may never have experienced before your baby arrived.

For example, if you strain your neck by frequently looking down to watch your baby in your arms, these routines will help you realign your spine, expand your chest, and broaden your potentially rounded shoulders. This is especially important for nursing mothers to read as you consider how much time is spent this way throughout the day (and night!), in potentially compromising positions.

As another example, if you sit or kneel on the floor to play with your baby, you might end up compressing your spine, hips, or other parts of your body. These exercises can help you decompress and restore your body to healthy, strong alignment. They can also be treated as a warm-up to prepare your body for the challenges each day brings.

Also, if you've developed a painful disorder such as diastasis recti, thoracic outlet syndrome, carpal tunnel syndrome, or sciatica as a result of being pregnant, giving birth, breastfeeding, or simply carrying around the weight of your baby, these exercises are likely to help you feel better, heal, and be better able to enjoy the time you'll be spending together.

None of these exercises take very long; you can typically perform a few solid repetitions in just a few minutes. Done properly, the exercises will likely have positive effects that last for hours afterward. Practiced with diligence and dedication, these exercises also will likely have positive effects on—and can even promote lasting changes to—the very root causes of your own movement dysfunctions.

As newish parents ourselves, we completely get that parents and caregivers don't necessarily have a lot of extra time, and your focus is primarily going to be on your baby. We encourage you to give yourself the gift of time spent on self-care, and not just to relax and check in with yourself, but to make sure that you don't get injured. Small moments that you take toward prevention will keep you from an injury that can keep you down for a week or more. Even if you feel completely okay now, if you allow your body to suffer continual small injuries every day without addressing the damage done, the chances are steadily stacking that you eventually will develop painful ailments that impair both your quality of life and your effectiveness as a caregiver.

In addition to health promotion and injury prevention, this physical self-care is backing you up like a form of insurance, in case you are called upon to become a superhero. As a new parent or caregiver, you might not want to imagine the worst-case scenarios, but—reality— kids do get into things and accidents do happen. As caregivers, we want to be able to respond quickly, to move with reflexive and coordinated agility and be there for our children if something presenting danger should occur. And it would be nice to make sure we don't get injured if we do need to jump. These exercises can help you to maintain your own physical well-being as well as prime your muscles and nerves to be readier for quick and efficient action should you need to rescue an endangered child. We hope that you'll never be in a scary situation requiring you to fully call upon the athleticism these exercises can help you develop and, instead, that you'll appreciate the security and peace of mind they can provide. Once you get in the habit of doing these exercises, you're likely to appreciate how they not only improve your comfort and quality of movement but also prepare you physically to be a stronger caregiver for your baby.

The next chapter first introduces you to five fundamental tools you'll be using across many or all FT exercises: Decompression Breathing, Measuring Sticks, Long Wing, Short Wing, Sphere of Tension.

It then describes the Foundation Training exercises that will most effectively help you meet both the normal daily physical challenges of parenting and the abrupt demands of the unexpected. These are: Supine Decompression, Prone Decompression, Standing Decompression, Founder, Kneeling Founder, Lunge Decompression, Woodpecker, Internal Leg Trace, Anchored Back Extension, Anchored Bridge, 8-Point Plank, Squat, Gorilla Lift.

For each exercise, you'll first see photographs showing you key poses of the routine and brief outlines of its various steps. You'll then be informed of the key benefits of the exercise so you can decide if it'll help meet your specific needs. Finally, you'll be pointed to a section of the Foundation Training website, found at Stream.FoundationTraining.com, that provides you access to a video that shows how to perform the exercise step-by-step.

If you care to dive deeper into the work, you can purchase a sub-scription that gives you access to the ever-growing library of FT content, including hundreds of workouts and poses for enhancing performance, eliminating pain, growing stronger, and feeling great. There is even a handy app you can use from your cell phone or tablet device.

As previously mentioned, at the end of Part III you will find a crossover chapter called "Growing Stronger Together," which in-cludes several delightful images that show parents incorporating el-ements learned in the previous chapters with their own practice of Foundation Training. We hope you will feel inspired and motivated to try weaving these activities into your own daily movements along-side your baby.

Key Tools for Foundation Training

Before you can start performing Foundation Training exercises, you will do well to become familiar with several fundamental tools that are used in many or all FT routines. These are Decompression Breathing, Measuring Sticks, Long Wing, Short Wing, and Sphere of Tension.

Decompression Breathing

When you breathe, you do so from one of two areas: your abdomen or your rib cage. Abdominal breathing takes relatively little effort, since it uses the soft tissue of your abs. It's most appropriate for low-energy activities, such as sleeping or resting. It's also the only way your baby breathes, as you can see by watching your little one's relaxed abdomen expand and contract while inhaling and exhaling.

When you're engaging in vigorous activity, though, it can be more effective to breathe using your rib cage. That's because your ab muscles have to maintain your

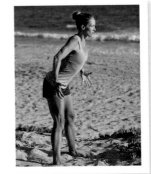

pelvis in a relatively static position, which limits their adaptability. In contrast, your rib cage is a tall, wide, deep structure with 360 degrees of circumference and expandability on all sides. So even though it's bony (as opposed to soft tissue), it's highly responsive to adjusting its size and positioning based on your movement and breathing needs.

When you neglect your body—for example, by too much sitting, lack of exercise, and excessive abdominal breathing—your rib cage may adjust its size and position, providing less room for your organs, and creating unhealthy compression points with nearby body parts such as your spine.

Decompression Breathing is the antidote. It leads you to take big 360-degree breaths that expand all the surface areas of your rib cage, giving your organs plenty of room to operate. It also lifts your torso to keep it high and powerful.

In addition, Decompression Breathing—in conjunction with specific hip movements—helps to lengthen and tighten a wide range of muscles, position them so they can communicate and work together most effectively as integrated chains, and prime them to disperse your body weight evenly across them to generate greater strength.

Further, Decompression Breathing helps to combat unhealthy compression points that may have developed throughout your body and contributed to creating degenerative disorders such as sciatica, thoracic outlet syndrome, carpal tunnel syndrome, cluster and tension headaches, and migraines. If left untreated, such issues cause pain and other symptoms that have the potential to last a lifetime. However, they can often be eliminated by using this breathing method in conjunction with the exercises you will encounter next in this chapter. Getting good at this practice will help to reestablish an appropriate amount of space between your rib cage, spine, and other joints of your body.

Decompression Breathing is also especially important if you're a new mom. That's because pregnancy expands your belly. If you engage in only abdominal breathing after you give birth, you're just making matters worse by further expanding your stomach. This risks your developing an abdominal distension disorder such as diastasis recti.

In contrast, Decompression Breathing will adjust your rib cage to fit your postpartum torso more effectively; and it'll help to pull your abdominal muscles back from their natural separation by training the transversus abdominis muscle in the deepest layer of your abdomen.

To sum up, Decompression Breathing is helpful for anyone and offers extra value if you have existing back pain or are a new mom.

This is the breathing technique you should use while performing Foundation Training exercises. And, heads up, it can be challenging. It may take a while to fully get the hang of it. But it's far more important that you do it at all than you start off doing it perfectly. With patience and practice, you're very likely to master this fundamental FT tool.

The step-by-step details of performing this vital component of Foundation Training are most effectively taught by a video demonstration, which you can find by going to FoundationTraining.com /parents and selecting the "Decompression Breathing" option.

Measuring Sticks

In Foundation Training, your "measuring sticks" are your fingers.

Specifically, for any Foundation Training exercise that you perform standing, start by placing your thumbs on the base of your ribs and your pinky fingers on the pointy bone of your pelvis (as shown at right). This allows you to continually feel where your rib cage and pelvis are, and more importantly, how much space you manage to create between them as a result of your Decompression Breathing and movements.

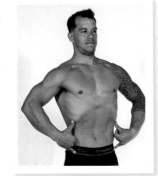

At the same time, set your elbows wide, pulling away from each other, and lift your chest up so it expands and makes it easier for you to breathe into both the front and back of your lungs.

As you inhale using Decompression Breathing, you should feel your rib cage lift up (which should occur equally at the front and back without the lower ribs pressing forward and sticking out). As the lower edges of your inhalation muscles find their contraction point, they'll pull hard, and your rib cage will pull away from your pelvis. The increased space from your pelvis that results is great for organs, such as your liver and pancreas, that reside under the dome of your rib cage and diaphragm. It's also terrific for your spine, and for the entire center of your body.

To watch a video showing how to use this tool, go to Foundation Training.com/parents and select the "Arm Positions" option.

Long Wing and Short Wing

Two positions you'll encounter in a number of Foundation Training exercises are Long Wing and Short Wing. In both cases, your fingers are extended apart from each other (see below). Long Wing has your elbows slightly bent and hands at roughly waist level, while Short Wing has your elbows fully bent and hands at roughly neck level.

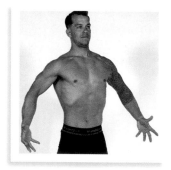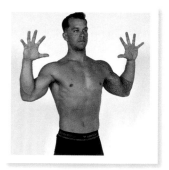

When using these positions, you should not be squeezing your shoulder blades together, but instead breathing very wide between them. The goal is to create a lot of space between your shoulder blades with every inhalation.

While the photos above are of standing poses, the Short Wing is most commonly used for anchoring exercises performed on your stomach. You can find an example in the "Anchored Back Extension" exercise later in this chapter.

And to watch a video showing how to use the Long Wing pose, go to FoundationTraining.com/parents and select the "Arm Positions" option.

Sphere of Tension

The Sphere of Tension (or SoT) is similar to the Long Wing pose just described, except instead of pulling your arms away from your sides, you place your arms in front of you (either at shoulder level or overhead), and press your hands toward each other by flexing each finger and touching your fingertips. This creates an upper body closed kinetic chain.

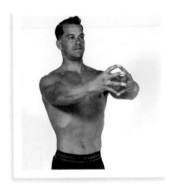 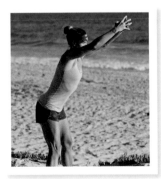

There's a lot of back-and-forth isometrics in this position. For example, your hands are pushing together but your wrists are pulling apart; and your elbows are pushing together but your shoulders are pulling apart.

At the same time, the pose opens you up to breathing deeply across the back of your rib cage.

The SoT expands and hones your muscles and teaches them to absorb force by lengthening against them. This primes your muscles to contract more effectively when they shorten.

To watch a video showing how to use the Sphere of Tension pose, go to FoundationTraining.com/parents and select the "Arm Positions" option.

Now that you have an understanding of some of the fundamental tools of Foundation Training, you're ready to start learning and performing complete exercises. These are covered next, starting with decompression routines.

Supine Decompression

Supine Decompression is an exercise you perform while on your back. It allows you to align your spine and lengthen your body with minimal interference from gravity.

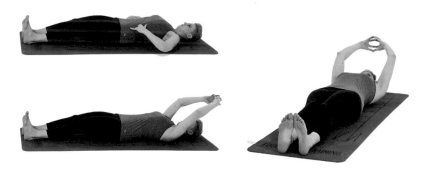

This is the best Foundation Training exercise for actively aligning your spine and body. It takes only a few minutes, and it's recommended that you perform it twice a day—in the morning to start your body off right, and at night to restore your alignment before going to bed.

While this is a relatively simple exercise, actively aligning your body is challenging. My husband, Eric, has seen some of the finest athletes in the world perform a Supine Decompression for the first time and in forty-five seconds end up trembling from the exertion. That's in part because this routine fires up muscles that most of us, including professional athletes, underuse. So if you initially find yourself struggling with this routine, take it slow and be diligent with the details.

To watch a video showing how to perform this exercise step-by-step, go to FoundationTraining.com/parents and select the "Supine Decompression" option.

Prone Decompression

Prone Decompression is very similar to Supine Decompression. The key differences are that it's performed on your stomach instead of your back; and it focuses on your anterior chain, which consists of the muscles along the front side of your legs and spine, which include the abs, quads, and pectoral muscles.

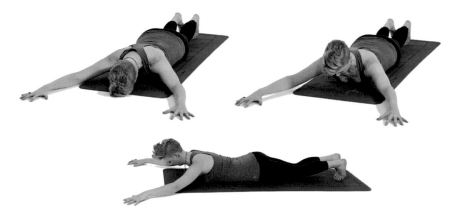

Prone Decompression teaches you to not extend your spine (the way you do in, say, a Cobra yoga pose), but instead use your transverse abdominal muscle to keep the back of your rib cage expanded, your abdomen tight and long, and your breath as big as possible.

Performing this exercise is a bit like hanging from the edge of a cliff with your fingers, pulling into where your hands are. If you do it right, you feel the back of your body engaged from your shoulders down your back; and you also feel your abdomen engage as it's trying to lift the back of your rib cage toward the ceiling.

As with Supine Decompression, it's recommended that you perform this routine at the start and the end of each day. More specifically, begin with Supine Decompression for one to two minutes, then flip from your back to your stomach and do Prone Decompression.

To watch a video showing how to perform this exercise step-by-step, go to FoundationTraining.com/parents and select the "Prone Decompression" option.

Standing Decompression

When you're holding your baby, you shouldn't feel the weight in your spine. Instead, you should feel it in the pads of your feet, the muscles of your legs, and the broadness of your back and shoulders.

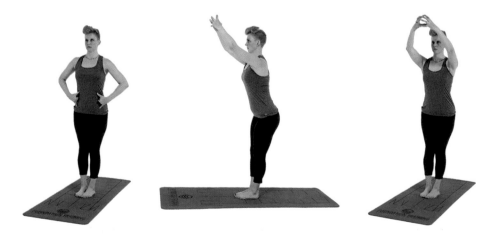

This Standing Decompression exercise helps make that happen. It teaches you to actively stand up tall, dispersing your force into the ground through your feet. It also helps you to create connections between your muscular nerve channels and your brain's neural network that build stability and strength.

Coupled with Decompression Breathing to expand your rib cage while holding Long Wing or SoT poses with your arms and hands, this is an exercise that creates a strong antidote to the time spent looking down to check in on and care for your little one.

Standing Decompression can also be performed with your baby in your arms to add a little extra weight to the exercise. See the "Growing Stronger Together" chapter for an image of this exercise being performed while babywearing.

This routine is best learned by watching it demonstrated. To see a video showing how to perform this exercise step-by-step, go to FoundationTraining.com/parents and select the "Standing Decompression" option.

Founder

The Founder is the most recognized of all Foundation Training exercises. It's become FT's signature routine because it's relatively quick and easy to do anywhere and anytime and is incredibly effective.

The Founder is a hip hinge exercise that will strengthen you. It activates and aligns your muscles, lines up your nerves, and trains you to breathe powerfully regardless of your body's tension and intensity. Your body remembers improvements you make to your posture and breathing, so it'll retain the positive effects of the Founder long after you've completed the exercise.

Every time you reach for your child, pick your child up, or put your child down, the Founder will help you feel more powerful, as it helps provide you with an active muscle alignment to accomplish these tasks with protection and stability. Also, if you throw yourself out of alignment, the Founder will help your body return to protected stability.

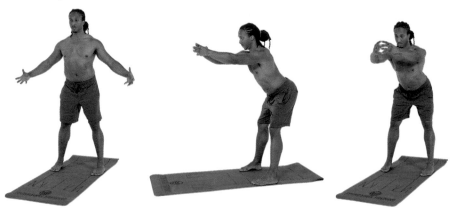

More specifically, the Founder bolsters the stability of your hips so that no matter how flexible your hips become, they'll be equally strong in every direction. Every motion of your body is ultimately guided by your hips, starting at your hip joints and your body's center at the pubic symphysis (a joint between the left and right pubic bones). The Founder strengthens every moment of a hip hinge, from the very beginning of it to the farthest range you can achieve.

It does so by loading your posterior chain, which consists of the muscles along the backside of your legs and spine, including the hamstrings, glutes, and calves; and it integrates your posterior chain with the other muscle chains in your body.

The Founder uses an isometric pose that incorporates Decompression Breathing, which challenges your respiration muscles and anchoring line (the middle line of your arches up your inner leg to your pubic symphysis). It employs pelvic anchoring, an isometric squeezing that gathers all the muscles of your inner leg to challenge the muscles on the back of your leg.

You'll know you're doing a Founder well when your heart rate increases and your body heats up. Most people start to sweat within a minute.

That happens because you're holding an isometric pose using over 80 percent of the muscles in your body. These muscles are all working together to provide you with zero focal points of pressure as they're dispersing your body weight evenly among the largest muscles of your body and dispersing the tension of your pose evenly out to your limbs.

The Founder is quickly becoming one of the most popular exercises in the world of corrective exercise and rehabilitation, and even in strength training.

To watch a video showing how to perform this exercise step-by-step, go to FoundationTraining.com/parents and select the "Founder" option.

Kneeling Founder

Over 70 percent of your core strength comes from the bottom of your pelvis and the big muscles that surround your bottom muscles. These include your hamstrings, which are the muscles at the rear of the thighs that play a key role in such activities as walking, running, and jumping; and your adductor muscles, which originate in the groin, are attached along the thighbone, and aid in drawing your thighs together, rotating and flexing your thighs, and maintaining your balance when you stand or walk.

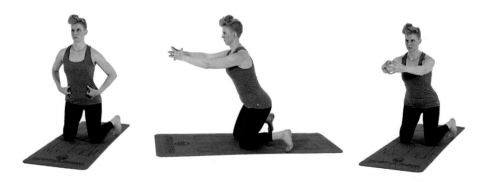

You want these muscles to be much stronger than the muscles in your abdomen and lower back. Otherwise you risk having your body get out of balance, which can result in lower back pain, hip joint pain, collapsed arches, and/or overall tightness and weakness.

The Kneeling Founder helps prevent such problems by teaching you how to move your entire torso against tension held at your bottom muscles and groin muscles. The result is a very high level of stability at the bottom of your pelvis.

In addition, the exercise strengthens the stability of your hips.

The Founder is actually great at creating these improvements too. But the Kneeling Founder has several advantages over the Founder.

As its name indicates, the Kneeling Founder is performed while on your knees rather than on your feet. It's therefore more convenient during those times when it's easier for you to exercise kneeling versus standing—which can occur frequently during child care.

If you get the leverage right, the Kneeling Founder takes all the weight off your feet. You perform it on your knees, and use your feet only to maintain balance. Consider placing something comfortable, such as a mat, under your knees to ensure they don't get sore as you engage your muscles through this activity. You'll know you're working the right muscles as you go if you almost instantly feel your gluteal muscles in your bottom activate.

The Kneeling Founder is especially effective at treating lower spine instability (e.g., spondylolisthesis). This is a common disorder for moms because the pelvis goes through dramatic changes during and after pregnancy, and recovering your previous stability won't necessarily happen automatically. This exercise is a direct remedy for the instability caused by such pelvis expansion.

To watch a video showing how to perform this exercise step-by-step, go to FoundationTraining.com/parents and select the "Kneeling Founder" option.

Lunge Decompression

While engaging in activities with your baby, you'll often have to kneel or assume some other position that compresses your legs. The Lunge Decompression exercise, along with the Kneeling Founder, is the ideal antidote, restoring your legs to a strong and functionally balanced state. It's also terrific at treating tight calves, tight psoas muscles, and overly tight abs.

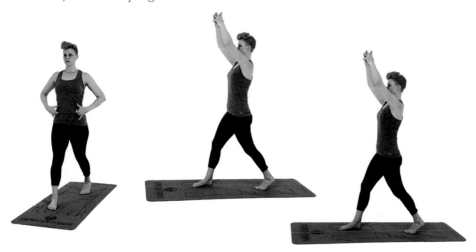

Many of the movements in this exercise overlap with Standing Decompression. The main difference between these two routines is that instead of keeping your feet together, in Lunge Decompression you set them a long step apart via a split stance. If training on one leg seems strange, consider that in real life you'll rarely move on both legs at the same time. Instead, you'll be on one leg or the other as you turn, walk, or run. This exercise therefore helps you develop single leg balance and single leg strength, allowing you to rely on either leg alone whenever you ever need to.

A key part of this exercise is trying to close your legs together without actually moving them. The scissoring tension that results from the back of your front leg to the front of your back leg stands you up even taller. It also triggers a line of stability in the very deep muscles of your spine and pelvis.

If you perform this exercise well, you'll feel as if your body has been lengthened; and that feeling will last for hours after you've completed the routine.

To watch a video showing how to perform this exercise step-by-step, go to FoundationTraining.com/parents and select the "Lunge Decompression" option.

Woodpecker

The Woodpecker is very similar to the Lunge Decompression. The key difference is that you perform the Woodpecker with a strong pelvic-driven hip rotation that muscularly guides the movement of your trunk along with it.

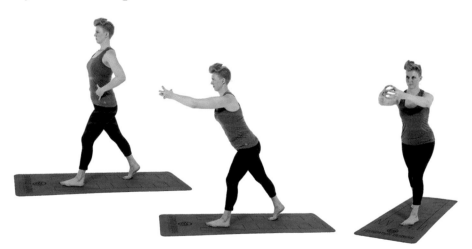

Because of this, the Woodpecker enhances your ability to quickly transition from asymmetry to symmetry, which can be incredibly beneficial when you consider the asymmetric forces your body is likely to encounter while holding your baby toward one side of your body throughout their first couple years as they grow heavier and heavier.

The Woodpecker is also great at treating hip pain, lower back pain, weakness, and plantar fasciitis, which are unfortunately quite common in life and especially during pregnancy.

To watch a video showing how to perform this exercise step-by-step, go to FoundationTraining.com/parents and select the "Woodpecker" option.

Anchoring

The next four workouts in this chapter are called "anchoring" exercises. These relatively simple but effective routines consist of the Internal Leg Trace, Anchored Back Extension, Anchored Bridge, and 8-Point Plank.

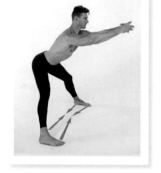

The vast majority of your core strength should ideally be coming from the muscles that directly connect to the bottom of your pelvis, which are your medial groin muscles, your adductors, and your medial hamstring. These muscles support your arches, your feet, your legs, and your groin, forming what's referred to as your anchoring line. And they all connect at your pubic symphysis at the base of your pelvis (about five inches, or three fingers, below your navel).

The muscles of your anchoring line work together to lift your arches and contract your inner legs toward your pubic symphysis, allowing you to stand tall. Your strength comes from these muscles, while your range of motion comes from the muscles by your ankles and wrists.

When your anchoring line pulls to raise your arches and support your feet and legs, there's a reciprocal pull from your posterior line. As a result, when your anchoring line is strong, it perpetually strengthens your posterior line.

Similarly, when your posterior line is strong and your anchoring line is accurately positioned, your posterior line perpetually strengthens your anchoring line.

This reciprocal strengthening is a great source of power, resilience, reflexiveness, and flexibility that helps your limbs move accurately and well.

The anchoring exercises that follow create bilateral centralizing contractions that pull your hips deeper into your hip joint, and pull the center of your pubic symphysis as close as it can get to its neutral center, maximizing stability. This provides all the muscles that surround your pubic symphysis—bottom, hamstring, back, abdomen, shoulder, neck—a better starting point from which to contract. The results are more efficient contraction, and your body weight is more evenly dispersed among your muscles; that in turn allows you to exert less effort while getting more done.

The Decompression Breathing tool you learned earlier in this chapter relies on the anchoring at your pelvis and below to your feet, creating equal and opposite pulls. This creates substantial extra room in the area where your sacroiliac joint is close to your pelvis, which can help prevent or eliminate a common source of lower back pain.

The anchoring process also helps protect your entire back and your hips, which are very common areas of degeneration (where most people develop arthritis).

As a parent, the anchoring exercises that follow will help give you the strength to more easily lift your baby, push a stroller, squat while playing with your baby on the floor, or make a quick dash getting to your little one should the need arise. The muscles of your anchoring line are designed to do most of the work for these activities, so training these muscles to be more effective will allow you to do all these things more smoothly and with posture that doesn't compromise your own physical well-being.

Now that you have a general understanding of what Foundation Training's anchoring exercises do for you, please read on to learn specific details about the Internal Leg Trace, Anchored Back Extension, Anchored Bridge, and 8-Point Plank.

Internal Leg Trace

When performing anchoring exercises, it's usually best to start with the Internal Leg Trace. This is a quick, easy routine that's terrific at activating (think: preparing!) the muscles in your anchoring line, warming you up for any subsequent and more challenging exercises that also incorporate anchoring.

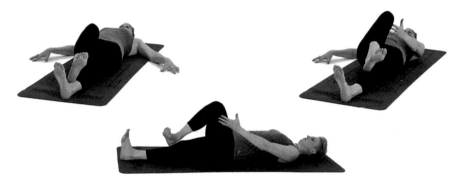

The steps for the Internal Leg Trace are simple. And it's a great one to do during the day when you're down with the baby because it can be done just about anywhere you find a smooth, flat surface to lie down upon. You can even do this with your baby practicing their tummy time atop your chest or abdomen when you get comfortable with it!

Begin on your back, legs extended straight ahead on the floor, with your big toes together and heels slightly apart. Rotate one leg inward from the hip, and place the heel on your other leg's ankle. Trace your heel up along the other leg, going just below or above its kneecap. Use the pinky side of your opposite hand, palm up, to press the inside of your first leg's knee for five seconds, applying roughly five to ten pounds of pressure. Let your hand relax, trace your leg back down your other leg, and return to your starting position.

Then switch legs and repeat.

This exercise helps prevent your hip joints from pointing outward, so that they instead point either straight ahead (i.e., are neutral) or point slightly inward.

It also efficiently activates your adductor muscles, which originate in the groin and are attached along the thighbone, and aids in drawing the thighs together, rotating and flexing your thighs. This big group of muscles helps in maintaining your strongly decompressed posture, helping to stabilize the bottom of your pelvis.

The Internal Leg Trace is especially helpful if you're suffering from a partial separation of the muscles that meet at the midline of your abdomen, a condition called diastasis recti. This occurs to an estimated 60 percent of mothers during or following pregnancy as a result of the uterus stretching the abdominal muscles to make room for the growing baby.

This condition can strike any gender, though, as other causes include lifting heavy weights the wrong way, or performing abdominal exercises excessively and/or incorrectly.

Symptoms of diastasis recti may include a bulge in your stomach, especially when you strain your abs; lower back pain; bloating; constipation; and bad posture.

Diastasis recti can be treated by stabilizing the bottom of your pelvis—and performing the Internal Leg Trace is one of the most effective ways to do that. As you heal, the back of your rib cage will become broad and powerful, and your abdomen will learn to stay tight (like a scroll closing toward its center).

The Internal Leg Trace is also useful if you have a painful disorder called sciatica. For more about this, see the "Anchored Bridge" section.

To watch a video showing how to perform this exercise step-by-step, go to FoundationTraining.com/parents and select the "Internal Leg Trace" option.

Anchored Back Extension

The Anchored Back Extension challenges you to support your spine in a mildly extended position. In addition, it improves the effectiveness of your adductor muscles, which will traction (decompress) your spine at the same time you're extending it.

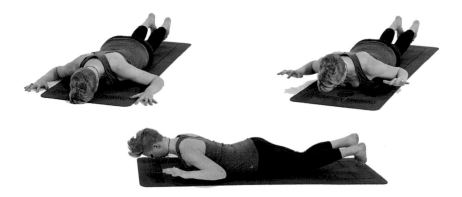

You begin this exercise on your stomach, with your legs out, ankles up, and big toes and knees together. You first muscularly engage your arms in a Short Wing pose (described earlier in this chapter), with your elbows bent and fingers spread apart.

You then raise your toes eight to ten inches off the mat, with your knees still on the mat and squeezing together as hard as you can manage. This tension will fire your hamstrings and get the middle of your legs burning. (Note that you're not driving your hips into the ground, only your knees, with your inner thighs squeezed toward each other. Otherwise you'd be squeezing your glutes, which isn't what's desired for this exercise.)

While continuing to squeeze your knees, raise the top of your body, with your chin, arms, and wrists at the same level. Lift just high enough that you're off the ground and feeling supported.

Your emphasis should now be directly ahead of you, as if you're climbing a ladder horizontally across a bridge. You're "anchoring" your legs, by squeezing and creating a contraction at the base of your pelvis that tractions your torso away every time you inhale.

Go as far as you can, as wide as you can, and as slowly as you can for a few deep breaths, expanding your rib cage in all directions as you inhale.

Then exhale, engaging your abdomen, and slowly lowering the top half of your body back to the mat.

This exercise isn't designed to be difficult. If you want to make it more challenging, though, while the top of your body is raised, you can slowly move your arms ahead of you until your hands meet in a Sphere of Tension. This bolsters your thoracic, oblique, and adductor strength.

To watch a video showing how to perform this exercise step-by-step, go to FoundationTraining.com/parents and select the "Anchored Back Extension" option.

Anchored Bridge

In this exercise, you're essentially trying to create a suspension bridge from your arches to your adductors by using your hamstrings and posterior chain to suspend your hips about an inch off the ground. Your focus is on the internal rotation and squeezing together of your knees, inner thighs, and big toes.

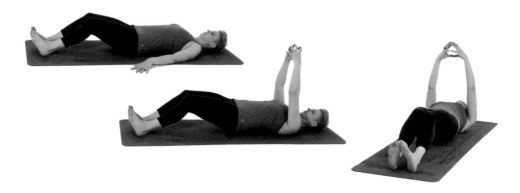

One of the challenges of the Anchored Bridge is that as you pull your hips up, your knees will naturally try to separate. However, the exercise depends on keeping your knees together while your hips are suspended off the ground.

Another common mishap is squeezing the bottom muscles during the exercise. This breaks the anchoring effect, and might even end up creating back pain, so take care to not do this.

You start the Anchored Bridge on your back, with your heels slightly apart, and your big toes together and pointing straight up. Your knees should be pressing together, wrapping toward each other with a subtle internal rotation from the hips as they're bent and raised, with about six inches between the back of your knees and the floor mat.

While keeping your knees squeezed together and raised, inhale deeply to fill your rib cage (similar to a decompression exercise). As you do so, try to feel your rib cage (not your spine) against the mat.

Pull your neck a bit longer, and squeeze your knees together a bit harder, so that your hips and your heels pull at each other. If you're anchoring properly, you should feel your adductor muscles and inner hamstring muscles on the back of your legs. Use these muscles to continue pulling your hips one to three inches off the ground. (Don't press your hips, because that will end up squeezing your butt muscles and cause you to lose the anchor.)

If you feel stable enough to do so, raise your arms straight up at the ceiling, then join your hands in a focused Sphere of Tension. This should feel difficult, like the entire back of your body is supported and lifting your hips above the mat.

While continuing to keep your arms straight and fingers pressing together, stretch your arms down to the floor, over your head, and take a few more deep breaths.

Finally, relax your arms and return them to the mat, and gently bring your hips back down.

The Anchored Bridge is especially helpful if you have back pain as a result of reaching for your baby, picking your baby up, putting your baby down, and other bending activities. The exercise's focus on squeezing your knees together will typically reduce or end your back pain, especially in the lower back.

The Anchored Bridge is also one of the best ways to treat a common ailment called sciatica, which is pain that radiates along the sciatic nerve from the lower back down the hip, butt, and leg (typically on just one side of the body).

Two ways a parent might unwittingly develop sciatica are by breastfeeding with rounded shoulders and slumpy posture, and by holding a baby on one hip with your weight shifted heavily over to one side (versus holding them strongly and symmetrically). Both can lead you to externally rotate your hips and potentially put excessive pressure on tiny muscles located very deep in your hip. The sciatic nerve happens to travel directly around and through several of these muscles. The more externally rotated your hips get, the tighter this becomes, and the less space is available for your sciatic nerve. When that nerve starts feeling cramped, it protests by sending pain signals to your brain.

The Anchored Bridge—and also the Internal Leg Trace—quickly create space for your sciatic nerve, which is likely to result in the nerve reducing, and eventually ending, its pain signals.

To watch a video showing how to perform this exercise step-by-step, go to FoundationTraining.com/parents and select the "Anchored Bridge" option.

8-Point Plank

A plank is an isometric exercise in which you hold a position similar to a push-up to build core strength.

Foundation Training's 8-Point Plank is so named because it's a plank with eight points of contact: your two wrists, two elbows, two knees, and two feet, all of which remain in touch with the ground throughout the exercise. In short, the goal of the 8-Point Plank is to get the back of your rib cage as wide and big as possible, and to tighten its front as much as possible.

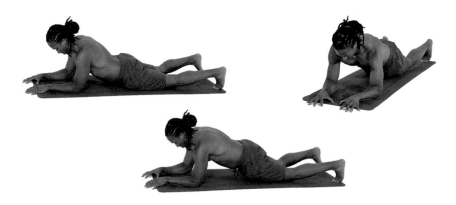

The 8-Point Plank is the most challenging anchoring exercise in this book. If you find yourself trembling and shaking, that probably means you're doing it well. So don't get discouraged if you can't get all the way through the complete exercise right away; that's normal. Performing the beginning portions of the exercise will be a great start to get you on your way. We encourage you to approach the 8-Point Plank with patience and diligence. With this, you're likely to master the entire exercise over time.

This is an abdominal chain exercise, creating a strong contraction of the transversus abdominis muscle, which is the deepest muscular layer of your abs. It also creates a strong contraction of the latissimus dorsi, which is the largest muscle of the upper body, stretching to both sides of the back and behind the arms.

Part of the challenge of the pose is to place your elbows at least two inches in front of your shoulders. It'd be a lot easier if your elbows were directly under your shoulders, but your body wouldn't benefit from that. The contraction of the latissimus dorsi comes from your elbows pulling toward your hips.

As for your rib cage, it's easy to let that just dip in. Therefore, keep focus to actively pull your rib cage up toward the sky. Almost immediately you'll feel the intense contraction of the latissimus dorsi, as well as other muscles.

After you've been doing the 8-Point Plank for a while, you may be surprised by how dramatically you've improved your abdominal strength. And to the moms out there working to heal their diastasis recti, the 8-Point Plank, like the Internal Leg Trace, is tremendously helpful for treating this condition.

To watch a video showing how to perform this exercise step-by-step, go to FoundationTraining.com/parents and select the "8-Point Plank" option.

Squat

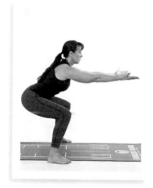

In the Squat the feet are turned a small few degrees outward from the center to allow the knee joint to comfortably achieve a ninety degree or more bend. The Squat draws the hips back to begin the motion, but quickly calls upon the knees and feet to lower the hips about as low as a chair would be. This backward and down motion is key. The Squat is healthiest when the hips actively pull backward through the entirety of the pose. It's a great glute builder and when done well will also strengthen your abdomen, psoas, hamstrings, and even the arches of your feet.

Squatting is something you are likely to do often during your baby's first year of life and into toddlerhood because floor play is such a big part of their early life. Performing this exercise with diligence will help program you to maneuver with your joints well protected.

Gorilla Lift

This exercise is purposeful in training the entire hip complex to remain stable and in power as the large thoracic spine is worked to improve its range of motion. The Gorilla Lift and the Squat are the only Foundation Training poses that ask you to begin with your feet facing subtly away from center instead of toward it. This small change allows the knees to have comfortable, stress-free motion as they approach the ninety-degree angle we hope they achieve. But close is close enough where that knee motion is concerned.

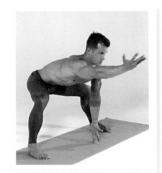

The bigger key to the Gorilla Lift is to maintain the important three points of contact between your feet and the ground; this protects the knees, ankles, and hips during the exercise.

Once you find a stable but challenging position with your hips and feet, draw your hips back into a squat, keeping your back and neck as expansive and muscularly decompressed as possible, then lift one arm at a time, in a motion called supination, as you challenge the latissimus dorsi muscle and the curvature of the thoracic spine to move while maintaining the broad expansion. To visualize supination, you can think of the palm of your hand holding a cup of soup. If your forearm is supinated, that cup won't spill as you lift your arm. (As opposed to the opposite of supination, which is pronation. If your arm were pronated with a cup in it, that cup would spill.)

This exercise is especially helpful to prepare you for floor play with your child; and, more specifically, for lifting and moving your child to and from the floor with a broadly expanded rib cage and long, strong spine.

Growing Stronger Together

Here are a few real-life examples of how you can incorporate things you've learned in the previous chapters—for both baby and yourself—to have a delightful time moving and grooving together.

Standing Decompression While Babywearing

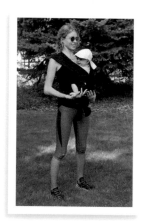

Here we see model mom Kelsey Dutton is standing tall with a strongly decompressed spine. Her chin is back, chest is up, shoulders are not rounding forward, and her elbows are pointing out widely to her sides. With one hand she is creating a platform for her baby's foot and with her other hand she is gently supporting under his bottom.

The baby boy here is nearly five months old and is showing off his strong upper spine as he turns to look over his shoulder.

With each breath his mom can lift and expand her rib

cage circumferentially as she uses the weight of her baby, on her torso and in her hands, as a weight to counterpressure and push against as she leverages her expansion.

Note: Mom is utilizing a wrap-style carrier (in a front wrap cross carry), which is less supportive than the Ergo-style carrier, but more supportive than the ring sling. There are many styles one can choose from, typically the only difference being the type of woven fibers making up the fabric. This style of carrier is simply a long piece of fabric you tie around yourself to create a pouch on your body (chest, hip, or back) where your baby can sit. The fabric is wrapped over your shoulders, across and around your torso in a way that is meant to distribute the baby's weight across the wearer's shoulders and hips.

As with other styles of carriers, we caution against wearing a baby on your back and advise strong diligence when performing asymmetrical side or hip carries.

Lunge Decompression While Babywearing

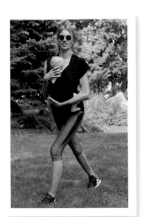

Mom models a strong setup that can be utilized for a Lunge Decompression or a Woodpecker, the latter of which is especially helpful for the act of walking around carrying a growing little bundle of joy. Mom is supporting both ends of her baby's spine well, and his feet are able to contact her legs for more feedback.

Lunge Decompression, Woodpecker, and Standing Decompression

Up next is a three-photo series, incorporating principles of the Lunge Decompression, Woodpecker, and Standing Decompression to safely lift the car seat with good mechanics, compliments of strong mom (and certified Foundation Training instructor!) Jessi Clemons.

This offers one biomechanically sound way to maneuver the heavy load of the car seat, which is something you may not consider, but are likely to do often in your life with your little one. Here we see strong model mom Jessi Clemons split her stance for this, keeping a long, decompressed spine as she hinges forward and weaves one arm through the top of the seat and around the handle while her other hand grasps the handle from the top. Once she has a solid grip on the seat, she anchors her legs and activates her posterior chain to return to an upright stance. Before moving her baby to the car, she takes a moment to balance her weight with this load using a Standing Decompression. Despite the asymmetrical load she is holding, Mom looks strong and well aligned, and you'll note that sweet baby Jorja has remained sleeping throughout this, which speaks to the smooth fluidity of Mom's motion.

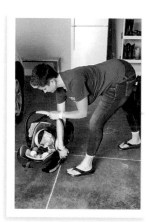 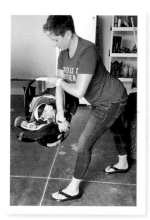 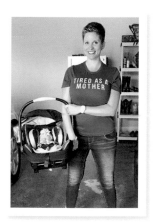

A split stance like this is beneficial in preparing the caregiver's body to then transition this load into the car, which, in itself, presents a bit of an awkward positioning challenge. As you lift and place the load, it can be helpful to place the knee and shin of your lead leg upon the seat and try to keep the car seat closer to your body as opposed to reaching your arms too far outstretched from your body. The more extended your arms, the longer the "lever" you create, which puts more weight and strain on your body to support it.

Once your child is safely locked and loaded in the car, it's well advised to follow this activity with a strong Founder and Standing or Seated (since you'll be in the car) Decompression to help reset your symmetry.

Strong Hinge Examples

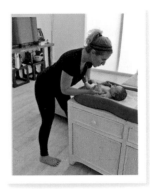

The Founder exercise in particular reinforces a strong hinge pattern. Here are some examples of how you can take that into your daily life.

Many hours are going to be spent changing diapers and clothes, bathing, and playing with a little one. Attention to the mechanics you bring within your own body as you do so is very important as you can build yourself up or break yourself down. Here we see model mom, sports chiropractor Dr. Sandy Doman, DC, exemplifying a solid forward hinge at her baby's changing table.

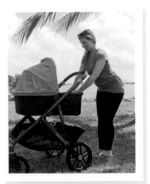

Here is the same idea at the stroller. This time Mom's stance is narrow, her legs internally rotate, and her big toes touch as she checks in on her daughter Sage. (Check-ins are very important to ensure that the movement and rattling that come with strolling do not shift the baby into potentially compromising positions.)

In the third image on this page our lovely model mom Kelsey is seen here practicing a strong hip hinge while wearing her nearly five-month-old son, Lew. She activates her posterior chain to pull her hips behind her; her toes subtly point toward each other; and her knees are unlocked and gently bending. She keeps her chin back and her neck long and aligned with the rest of her spine as her arms come under and behind her baby's pelvis and torso to support his hips, bottom, back, neck, and skull. His feet gently press into Mom's upper legs, which gives him cues

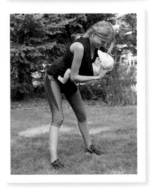

that help organize his body's understanding of where he is in space. Mom uses the weight of the baby's body as leverage against which to strongly expand as she breathes.

Wearing a baby like this as one hinges also provides additional work for the muscles of the posterior chain. This activity gives the baby a fun ride that allows a hidden challenge to his own alignment as he works against gravity not to let his head, neck, or upper back flop backward.

HINGE AND SQUAT

Here are two strong seaside movements for FT's founding dad giving his baby girl a bird's-eye view of the beach. Dad's hands broadly spread the span of her torso, giving her added trunk stability to feel secure at such a height. Her weight atop his shoulders in this way creates added challenge and strengthening potential for his entire posterior chain.

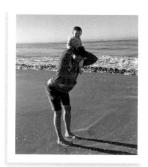 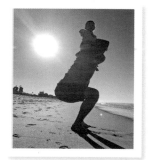

SQUAT

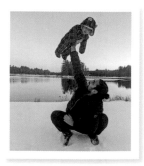

Here we see another strong chiropractor dad, Georges Dagher, DC, CSCS, founder of Dagher Strength, exemplifying a deep squat. Georges has made movement part of his daily life practice and is strong in his thoracic rotation with a well-stabilized spine and pelvis, allowing him to powerfully lift his young son in this manner. In this position, baby boy Will gets a great view along with some challenging tummy-time practice. He responds beautifully, lifting his head with a big smile and a well-aligned spine.

Kneeling Founder and Modified 8-Point Plank

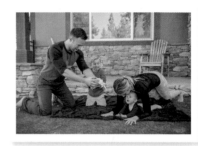

Here is a great family shot, compliments of one of the members of Foundation Training's team of core educators, Los Angeles County Fire Department Captain Evan Halquist.

Here we see Dad is in a Kneeling Founder with his Sphere of Tension low and surrounding a toy to attract his young son to lock his eyes and visually track as his dad shifts his sphere higher. This makes the exercise more dynamic for Dad and the tummy-time propping more dynamic for baby. Mom, nurse Kristin, is in a modified 8-Point Plank, with her knees lifted off the surface and her forearms providing stability for her young one's tummy-time experience. Big brother William is following Dad's modeling of a Kneeling Founder while cheering on baby bro Everett (who is so enamored with his mama that his attention, head, and neck are strongly upright). Everyone is doing awesome, exemplifying that exercise can absolutely be a family affair that is woven into floor play, anytime, anywhere.

8-Point Plank

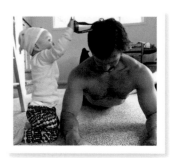

Dad Eric is in the process of pulling his rib cage toward the back of his body, muscularly pulling up into an 8-Point Plank. Daughter Sunny began kneeling with her bottom resting on her legs and when Dad elevated, she began to elevate with him. She was given sunglasses and told "put them on Daddy's head." So here you see her working to do that. Any leaning into his head meant his muscles were working extra to maintain his stability!

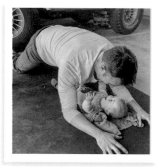

You could also give kiddo a hat, stickers, a brush, any number of playful or practical things to entice them to playfully engage with their caregiver.

Here we see another dad doing the same exercise with his six-month-old on his back. This is a win-win. They get excellent bonding eye-contact and face-to-face time while Dad gets to do his exercise and baby boy gets to practice reaching up for his dad.

Gorilla Lift

Mama Jen is seen here in front of a gorilla statue modifying the Gorilla Lift while wearing her baby gorilla forward facing in her Ergo carrier.

Mom is using her left arm to lock her daughter in a strong hold under her torso and left arm in a way that the baby feels supported enough to look up toward her grandma who was calling her name. Mom's right arm is reaching forward as in the Gorilla Lift exercise, expanding her rib cage and challenging the mobility of her thoracic

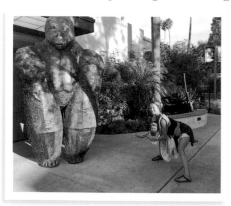

spine while effectively creating a platform for the baby to reach out, hold on to, and press her own body up from as she works to lift her head, neck, and upper body. Mom can focus on utilizing this frame of support for her baby as her own leverage point to push the work of holding her baby's weight into her lats, glutes, and hamstrings, while she keeps her heels firmly planted to engage her anchor.

Conclusion

Being a parent is among the most wonderfully rewarding experiences life has to offer, but it carries with it a lot of potentially challenging responsibilities. At times this is likely to feel overwhelming, and when it does, please try to give yourself grace over shame. You don't have to be perfect, and, to the tiny human in your care, you already are! Use these fundamentals as a resource for this one area of physical development and just keep showing up, meeting your baby with love and encouragement exactly where they are, and trying your best. With that, you're likely to do a great job as you guide your growing little one and help them to thrive.

Try to keep in mind that in the process of caring for your child, you're likely to be in physical positions that can potentially wreak havoc on your own postural health and comfort. Rather than letting this break you down over time, remember there are many small things you can do daily that can build you up and yield tremendous health-benefiting results. So give it your best go! Perhaps the most beautiful perk is, because children are ever-watching, ever-learning little sponges, if you keep at it as your little one grows, you're likely to find that you've helped to establish exercise and healthy movement habits as an important part of daily life. And that in itself is likely to result in priceless benefits for the rest of your child's life.

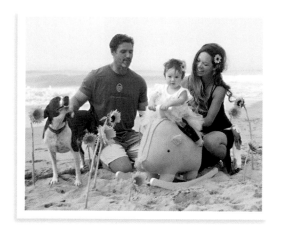

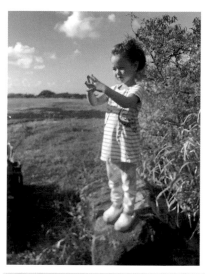

Acknowledgments

So many wonderful folks, more than listed here, contributed to this book's creation, and within its pages there is a collective drive to help as many folks as possible with this compilation of info. Thank you all for the support!

MY SWEET SUNNY SKY: You are now almost three and a half as I write this! Thank you for making me a mama and the incredible joy you bring all of us who love you. You are the brightest light and grandest teacher I've ever known, and 100 percent my muse for this book! I will love you to infinity and beyond!

ERIC GOODMAN: Dear, goofy husband, thank you for seeing me, supporting me, and standing beside me. You heard my earliest thoughts about this stuff and encouraged me from the start. Thank you for your love and our beautiful daughter. Words will never capture how full my heart is.

KAREN RINALDI: Thank you, as a mother yourself, for recognizing the genuine need for this resource. I am forever grateful for the opportunity to have a voice to share a few key things that I suspect *every* peds therapist has wished parents and caregivers knew. Thank you for your patience, encouragement, support, and faith.

REBECCA RASKIN: You helped bring this book to life! Thank you for your support—technical and creative—in the process of this coming to tangible form.

HY BENDER: Thank you for helping to structure the flow of images in journalistic fashion and for attempting to make my "clinical speak" more user-friendly.

DR. IRIS CASTANEDA-VAN WYK: Our beloved integrative pediatrician in Santa Barbara, California. Thank you for your holistic care for our precious baby and supportive kindness for us as new parents. We have the deepest appreciation for you, Doctora, and are honored to have your beautiful words greeting our readers as they dive into the pages of this book.

DANI RHOADES, NC, PERINATAL AND PEDIATRIC NUTRITIONIST, CO-FOUNDER OF HAPPY HEALTHY LITTLES: Thank you for your support during my pregnancy and Sunny's first years of life, and for the pearls you've interjected into this book.
(If you're looking for guidance in perinatal, infant, toddler, and/or postpartum nutrition, we encourage you to visit happyhealthylittles.com.)

ALLI COST, OT: Thank you for bringing your energy to Foundation Training. Your presence has brought so much to the team! And thank you for proofing this text and contributing important insights on development from the lens of a peds OT. Parents need to know this important stuff.
(Ms. Cost has more than ten years of experience treating babies and children. She has a passion for embedded coaching, having developed trainings for families, practitioners, and communities both in the United States and abroad. She has been a PT, part of FT's core leadership team since 2019.)

AMANDA SHERFIELD, PT: My dear PT school sister, thank you for proofing this book. Your experience as a mom of five gives you legit insight that I respect deeply. I love you to *CHICAGO* and back!
(Mrs. Sherfield, MSPT, has been in pediatric practice for nearly two

decades. She practiced for eleven years with United Cerebral Palsy, in Orlando, Florida, and now offers her services via Florida's Early Steps early intervention program.)

AMANDA VARGAS, OT: In the spirit of Lez and Suz, thank you for proofing and helping us polish the fine motor and sensory details with some of your magic!

(Mrs. Vargas, MOT, OTR/L, SCFES, CBS, is the co-owner of Bold Child Co., a pediatric private practice in Jacksonville Beach, Florida. She's passionate about empowering families in the areas of feeding and development, specializing in the pre/post-rehab of tethered oral tissue—tongue and lip ties—and helping families with feeding from birth.)

LAURA, LANE, CHEYNE, AND MATT JOSLIN, ROBERTA NEVES, PT, MSPT, TANJA VANWELL-MCARTHY, PT, ALESHA CONKLIN—THE ORIGINAL CREW OF ABILITY PLUS THERAPY IN MELBOURNE, FLORIDA: Thank you for opening your clinic and hearts to me as a curious student PT. Your mentorship went above and beyond any clinical affiliation I could have dreamed of and was incredibly formative in my life and career. The hearts with which you approach the care of all the special individuals you are in service to are simply beautiful, and I'm eternally grateful to have had the experiences I did with you all.

(Ability Plus Therapy is a pediatric therapy center that specializes in providing intensive therapies to children from all over the world with neurological and genetic conditions. They also offer traditional PT, OT, and speech therapy services. What began as a clinic started by parents seeking to provide the services their child and others needed has grown into a special school called No Limits Academy. This school provides innovative education to children with complex physical disabilities, such as cerebral palsy and spinal cord injuries, among others. Their methodology provides each student with high-tech lesson plans, personalized educational adaptations, and physical modifications that empower them to learn, thrive, and increase opportunities for advanced achievement.)

Models/Photos/Production

Sunora Sky Goodman, parents, and grandparents
   Sandy and Jess Salas

Sage Wolf Kaplan and parents Dr. Sandy Doman and Eric Kaplan

Arrow Adams and mom Melika

Ruthe Harley Peterson, parents Alli and Brian Peterson,
   and grandfather Stuart Blum

Allison Cost, Jessie Salas, Josh Holland, Adrienne Smith,
   Gail DeSart, Martin Reader, and Dustin DeRyke

Lewis Garrett Dutton, IV, and mom Kelsey

Evan, Kristin, William, and Everett Halquist

Georges, Sarah, and Will Dagher

Jessi and Jorja Clemons

Paul Mathieu

Sarka Holečková

Marisa Matluck

Trang Sage

Chau Leminh

Ryne Swanberg

Notes from a Pediatric OT

Nothing develops in solitude, and the body is a beautiful network of interrelated systems that must all function well together to help it truly thrive. As your little one develops, there are multiple "domains" of development you are likely to read about in addition to "gross motor." These include the cognitive, communicative, and social-emotional domains, to name a few. All these aspects of development contribute to establishing a foundation for a child's health and wellness. This book has been centered around the gross motor domain, but another intimately interwoven field that we've lightly touched on, the fine motor domain, deserves a separate introduction here.

Respecting that this area is outside our scope of practice, we have turned to pediatric occupational therapist Allison Cost, MS, OTR/L, who is part of Foundation Training's Infant and Early Childhood Development Team. She has provided a wonderful breakdown of the first year's fine motor development with some focal pearls for our readers to keep in mind.

HAND DEVELOPMENT IS braided together with muscular coordination and sensory self-regulation. Nothing builds in isolation. As the core muscles and joints stabilize, the fine motor skills of the limbs can specialize. Babies need their big muscles (which they develop within their budding gross motor skills) to get strong before their smaller muscles can develop and learn their role. The input your baby is provided into their hands through big movements like pressing, pulling, and crawling is the precursor to developing their fine motor skills. Your baby is not only experiencing the world around them but also discovering their own body. Remember that each experience your baby has (whether on their belly, side, back, or in your arms) is a way for them to learn and grow.

IN THE FIRST months of your baby's life their arm and hand movements are determined primarily by reflexes. Hands remain mostly closed, opening occasionally then squeezing shut when pressure is put on the palm. Remember that this "strength" felt in your baby's grip is not stabilized muscular strength but a reflex. Therefore, it is not safe to hold your baby up with their grip since their muscles and tissue lack the actual ability to support their body weight.

AS YOUR BABY approaches two months of age, the thumb will no longer be held tightly in the palm. Their arms now begin to respond with some intentional, albeit still uncoordinated, movement to display excitement at the sight of a toy. Colors are now visible, so switch from the high-contrast black-and-white pictures to bright toys to encourage those happy wiggles.

AROUND THREE MONTHS, a baby's hand will remain open about half of the time. They will start to reach for toys intentionally with arms extended toward a desired item. Your baby can bring their hands to midline and visually follow moving objects as well. Offer toys from all angles to encourage reach, press, and pull. Sensory input along their open hands increases not only their motivation but also body awareness, so add in texture-rich toys. Along with touch, sound awareness is increasing with the ability to start associating sounds with familiar objects. Bring in sounds to which the baby responds positively such as maracas and silly noises you can make.

AT FOUR MONTHS, your baby has the capacity to see tiny objects one to two feet away and to track those objects more with their eyes (instead of with moving their head). Help your child learn visual searching and tracking by placing their favorite toy in sight and moving it around as if it's flying (with silly sounds, of course). Add in tactile input by gently tapping on their hands or feet or lips, which are the areas with the highest amount of sensory receptors. This is the age of building shoulder joint stability with practice holding themselves up on their forearms while on their belly. These moments are the cornerstone of stabilized reaching for the coming months and years. Your baby's weight is shifted onto their arms mostly due to their head movements of lifting and rotation. It is important to provide toys both from the left and right sides equally to prevent any imbalance in the neck and back musculature. Grasp development initiates around this time with small objects held in the palm using middle, ring, and pinky fingers, and a flexed wrist. This is referred to as "ulnar grasp" since the items are near the pinky side of the palm toward the ulna bone.

AT FIVE MONTHS the grasp develops further with all five fingers holding items in the palm in a "palmar grasp." Reaching is done with two hands clumsily, but intentionally, moving together. Babies now have an increased motivation to get to desired out-of-reach objects, so place those items out of arm's reach to promote increasingly complex patterns of movement. Movements integrate into communication with arm and hand actions, such as wiggling to continue a song and arms held up on prediction that they will be picked up. Imitate their movements and demonstrate with your body how to maneuver to items out of their reach. How we move is imprinted on our children.

Move with intention, knowing they are writing what they see into the groundwork of their own patterns.

SIX MONTHS IS a big milestone for babies as they acquire confidence in their ability to weight bear on their hands while lying on their belly. This provides the increased sensory input and joint stabilization to coordinate reaching for an object with just one arm. With the Grasp Reflex completely gone, your baby can open their hands fully with the intention to grab something, maintaining that grasp with their index, middle finger, and thumb pressing small items into the palm. This is a "radial-palmar grasp," with items held more toward the thumb side of the palm, near the radius bone. Since babies are now looking at objects both close by and a few feet away, they will attempt to pick up tiny objects nearby and search out ones that are out of their reach. This adjusts the child's interest from being in their own hands to the larger world around. Place toys both in reach and slightly out of reach to encourage searching. Babies now have an increased response to facial expressions and are able to identify the directions sounds are coming from. A good sensory experience for this age is to move around them making sounds and silly faces, or you can bring them in front of a mirror so they can see themselves and their own facial expressions. Your actions entertain, engage, and motivate more movement exploration.

AROUND EIGHT MONTHS the elbow extends with more control for reaching, allowing the hand to rake objects with bent fingers. The thumb starts opposing the other fingertips in a "radial-digital grasp," which is a precursor to the more complex fine motor skills to come. This is the perfect opportunity to have your baby "rake" their fingers through textures like sand or dry beans to get a little toy. If your baby is endeavoring into solid foods, you can preload flat utensils or short silicone spoons with avocado or other mash-able foods to encourage this new ability.

EIGHT MONTHS IS the age when your baby is likely able to transfer objects between hands and start to use movements to manipulate toys. Cooperative back-and-forth games are a perfect challenge with items at different angles. For example, have your baby pick up items and pass them to your hand at different levels. This is also the age to start experimenting with the amount of force needed to push/pull objects, which builds proprioceptive sensory awareness. You can fill up plastic eggs with different amounts of water to provide differently weighted objects for them to pick up. This skill will soon build into learning the appropriate force of using eating utensils, and later into throwing a ball. You can continue to offer touch input by having your baby turn pages of a firm board book. This is a good age to allow exploring smells by wrapping foods (like a cut lemon placed briefly in a washcloth) and having them sniff at their desire.

DURING MONTHS NINE AND TEN, the wrist will begin to voluntarily extend to get an item. As the wrist establishes this control, the index finger gains isolated movement in relation to the rest of the other digits. This sets up the ability to poke and use a thumb-to-index-finger "pincer" grasp. Encourage high-fives and start using pointing to indicate locations of body parts and objects in a book. An extra bonus of learning body parts is that it also builds body awareness. Sensory poking tasks are a hit at this age. This can be integrated into food play tasks such as pushing fingers into soft foods. A less messy option is to place paint in a ziplock bag, tape the edges to a flat surface, and use an isolated index finger to make dots or lines. You can also encourage exploring with the index finger by pushing items through holes in the back of empty cardboard egg cartons.

YOUR BABY IS now fully in control of dropping objects voluntarily. Their two arms are now functioning as unique limbs but able to work for common goals such as banging blocks together. An important play pattern to encourage at this age is dropping and finding toys. It provides not only sensory input on the sounds of the drop, but visual searching and motor planning challenge. As your baby masters crawl-ing, ask them to bring toys to you or take toys across the room to put in a container. Carrying items in the hand while crawling contributes to the development of palmar arches. These arches are the building blocks for holding writing utensils in the future and having control of tools like scissors. Work to provide novel and varied textures to crawl over by placing preferred items on the other side of a safe, age-appropriate obstacle course (think pillows and blankets rolled up).

AS YOUR BABY nears their eleventh and twelfth months, their arms have been isolated as two separate movement levers and their hands are now ready to follow this pattern. Babies now use each hand inde-pendently of the other. Those blocks they were banging together last month can now be stacked on top of each other. Your baby now has the coordination to put objects into containers with wide openings and use one hand to stabilize while the other manipulates. Fill up those empty tissue boxes with toys and have your child take them out. Your baby can turn the palm upward, called forearm supination, to reach for an offered item. This builds a healthy posture pattern with shoulders in socket and midsection engaged. You can integrate play tasks such as holding bowls from the bottom and placing Velcro pictures on the underside of play forts to encourage this arm and wrist rotation.

FINE MOTOR SKILLS should be done in sitting, standing, kneeling, ly-ing on the belly, lying on the side, and just about any other way your baby feels motivated to try. More positions mean more problem solv-ing to complete the task. This then leads to stronger, coordinated, and more balanced kids. It is important to note that if a fine motor task is difficult at this age, your baby may indicate this by bending their elbows and keeping arms glued to the side of the body. If you see this, offer some increased core stabilization and work on building tummy and trunk muscles.

FINALLY, SOME NOTES on sensory skills. Babies are born functioning on reflexes. Truly codependent, their sensory experiences are rooted in responses that they don't have control over. Babies cry when discomfort arises, coo when pleasure arises. There is no such thing as spoiling your baby these first months of life, as your baby literally relies on caregivers to regulate themself. The focus of the first couple months is allowing the brain to learn that basic needs will be met, and that the child is safe. Pay attention to what calms or alerts your baby, understanding that all babies need different input at different times. Self-regulation in toddlers, children, and even adults is built from these formative experiences of trusting that their needs will be met. It teaches their brain that they are safe and can get through discomfort. Embrace the healthy functional codependency with your baby.

YOUR BABY IS learning self-regulation from the moment they are born. They are learning how to self-soothe, shift attention, maintain a routine, and tolerate the variety of sensory experiences that you are exposing them to. As they approach a year, they will start learning how to adjust their behaviors and regulate strong feelings. This is a wonderful opportunity to learn more about yourself too. What calms you? What sensory experiences do you crave or avoid? A couple key items to remember as your child builds their sensory self-regulation is to praise effort (not the end result) to build a growth mind-set. Teach your children how to deal with strong feelings by labeling the emotion or feeling and demonstrating calming practices.

ALSO KEEP IN mind that in terms of sensory experiences, everything baby sees, smells, hears, touches, and tastes will garner some sort of input for their sensory system. Movements like rocking and swinging are two favorites of babies in their first year that provide calming sensation for their vestibular system (which contributes to the body's balance and spatial awareness). Enrich your baby's play sessions with mindfulness to the details of their play environment, activities, and selection of toys. What materials are things made of? What textures, colors, sounds, smells, tastes is your baby experiencing? And don't neglect that some of the most rich sensory experiences of the first year revolve around baby's budding eating skills. All new flavors and textures combined with figuring out how to get food into the mouth (hand skills of grasp, release, and reaching!), and coordinating mashing or chewing the food up and swallowing it while also focusing on sitting upright. Of course, this is only in the later half of the year. In the first half, there is a whole sensory and oral motor dance to learn around feeding whether it is by breast or bottle. We aren't diving deep into any of these topics here, but I do hope you will be aware of and consider these sorts of details. Sensory seeking or sensory aversive behaviors can absolutely impact a baby's willingness to participate in movement and it's always important to keep in mind that everything is working and learning together. Every day provides new opportunities for both you and your little one to grow further into a healthy mind and body. Enjoy the ride.

Glossary

If you're not sure of the meaning of a term in this book, you can probably find a definition of it in this glossary, which is organized in alphabetical order.

Heads up: In the movement world there are certain words (words you already know and likely use in other ways), such as *opening* or *cruising*, that have different and specific meaning as it relates to the body and its movement.

ABDOMEN: The part of the body between the chest and pelvis, which includes the abdominal muscles and the organs that lie underneath them.

ABS: Short for abdominal muscles.

ACCESSORY MUSCLES: Muscles that assist, but don't play a primary role, in a particular action.

ADDUCTOR MUSCLES: A group of muscles in the upper inner thigh originating in the groin and attached along the femur (thighbone). The primary job of these muscles is drawing the legs inward toward the midline. They also aid in rotating and flexing the thighs and maintaining the body's balance when kneeling, standing, or walking.

ALIGNMENT: How bones and body parts sit in relation to one another while in any given position (lying, sitting, kneeling, standing). We focus on alignment as a way to guide how children utilize their muscles during any given activity. It is by strengthening the muscles with controlled actions that we can help to guide the developing alignment of a child's body.

ALL FOURS: Being positioned on both hands and both knees while the tummy is turned to the ground. Before babies will crawl on all fours, they typically exhibit practicing rocking back and forth on all fours first (an act that primes their muscles and joint surfaces for more movement).

ANCHORED BACK EXTENSION: A Foundation Training exercise performed on the stomach that supports the spine in a mildly extended position. In addition, it improves the effectiveness of the adductor muscles, which will traction (decompress) the spine at the same time this exercise is extending it.

ANCHORED BRIDGE: A Foundation Training exercise that effectively creates a suspension bridge from the arches to the adductors by using the hamstrings and posterior chain to suspend your hips about an inch off the ground. This exercise can be helpful for treating lower back pain resulting from bending activities, and (along with the Internal Leg Trace) for treating sciatica.

ANCHORING LINE: Formed by arches, feet, legs, and groin. The associated muscles—medial groin, adductors, and medial hamstring—directly connect to the bottom of the pelvis and work together to lift the arches and contract the inner legs toward the pubic symphysis, allowing the body to stand tall. Foundation Training exercises that work the anchoring line include the Internal Leg Trace, Anchored Bridge, Anchored Back Extension, and 8-Point Plank.

ANTERIOR CHAIN: The muscles along the front side of the body (e.g., abs, quads, pecs).

BALANCE: The ability to keep the center of mass within one's base of support, whether moving or still. Balance keeps us upright so we don't fall over. (Not synonymous with *stability*.)

BASE OF SUPPORT: When sitting, the points of contact of the lower body—bottom, legs, feet—on which body weight is being supported (also called the *seated base*). When standing, the support formed by the feet and how the legs are positioned (e.g., close together, wide apart).

BODY WEIGHT: The overall weight of a body.

BOPPY PILLOW: A C-shaped pillow that can be helpful for positioning baby for certain activities. The cushioning provides some stability for the baby's body, cues to guide their posture, and a bumper in case the baby begins to topple over. There's an opening at the front that makes it easy for the baby to reach out and interact with whatever's before the pillow. This allows the baby to operate with some independence while enjoying a level of protection. If you don't have a Boppy pillow available, you can instead use anything that provides comparable padding for a baby's back and sides—for example, a long, thick, rolled-up towel placed into a C shape.

BUMPER ROLL: A cushion, typically created from a rolled-up towel or receiving blanket, used to help control the body's alignment when a baby lacks the muscular strength and skills to do so.

CENTER OF GRAVITY: For an adult, the center of gravity is the pubic symphysis, but this is not the same for a baby since they have yet to develop the muscular strength or stability to hold their weight as upright as an adult. In fact, you'll notice most babies stand and begin walking with their belly protruding in front of them, jutting forward and making their center of gravity fall in a different area than a more matured, developed body. They have not yet learned to fully engage the muscles that hold them upright and pull their central point of weight backward.

CORE: The center of a body's movement and stability. The core includes all muscles directly connected to the pelvis (e.g., muscles of the abdomen, back, upper legs, glutes).

CRAWLING: Baby's first real mobility (beyond rolling) from point A to point B. The typical visual for crawling is that of baby on their hands and knees with their stomach hovering over the floor, but that is actually advanced. Most babies will exhibit an immature (less strong) version first that is much lower to the ground; their belly may even be dragging, as they push and pull with their arms low to the ground and push with their legs often externally rotated and in more contact with the floor than just being atop the knees. Crawling gets the baby moving with reciprocal arm and leg action as well as some side-bending and rotational movement in the lower trunk—all of which strengthens and prepares their body for more upright mobility such as cruising and walking.

CRUISING: For a baby, standing in front of a support structure, such as a couch, and taking side steps to move along the structure. This is typically done while holding on to the structure with one or both hands for extra stability and balance, and sometimes even leaning the chest or abdomen into the surface for additional help before the muscles are strong enough to support a more upright stance. Aka *sidestepping*.

DECOMPRESSION BREATHING: Breathing that expands the rib cage and strengthens respiratory muscles. This tool is a component of every Foundation Training exercise.

DIASTASIS RECTI: A partial separation of the muscles that meet at the midline of the abdomen. This occurs to an estimated 60 percent of mothers during or following pregnancy as a result of the uterus stretching the abdominal muscles to make room for the growing baby. It can also result from lifting heavy weights the wrong way, or performing abdominal exercises excessively and/or incorrectly. Symptoms may include a bulge in the stomach, especially when straining abs; low back pain; bloating; constipation; and bad posture. The 8-Point Plank and Internal Leg Trace exercises can help treat this condition by stabilizing the bottom of the pelvis.

DISTAL: Farther from the body's central midline; the opposite of proximal, which is closer to the midline.

8-POINT PLANK: A Foundation Training exercise performed on the stomach that helps get the back of the rib cage as wide and big as possible and tighten its front as much as possible. This abdominal chain exercise creates a strong contraction of the transversus abdominis muscle, which is the deepest muscular layer of the abs. It also creates a strong contraction of the latissimus dorsi, which is the largest muscle of the upper body, stretching to both sides of the back and behind the arms. This exercise is helpful for treating diastasis recti.

EXTEND: To straighten, increasing the angle between two body parts (e.g., a baby extends their elbow to straighten their arm and reach outward for a toy). The opposite of *flex*.

EXTERNAL ROTATION: A term describing movement of a joint. See *opening*.

FEMUR: The thighbone. This is the longest and strongest bone in the body, extending from the hip to the knee.

FLEX: To bend, decreasing the angle between two body parts (e.g., a baby flexes their knees and hips to lower down in a squat). The opposite of *extend*.

FOREARM: The lower arm, between the wrist and the elbow.

FOUNDATION TRAINING: A process that gives you the means to change the way you move and correct the imbalances caused by our modern habits. Through a series of body weight exercises, Foundation Training activates your posterior muscle chain, anchors your hips, decompresses your spine, and teaches you to take the burden of supporting the body out of your joints and put it where it belongs—in your muscles.

FOUNDER: A hip hinge exercise that activates and aligns your muscles, lines up your nerves, integrates your posterior chain with the other muscle chains in your body, bolsters the stability of your hips, and trains you to breathe powerfully. This is Foundation Training's most appreciated exercise because it's relatively quick and easy to do anywhere and anytime, and is incredibly effective.

GLUTES: The muscles of the buttocks. They are responsible for extending, abducting, and outwardly rotating the hips and add stability to the low back, hips, and legs.

HALF KNEELING: Kneeling atop one knee and one foot. See also *kneeling*.

HAMSTRINGS: A powerful group of muscles at the back of the thigh that extends the hips and flexes the knees. Part of the posterior chain.

HIGH GUARD: Self-stabilizing position of the upper extremities during gait in which the arms are not freely moving; rather, they are flexed at the elbow and the hands are held at the level of the shoulders or above. This is an arm position that gives cues as to the balance and control of the body while walking. See also *low guard, mid guard, reciprocal walking*.

HINGE: Hip flexion and extension. Hip flexion as you draw your hips back, hip extension as you pull your hips forward to return to standing.

HIP JOINT: The ball-and-socket joint connecting each leg to the torso.

INTERNAL LEG TRACE: A quick and easy Foundation Training exercise that's terrific at activating the muscles in the anchoring line, warming the body up for any subsequent and more challenging anchoring exercises. In addition, like the 8-Point Plank, this exercise helps stabilize the bottom of the pelvis, which can be effective for treating diastasis recti; and like the Anchored Bridge exercise, it can be helpful for treating sciatica.

INTERNAL ROTATION: A term describing movement of a joint. See *opening*.

JOINT: A point where two or more bones of the skeleton come together to allow motion.

KINETIC CHAIN: Interrelated groups of muscles, connecting joints, and body segments operating together to perform movements.

KNEELING: Positioning the body such that it is seated atop both knees, which are flexed, with both lower legs and feet on the floor behind the torso. Kneeling can be low or high depending on how the trunk positions in relation to the hips. Playing in this position strengthens and adds stability to baby's core-pelvis-hips, further enhancing development of the lower regions of the spine's curve. See also *half kneeling*.

KNEELING FOUNDER: A Foundation Training kneeling exercise that teaches how to move the entire torso against tension held at the bottom muscles and groin muscles. The results are increased stability at the bottom of the pelvis and at the hips, helping to treat such ailments as lower spine instability (spondylolisthesis).

KYPHOTIC CURVE (OR KYPHOSIS): A curve that is convex at the back of the spine and concave at its front (so rounds outward toward the back).

LATISSIMUS DORSI: The largest muscle of the upper back, and the facilitator of shoulder protection and rib cage stability. Part of the posterior chain.

LIMBS: The arms and legs.

LONG WING: This is a variation of arm position utilized in a number of Foundation Training exercises that involve standing, including the Founder, Standing Decompression, and Lunge Decompression. See also *Short Wing*.

LORDOTIC CURVE (OR LORDOSIS): A curve that is concave at the spine's backside and convex at its front (like a backward C).

LOW GUARD: A self-stabilizing position of the upper extremities during gait in which the arms are not freely moving; rather, they are kept closer to the body, and in this case the elbows are extended and the hands are held at roughly the level of the lower abdomen/hips. This is an arm position that gives cues as to the balance and control of the body while walking. See also *mid guard*, *high guard*, *reciprocal walking*.

LUNGE DECOMPRESSION: A Foundation Training exercise that's great for unwinding compressed or tightened-up parts of the body, such as the legs, calves, psoas muscles, or abs. It's similar to Standing Decompression, but instead of keeping the feet together, in this exercise you set them a long step apart via a split stance, and then try to close your legs together without actually moving them. The scissoring tension that results from the back of your front leg to the front of your back leg stands you up taller and triggers a line of stability in the very deep muscle of your spine and pelvis.

MEASURING STICKS: A built-in tool that we all carry around with us—a mini Measuring Stick created by placing your thumbs on the base of your ribs and your pinky fingers on the pointy bone of your pelvis. Using your fingers in this way allows you to continually feel where your rib cage and pelvis are, and more importantly, how much space you manage to create between them as a result of your decompression breathing and movements. This is encouraged with every Foundation Training exercise.

MID GUARD: A self-stabilizing position of the upper extremities during gait in which the arms are not freely moving; rather, they are flexed at the elbow and the hands are held at roughly the level of the chest to waist. This is an arm position that gives cues as to the balance and control of the body while walking. See also *low guard*, *high guard*, *reciprocal walking*.

MIDLINE: An imaginary vertical line that divides the body down its center into symmetrical halves.

MORO REFLEX: See *Startle Reflex*.

NEUTRAL ALIGNMENT: The optimal position in which the spine or joints are lined up to move without causing damage or pain. No segments of the body are oddly rotated, bent, or compressed. Neutral alignment of the spine facilitates healthy communication between the nerves that send signals between the brain, spine, and body parts; and it also promotes unrestricted blood and lymphatic flow. See also *alignment*.

NEWBORN: A baby zero to two months old.

OBLIQUES: The internal and external abdominal oblique muscles are portions of the abdominal muscles that help to flex, side-bend, and rotate the trunk. They also play a part in respiration, during exhalation. They span from the low back, over the crests of the hip bones, to a common tendinous insertion shared with other abdominal muscles along the central line of the abdomen.

OPENING: In the context of joints, rotating outward (away from the midline, also called *external rotation*) as opposed to inward (toward the midline, also called *internal rotation*). Also, when a baby is in front of and facing a support structure, *opening* the hip or torso means turning *away* from the structure.

PECTORAL MUSCLES: The muscles of the chest connecting the ribs with the shoulders and upper arms. These are also abbreviated as "pecs" and are part of the anterior chain.

PELVIC GIRDLE: The bony structures and surrounding muscles that attach the legs to the rest of the skeleton. It is home to the pelvic floor muscles, which are present in both males and females, and can be a source of dysfunction (for which FT exercises can be beneficial!) during pregnancy and after.

PELVIS: The bowl-shaped bone structure below the waist and at the top of the legs, and which connects the legs and spinal column. During hip hinging, and at other times, the two regions dissociate and move separate from each other, such as in rolling. The pelvis is the central hub of the body; it houses the center of gravity.

PLANK: A position similar to a push-up that extends the entire body, making it resemble a long, straight wooden plank.

POSTERIOR CHAIN: The muscles along the backside of the body from head to feet, which include the neck and back extensors, the glutes, the hamstrings, and calves. These muscles play a vital role in many forms of movement, including standing, walking, running, and jumping. They're also important for creating stability in the legs, hips, pelvis, and spine. These muscles get their first call to action when a newborn baby tries to lift their head to latch and nurse. "Tummy time" is crucial for babies as it challenges their posterior chain.

POSTPARTUM PERIOD: The first six weeks following childbirth. The uterus is healing; organs are shifting back after being displaced to make room for the growing and developing baby; and the spine is experiencing significantly different forces because of the last nine to ten months of changes in the center of gravity. If the birth was a cesarean section, there is also healing of several layers of tissue that must occur during this time. There are also major shifts in several hormones of the body (which will continue to happen as long as the mother is breastfeeding), causing shifts in everything from sleep to digestion to ligament laxity. If any trauma occurred during labor and delivery, the body may have additional healing taking place within this period and potentially beyond.

POSTURE: The positioning of the body. See also *neutral alignment*.

PRONE: Positioned lying on the stomach (aka *tummy time*).

PRONE DECOMPRESSION: A Foundation Training exercise performed on your stomach that teaches you to not extend your spine (the way you do in, say, a Cobra yoga pose), but instead use your transverse abdominal muscle to keep the back of your rib cage expanded, your abdomen tight and long, and your breath as big as possible. Performing this exercise is a bit like hanging from the edge of a cliff with your fingers, pulling into where your hands are. If you do it right, you feel the back of your body engaged from the shoulders down to the back; and you also feel your abdomen engage as it's trying to lift the back of your rib cage toward the ceiling. See also *Supine Decompression*.

PROPPING: Supporting the body's weight via one or both arms pushing into the ground. For example, a newborn on their stomach will initially prop themselves a bit up from the ground on their lower arms with elbows bent. Once their body develops sufficient strength and muscle control, they'll prop themselves up higher from the ground on open palms with elbows extended. Propping in this manner helps activate the posterior chain and is a key developmental skill that precedes crawling.

Propping is also part of early sitting skills before trunk control develops. Using the arm as a tripod with sitting is not the same as *reflexively* using the arms as a safety response to catch the body if it's off-balance and falling.

PUBIC SYMPHYSIS: A joint located between the left and right pubic bones, joined by a cartilaginous disk. It is an adult's center of body weight, and it helps act as a shock absorber during movement. It also shifts, allowing more space in the pelvis for baby during childbirth. This is a common site of pain for many women during pregnancy because of the added weight, stretch, and pressure to the abdominal muscles (which attach here) while the hormones are fluctuating and causing ligaments to be more lax than usual.

QUADS: The quadriceps are a group of powerful muscles in the front of the thigh that flex the thigh at the hip and extend the leg at the knee. They are considered in the anterior chain of muscles.

RANGE OF MOTION: A joint's potential for movement. Clinically this is measured (in degrees or percentages) to assess baseline function and measure progress. Range-of-motion activities can be done with the intent of teaching the joints (and muscles and brains) about movement. With a newborn this type of activity is more passive, with a caregiver leading the movement. As the child gains strength and mobility they will naturally take their own joints through their available ranges of motion as they experiment more with movement.

RECIPROCAL WALKING: Advancing the left arm in sync with the right leg followed by the right arm with the left leg. This advanced gait is what adults typically use. It will develop sometime during toddlerhood, once the muscles of the torso and pelvic girdle are sufficiently strong and stable enough during movement that the limbs can move freely while the torso remains upright and balanced. See also *low guard*, *mid guard*, and *high guard* to better understand postures your child may exhibit on the path to walking reciprocally.

RING-SITTING POSITION: Sitting with the feet together in front of the body and knees bent such that the legs form a shape resembling a circle, or "ring."

ROTATING: Turning a joint (e.g., hip joint, shoulder joint) around an axis. Rotating inwardly or internally is rotating a joint toward the midline; rotating outwardly or externally is rotating a joint away from the midline.

SCIATICA: A condition manifested by pain that radiates along the sciatic nerve from the lower back down the hip, bottom, and leg (typically on just one side of the body). Sensation and movement issues can both come along with this condition, which is likely rooted in a history of poor movement patterns. Sciatica plagues many different shapes and sizes of bodies, male and female alike, and some are especially vulnerable during pregnancy. Exercises that help treat sciatica include the Anchored Bridge and Internal Leg Trace, which can restore enough space near a sciatic nerve that's become cramped to reduce, and eventually end, its pain signals.

SEATED BASE: The points of contact within the lower extremities (bottom, legs, feet) through which a baby's body weight is being supported while sitting. See *base of support*.

SHIFT: Move a short distance. For example, you might shift your hand from your baby's hip to their thigh; your baby might shift a foot six inches to the left; or your baby might shift their weight from their flat foot to their toes.

SHORT WING: A variation of arm position used to activate the posterior capsule of the shoulder and the latissimus dorsi. This is a component of a number of Foundation Training exercises, which you can see in the "Foundation Training Exercises for Parents." See also *Long Wing*.

SHOULDER GIRDLE: The bony structure and surrounding muscles that attach the arms to the rest of the skeleton.

SIDE-LYING: Lying horizontally on one's left or right side.

SIDE SITTING: Sitting with weight shifted over to one side of the body. Typically the leg on that side of the body will be flexed at the hip and knee to create a broad base of support on that side.

SOT: See *Sphere of Tension*.

SPHERE OF TENSION: This is a component of a number of Foundation Training exercises. Abbreviated as *SoT*. A position for the upper body in which the arms are in front of the torso and the hands are pressed against each other at their fingertips, creating an upper body closed kinetic chain of muscular engagement.

SQUATTING: Shifting the body toward the ground, with hips and knees bending to lower the bottom while the torso remains upright.

STABILITY: The ability to control the body against forces during movement to remain balanced (not synonymous with *balance*.)

STANDING DECOMPRESSION: A Foundation Training exercise that teaches you to actively stand up tall, dispersing your force into the ground through your feet. This exercise also helps you to create connections between your muscular nerve channels and your brain's neural network that build stability and strength. It allows you to practice

Decompression Breathing to enlarge your rib cage while holding Long Wing and Sphere of Tension poses.

STARTLE REFLEX: A natural reflex of a baby in reaction to a loud noise (such as a dog bark or door slam) or sudden perceived change in environment (such as an abrupt alteration in position). For some sensitive babies, even a light touch that was unexpected or a change in temperature can be a trigger. The baby will respond with arms, and possibly legs, flinging outward. The limbs then retract back toward the body. This is typically accompanied by crying and increased heart rate, and changes to breathing pattern. The Startle Reflex becomes milder as a baby becomes more acclimated to various sensory stimuli, and it typically disappears within three to six months of age. Also called the *Moro Reflex*.

STRADDLING: Positioned with one leg on either side of something—for example, a baby astride a parent's leg or arm.

SUPINE: Positioned lying on the back, belly up.

SUPINE DECOMPRESSION: A Foundation Training exercise performed on your back that allows you to align your spine and lengthen your body with minimal interference from gravity. See also *Prone Decompression*.

SUPPORT STRUCTURE: Any structure that a baby can press into or hold on to for external support for the sake of sitting, standing, or walking. It adds an external source of stability to the baby's body. Just about anything stable can serve as a support structure and easy examples include pieces of furniture such as a couch, a bed, a table, or an ottoman; and they can also range from a wall to a turned-over laundry basket to a parent's body.

SUPPORT SURFACE: The surface of a *support structure* (see directly above). In this book's activities, toys are placed on these elevated surfaces to entice a baby to move toward and reach for them. The height of the support surface is an important detail addressed within related activities.

SWADDLING: Wrapping a baby tightly in a blanket to restrict their limbs from moving.

THIGH: The upper part of the leg, between the hip and the knee.

TORSO: The upper body between the neck and the pelvis, not including the limbs. Also called the *trunk*.

TOY WALKER: A wheeled toy that a baby can use as a support tool for walking (with constant adult supervision to ensure safety). A variety of walkers are available, but the type referred to in this book has four wheels (optionally with controls that let you set how quickly or slowly the toy rolls), and a handlebar that the baby can stand in front of and hold on to with both hands. For further details, see the "Introducing a Toy Walker" chapter.

TRANSVERSUS ABDOMINIS MUSCLE: The innermost muscular layer of the abdominal muscles. It runs from portions of the rib cage near the diaphragm to portions of the pelvis and shares the same common tendinous insertion as other ab muscles in the midline of the abdomen. When it contracts, it compresses the ribs and organs, adding a muscular bracing stability to the pelvis and spine.

TUMMY TIME: The time a baby spends lying on their stomach. As baby gains strength and mobility, this will be characterized by rising from the floor via propping with the arms and eventually pushing back onto hands and knees.

VISUAL TRACKING: Focusing on and visually following a moving object with the eyes.

WOODPECKER: A Foundation Training exercise similar to the Founder but performed in a split or lunge stance. It teaches you to integrate the posterior chain on one side of the body at a time. This exercise helps you develop single leg balance and single leg strength, allowing you to rely on either leg alone whenever you need to. It makes an excellent "reset" exercise for caregivers after carrying baby, as the act can often lend to using one arm or side of the body for other needs and therefore using the body asymmetrically.

About the Authors

JEN GOODMAN, PT, MSPT, mom to one delightful little girl, is a licensed physical therapist with nearly two decades of experience in pediatric practices, helping babies and children of all ages and abilities to achieve improved movement. Jen has worked clinically in the medical model of pediatric physical therapy in private practice clinics and hospital-based outpatient settings, United Cerebral Palsy and Easterseals charter schools, as well as home health early intervention services with babies zero to three years old. She is passionate about empowering parents to guide the positions and movements of their babies, to help them establish physical foundations that grow well during and beyond their first year.

Since 2015 Jen has been part of the Infant and Early Childhood Development Team of the well-respected Foundation Training organization, founded and led by her husband, Dr. Eric Goodman (to whom she was married in 2017).

HY BENDER is a *New York Times* bestselling author of more than twenty books, including several in the popular Dummies series and a Complete Idiot's Guide, which have sold more than one million copies. Bender has also written for such diverse national publications as the *New York Times*, *American Film*, *Advertising Age*, *Spy*, and *Mad* magazine.